Sexual Minorities and Mental Health

Joanna Semlyen · Poul Rohleder
Editors

Sexual Minorities and Mental Health

Current Perspectives and New Directions

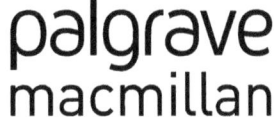

Editors
Joanna Semlyen
Norwich Medical School
University of East Anglia
Norwich, UK

Poul Rohleder
Psychosocial and Psychoanalytic Studies
University of Essex
Colchester, UK

ISBN 978-3-031-37437-1   ISBN 978-3-031-37438-8   (eBook)
https://doi.org/10.1007/978-3-031-37438-8

This Palgrave Macmillan imprint is published by the registered company Springer Nature Switzerland
AG
The registered company address is: Gewerbestrasse 11, 6330 Cham, Switzerland

Paper in this product is recyclable.

We dedicate this book to the memory of Professor Michael King.

Foreword

I am honored to have been asked to offer some introductory comments to this timely volume dedicated to the memory of Professor Michael King. I don't exactly remember when Michael and I first met. I imagine it was during an annual meeting of the American Psychiatric Association (APA) in the US, probably at one of the events of APA's allied organization, AGLP (formerly the Association of Gay and Lesbian Psychiatrists, now AGLP—The Association of LGBTQ+ Psychiatrists).[1]

However, I vividly remember Michael's invitation to me in 2009 to speak as a panelist at the Royal College of Psychiatrists annual meeting in Liverpool on "The Status of Sexual Conversion Therapies in the United States.[2]" I spoke on a panel entitled, "Therapies that Claim to Change Sexual Orientation: Historical and Current Perspectives."

Michael asked if I would come to Liverpool. Having been raised on Beatles music and what we refer to as "the British invasion," I was excited about the prospect of visiting Liverpool for the first time. Even before traveling to the UK, I reached out to my colleague Professor Andrew

---

[1] http://www.aglp.org/.
[2] See Drescher, (1998) and Drescher et al., (2016).

Samuels, originally from Liverpool, who advised me that while there I should "take the ferry cross the Mersey." I never imagined hearing those words in a conversation that was not about a 1965 song by Gerry and the Pacemakers![3]

Yet the highlight of my Liverpool visit was spending time with Michael King and getting to know each other better. As many know, he was a pioneer and leader in British psychiatry's efforts to change its clinical attitudes and approach to LGBTQ people (King & Bartlett, 1999; King et al., 2004; King, 2019). I was deeply saddened to learn when I was in London in November 2021 that Michael had passed away two months earlier.

Which brings me to the importance of this volume and the work that still needs to be done in educating professional organizations, the general public, journalists and policy makers in both the UK and elsewhere.

What kind of work is needed? More than a decade ago, the prestigious Institute of Medicine (2011) of the National Academies laid out a framework for the kind of research needed in the US at that time and perhaps even today. Their recommendations included:

- A national research agenda designed to advance knowledge and understanding of LGBT health.
- Data on sexual orientation and gender identity should be collected in federally funded surveys.
- Data on sexual orientation and gender identity should be collected in electronic health records.
- The federal government should support the development and standardization of sexual orientation and gender identity measures.
- The federal government should support methodological research that relates to LGBT health.
- A comprehensive research training approach should be created to strengthen LGBT health research at research centers like the National Institute of Health (NIH).

---

[3] https://www.youtube.com/watch?v=08083BNaYcA.

Despite having published these recommendations more than a decade ago, few of them have come to fruition. It should also be noted that 2023 marks the fifty-year anniversary of APA removing homosexuality from the DSM-II in 1973 (Bayer, 1981; Cochran et al., 2014; Drescher, 2010, 2015a, 2015b). Yet it is only four years since gender diagnoses were removed from the World Health Organization's International Classification of Disease (ICD-11) in 2019 (Drescher, 2015a; Drescher et al., 2014; Reed et al., 2016). While Professor Michael King did much groundbreaking work to change attitudes in the UK, there is still work to be done. The contributors to this volume are continuing his legacy of fighting prejudice against and dispelling mental health myths about LGBTQ+ people.

Jack Drescher, M.D.

References

Bayer, R. (1981). *Homosexuality and American psychiatry: The politics of diagnosis.* Basic Books.

Cochran, S. D., Drescher, J., Kismodi, E., Giami, A., García-Moreno, C., & Reed, G. M. (2014). Proposed declassification of disease categories related to sexual orientation in ICD-11: Rationale and evidence from the Working Group on Sexual Disorders and Sexual Health. *Bulletin of the World Health Organization, 92*, 672–679.

Drescher, J. (1998). I'm your handyman: A history of reparative therapies. *Journal of Homosexuality, 36* (1), 19–42.

Drescher, J. (2010). Queer diagnoses: Parallels and contrasts in the history of homosexuality, gender variance, and the *Diagnostic and Statistical Manual* (DSM). *Archives of Sexual Behavior, 39*, 427–460.

Drescher, J. (2015a). Queer diagnoses revisited: The past and future of homosexuality and gender diagnoses in DSM and ICD. *International Review of Psychiatry, 27* (5), 386–395.

Drescher, J. (2015b). Out of DSM: Depathologizing homosexuality. *Behavioral Sciences, 5*, 565–575.

Drescher, J., Cohen-Kettenis, P. T., & Reed, G. M. (2016). Gender incongruence of childhood in the ICD-11: Controversies, proposal, and rationale. *Lancet Psychiatry, 3*(3), 297–304.

Drescher, J., Schwartz, A., Casoy, F., McIntosh, C. A., Hurley, B., Ashley, K., Barber, M., Goldenberg, D., Herbert, S. E., Lothwell, L. E., & Mattson, M. R. (2016). The growing regulation of conversion therapy. *Journal of Medical Regulation, 102*(2), 7–12.

Institute of Medicine. (2011). *The health of lesbian, gay, bisexual and transgender people: Building a foundation for better understanding.* The National Academies Press.

King, M. (2019). Stigma in psychiatry seen through the lens of sexuality and gender. *BJPsych International, 16*(4), 77–80.

King, M., & Bartlett, M. (1999). British psychiatry and homosexuality. *The British Journal of Psychiatry, 175*, 106–113.

King, M., Smith, G., & Bartlett, A. (2004). Treatments of homosexuality in Britain since the 1950s—an oral history: The experience of professionals. *British Medical Journal, 328*(7437), 429. https://doi.org/10.1136/bmj.37984.496725.EE

Reed, G. M., Drescher, J., Krueger, R. B., Atalla, E., Cochran, S. D., First M. B., Cohen-Kettenis, P. T., Arango-de Montis, I., Parish, S. J., Cottler, S., & Briken, P. (2016). Revising the ICD-10 Mental and Behavioural Disorders classification of sexuality and gender identity based on current scientific evidence, best clinical practices, and human rights considerations. *World Psychiatry, 15*, 205–221.

Shame's Stone

ages five to twenty six   when a boy
stares   smirks   smiles   kisses   my face
flushes as blood rushes   pushes my shame
to the surface   a stone   at the centre of my
cherry   tart flesh surrounds a pit with a kernel inside
the drilling worm that turns green apple red
I'm five a day   cricket ball small
shame rises   bobs on my body of
water   it unfolds like
a note passed around class   is my shame like
that boy from school   who passed that note around
who I didn't like then and don't like now
is my shame like the first boy I
dated   who made me hard   who sucked me dry
who shoved me to the side of my life   who
made me put pen to paper   to write him
sonnets   does my shame feel like
nineties comics   Judge Dread   Dandy
from my childhood   juxtaposed images
actions   snatches of dialogue   something

I hang on to   but mean to throw away
a comic book baddy   nobody
can destroy   The Joker   hell bent
on taking me hostage   taking over
the city of my mind   a comic book
super hero   who has a unique view
of themselves   the universe   who
can turn shame's poison into petrol
into medicine   into poetry   all
these shamed selves live in me like annual rings
in sweet chestnut   I can't remember
who first threw shame's stone in the sea of me
but I remember each ripple

James McDermott

(Poem published in *Green Apple Red*, by James McDermott, published by Broken Sleep Books, 2022. Reproduced here with permission from James McDermott and Broken Sleep Books)

Contents

Notes on Contributors

Dr. Claire Bloxsom is an Assistant Professor in Counselling and Psychotherapy at the Centre for Lifelong Learning at the University of Warwick in the United Kingdom. She is a UKCP registered integrative psychotherapist and her research focuses on integrating the landscape of theory and practice between psychology and relational humanistic psychotherapy.

Melissa Brown is currently enrolled on the Clinical Psychology Doctorate at the University of Birmingham. Prior to training, she was a qualified teacher who taught A Level and GCSE Psychology for seven years across various schools and sixth forms in Birmingham. Her research areas focus on marginalised groups and ethnic minorities.

Dr. Catherine Butler is a clinical psychologist and systemic psychotherapist whose clinical background is in HIV, sexual health and adult mental health. For the past decade, she has worked as an academic on Doctorate in Clinical Psychology training programmes and as Course Director on Systemic Foundation and Intermediate training courses. She previously worked as the Clinical Director and Deputy Head of Department at the

University of Bath, and she currently works as the Academic Director, Selection Director and Equity, Diversity and Inclusion Lead at the University of Exeter. Catherine's research area is in LGBT discrimination and anti-racism practice.

Dr. Jake Camp is a queer clinical psychologist, DBT therapist and developing clinical academic based at a national DBT programme for adolescents within South London and Maudsley NHS Foundation Trust and the Institute of Psychiatry, Psychology and Neuroscience, King's College London. They are dedicated to improving equity of psychological therapies and reducing the impact of societal oppression on gender- and sexuality-diverse individuals, clinically and academically, with experience supporting these individuals using intervention models such as DBT in multiple contexts and advocating for structural change in clinical services.

Jordan Dixon is a COSRT registered psychosexual and relationship psychotherapist working in her busy private practice in Central London. Born North Yorkshire with Chinese-Spanish heritage and background in Social Policy, Jordan's awareness of intersectionality positions her at the centre of understanding the barriers people face in accessing their erotic potential. Jordan specialises in trauma, sex, gender, relationships, immigration, queerness and loss.

Dr. Brendan J. Dunlop is a Principal Clinical Psychologist in the NHS and Deputy Director of Research and Clinical Lecturer in Clinical Psychology on the University of Manchester clinical psychology training programme. In addition to NHS work, he works in an independent capacity providing psychological therapy to young people and adults, many of whom are from the LGBTQ+ communities. He is Associate Editor of the academic journal *Psychology and Psychotherapy: Theory, Research and Practice* and author of the book *The Queer Mental Health Workbook* (the first-of-its-kind LGBTQ+ self-help resource) published in 2022.

Dr. Sonja J. Ellis is Associate Professor in Human Development at The University of Waikato, New Zealand. She is an established researcher in LGBTIQ+ psychology, and lead author of the textbook *Lesbian, Gay, Bisexual, Trans, Intersex, and Queer Psychology: An Introduction* (2nd Edition).

Dr. Nicola Gunby achieved her Doctorate in Clinical Psychology from the University of Bath in 2021. She now works as a clinical psychologist in Early Intervention in Psychosis Services. Her research interests are in inclusivity and diversity, particularly improving understanding, inclusion and access to services for the LGBT community and those who present as neurodiverse. She is also passionate about psychosis and trauma-informed care.

Professor Rusi Jaspal is the Pro Vice-Chancellor (Research and Knowledge Exchange) and a Professor of Psychology at the University of Brighton in the United Kingdom. Much of his research focuses on identity processes in gay and bisexual men. He is the author of *The Social Psychology of Gay Men* (Palgrave, 2019).

Joshua W. Katz is a Ph.D. candidate in psychology at the University of Saskatchewan. His research interests revolve around gender and sexualities, disability studies and film studies. He has published in numerous outlets including *Sexuality & Culture* and *The Oxford Handbook of Sexual and Gender Minority Mental Health*.

Tirtha Kotrial has recently completed her second postgraduate qualification in Health Psychology and has worked with those who present as neurodivergent in healthcare. Her research interests lie primarily in the area of body image, LGBTQIA+ psychology, gender identity and eating disorders.

Dr. James Lea is a Principal Clinical Psychologist, accredited supervisor in Dialectical Behaviour Therapy (DBT), groupwork practitioner with the Institute of Group Analysis (IGA) and clinical supervisor. At present, they work as admissions director and clinical tutor in Clinical Psychology at The University of Manchester and has a private practice offering psychotherapy and supervision to individuals, groups and teams. James previously held the post of clinical lecturer at Bangor University and has worked in a variety of NHS services with children and families. His research focuses on qualitative exploration within Gender, Sexuality and Relationship Diversity (GSRD) groups, psychological distress, self-harm and suicide.

Dr. Alexander Margetts formed his career in HIV & Sexual Health at Chelsea & Westminster Hospital, including Lead Psychologist at their 'Club Drug Clinic'. He's now a Senior Clinical Tutor for the Leicester Clinical Psychology Doctorate and CNWL IAPT Diploma (including Course Director for Long Term Conditions). His life outside of psychology centres around tennis, board games and cats.

Dr. Samantha Martin is a Lecturer in Psychology at Birmingham City University and a qualitative researcher. Her research has developed online resources that support and empower trans and gender diverse young people with healthcare decision-making and responding to prejudice. She has a background in LGBTQ+ psychology, supporting victims of crime, psychotherapy and counselling and trans youth work.

Dr. Hazel Marzetti is a Research Associate in the School of Health in Social Sciences at the University of Edinburgh. She works on the topics of suicide and suicide prevention, with a specialism in LGBTQ+ mental health. Her current work focuses on using the arts to explore UK suicide prevention policies, politics and practices.

Professor Daragh T. McDermott is the Associate Dean for Psychology and Professor of LGBTQ+ and Social Psychology at Nottingham Trent University. His research focuses on issues pertaining to prejudice and discrimination towards sexual gender minorities.

Professor Elizabeth McDermott is Professor of Mental Health & Society at Birmingham University where she is the Deputy Director of the Institute of Mental Health. Over the last two decades, her research has concentrated on understanding why LGBTQ+ young people have elevated rates of poor mental health and developing ways of preventing these mental health inequalities. Most recently, the Queer Futures 2

Study has resulted in the first NHS Commissioning Guidelines for the provision of early intervention mental health support for LGBTQ+ young people https://queerfutures2.co.uk/resources/.

Professor Jim McManus is Director of Public Health for Hertfordshire, a county of 1.2million people and President of the UK Association of Directors of Public Health, which represents the professional voice of senior public health leaders to government. He is a Chartered Psychologist, Fellow of the British Psychological Society and a Fellow of the Faculty of Public Health. He has been working in public mental health and LGB health for thirty years.

Silva Neves is a COSRT-accredited and UKCP-registered psychotherapist specialising in sexology and intimate relationships. He is a Pink Therapy Clinical Associate. He is a Course Director for the Contemporary Institute of Clinical Sexology (CICS), an international speaker and broadcaster. He is the author of *Sexology: The Basics* (Routledge).

Professor Damien W. Riggs is a Professor in Psychology at Flinders University and psychotherapist in private practice working with trans young people. He is the author of over 200 publications on gender, family and mental health, including *Working with Transgender Young People: A Critical Developmental Approach* (Palgrave).

Dr. Katharine A. Rimes is an academic clinical psychologist and BABCP-accredited cognitive behaviour therapist. She undertakes transdiagnostic research into cognitive and behavioural processes involved in mental health problems and applies the findings to improve interventions. She co-leads the King's College London LGBTQ+ Mental Health Research Group.

Professor Ian Rivers is Associate Principal and Executive Dean of the Faculty of Humanities and Social Sciences at the University of Strathclyde.

Dr. Poul Rohleder is a clinical psychologist and psychoanalytic psychotherapist in private practice. He had a previous academic career for many years and is currently an Honorary Senior Lecturer at the Department of Psychosocial and Psychoanalytic Studies, University of

Essex. He is co-author of *A Clinical Guide to Psychodynamic Psychotherapy* (Routledge) and co-editor of *Qualitative Research in Clinical and Health Psychology* (Palgrave).

Dr. Michael Rolt is an early career clinical psychologist who recently graduated from Royal Holloway, University of London. He is currently working on the neuro-developmental and low-mood / anxiety pathways in Hampshire CAMHS. His research interests include substance use in men who have sex with men and behaviour-change approaches to service development. Before his mid-life crisis career change, he worked as a chartered accountant and business analyst. He loves living on the south coast and enjoys spending his free time running (no hills on the seafront!), and sea swimming and is an aspirational, but procrastinating, novelist.

Shoshana Rosenberg is an independent researcher currently based in Naarm/Melbourne, Victoria. Their research has focused on trans peoples' experiences of pleasure, embodiment and sexual health. Shoshana is an Associate Editor at the International Journal of Transgender Health and has recently published a co-authored book *Queer Entanglements: Intersections of Gender, Sexuality and Animal Companionship* through Cambridge University Press.

Dr. Joanna Semlyen is an academic health psychologist, Associate Professor of Psychology at University of East Anglia and leads the Diversity in Psychology and Medicine Research Group at UEA. She undertakes interdisciplinary, mixed methods research in sexual minority health and inequalities, and has been working in LGB mental health for 20 years.

Dr. Joshua K. Simpson holds a Ph.D. from the School of Education at the University of Strathclyde and is currently a Learning, Teaching and Quality Enhancement Project Officer at the University of Worcester.

Dr. Sue Westwood is a social gerontologist and socio-legal scholar, interested in ageing, diversity and equality in regulatory contexts and the equitable delivery of health and social care to older LGBTQ people. She has conducted several research projects on LGBTQ health and social care and published extensively on the topic.

Dr. Paul Willis is a social gerontologist and social work scholar. His research areas include: ageing, men and social relations; loneliness in later life; inclusive housing and social care for older LGBTQ people; social work with older people; and, sexuality and ageing. Paul has published extensively on LGBTQ ageing, housing and social care.

List of Figures

List of Tables

1

Introduction

Joanna Semlyen and Poul Rohleder

Sexual minorities (e.g. lesbian, gay and bisexual (LGB) people) remain a specific population that faces significant threat and discrimination. As will be shown in Chapter 2, sexual minority persons manifest greater prevalence of poor mental health, health risk behaviours and psychological distress when compared to the general population or when compared to heterosexual groups. As will be shown in this book, structural inequality means that psychological threat and minority stress is a common experience for sexual minorities. There is a compelling evidence base, and an emerging one from the UK, for mental health disparities in the LGBT population.

J. Semlyen
Norwich Medical School, University of East Anglia, Norwich, UK
e-mail: j.semlyen@uea.ac.uk

P. Rohleder (✉)
Department of Psychosocial and Psychoanalytic Studies, University of Essex, Colchester, UK
e-mail: p.rohleder@essex.ac.uk

J. Semlyen and P. Rohleder (eds.), *Sexual Minorities and Mental Health*, https://doi.org/10.1007/978-3-031-37438-8_1

About the Book

Our aim for this edited volume, is to provide an insightful consideration of research, challenges and perspectives in mental health in sexual
minority populations in the UK relevant for *all* professions working with
this population, students studying applications of psychology for sexual
minority health and, we hope, a wider, general audience who want to
understand this complex and compelling issue. In addition, we offer a
consideration of interventions for addressing this mental health disparity
in this population. While the focus is specifically the UK, the issues
highlighted are pertinent for other, international contexts. Drawing on
clinical, counselling, social, health and community psychology perspectives, as well as public health, this book highlights the urgency of this
topic in this population, and, we hope, provides an insight into some of
the ways we can understand and make sense of the increased prevalence
of poorer mental health in this population, whilst offering perspectives
and recommendations on ways to address the disparities they face.

Terminology, Inclusions and Initialisms

As sexual identity is often coupled with gender identity, readers may
ask why the book focuses primarily on sexual minorities, rather than
looking at "LGBT" mental health. *LGBT* is an initialism that describes
the lesbian, gay, bisexual and trans/gender non-conforming (TGNC)
population(s). Often this initialism can be written in the variant *LGBTQ*
with the addition of the letter Q for queer-identified, or *LGBT+* where
" + " indicates the inclusion of other diverse gender and/or sexual identities. *Q* is sometimes also used to denote *questioning*, especially in studies
of young people.

  Although TGNC populations experience widespread discrimination
that unarguably impacts on their mental health, we felt that their particular lived experience, based in gender identity, and the specific pathways
to poor mental health in this population, are likely fundamentally
different, and requires its own dedicated attention. Not least because of
the very real struggles this population have with gender identity services

and medical interventions, along with other particular issues related to their own context within society and public policy.

Moreover, importantly, we consider that sexual minority populations are themselves complex and diverse, impacted by varying social, cultural and other wide determinants of health, and differing in age, sex, and other historical and contemporary experiences that this book wishes to explore in detail. Mental health is also a complex and multi-dimensional health issue and this book intends to focus carefully and intentionally on the specific and particular aspects that disproportionately affect sexual minorities. However, while we feel a dedicated focus on sexual minorities is warranted, our purpose is not to exclude people who may identify as gender diverse. Thus, at various times, the book takes an intersectional approach, acknowledging that some sexual minorities also identify as trans/gender non-conforming.

There are other initialisms present in the book. In some epidemiological studies the term *LGBO* is used where *O* refers to a category 'other' than the offered categories of lesbian, gay, bisexual or heterosexual. The term *LGB* refers to lesbian, gay or bisexual identified individuals and is used in studies that focus on sexuality, or sexual minorities rather than gender identity, but the intersection with gender remains important to distinguish between gay men and gay women, bisexual men and bisexual women.

Outline of the Book

We have invited contributors from primarily the discipline of psychology, or closely aligned professions such as sociology and public health, each highly experienced and experts in their topics. While we had a prescribed focus and basic structure for the book, we invited contributors to express themselves as authors in the way they wished. A range of contributors bring different positions and ideas, thus representing a plurality of voices and views, rather than aim for a unified agreed position. There are also different styles of writing, and we invited the key author of each chapter to collaborate in writing their chapter, particularly with junior colleagues where possible. We have chosen not to adopt a unified approach to the use of descriptive labels, initialisms or categories, leaving authors to choose their own, in the recognition that there may be varying views on language and terminology used.

We have organised the book into two parts. Part 1 focuses on presenting a picture of the various mental health problems that impact on sexual minorities. The first chapter (Chapter 2) details the incidence and prevalence of mental health problems set within a broader consideration of causal pathways and treatment approaches positioning itself as an overview chapter. A second chapter (Chapter 3) looks specifically at social prejudice, providing a broad historical context for the lived experience of sexual minorities still evident today. The third chapter (Chapter 4) looks in detail at the issue of coming out, where the pertinence of navigating disclosure ties in closely with the ideas and challenges threaded throughout the rest of the book. The other three chapters explore some of the intersections with sexual minorities that are important, age (Chapter 5), ethnicity (Chapter 6) and gender diversity (Chapter 7). These are included not only as topics of their own importance but serve to remind us that sexual minorities are not one homogenous group but a diverse intersecting set of identities with their own particular and specific lived experiences.

Part 2 includes ten chapters that look at intervention practices and approaches to treatment. It is beyond the scope of the book to include chapters on all forms of interventions and therapeutic modalities and so we have included what we felt to be some of the approaches that might be regularly found in mental health services. We have had to be selective, and acknowledge that there are many other helpful and important approaches that could be considered (e.g. person-centred counselling, narrative therapies, existential psychotherapy, group therapies, to name just a few). We do not intend for Part 2 to be prescriptive about what helps, and hope that readers who practice in other modalities may draw from the issues raised and explored in these chapters and be able to transfer some of the thinking to their own particular modalities.

Part 2 includes a chapter (Chapter 8) on clinical formulation and the different issues that need to be kept in focus when formulating a sexual minority client's presenting difficulties and needs. The next six chapters present a range of approaches to therapy that offer a wide range of perspectives to treatment and offer a broad consideration of ways to address mental health for sexual minorities: Affirmative therapy (Chapter 9), therapeutic practice with queer trans people (Chapter 10), cognitive behavioural therapy (Chapter 11), dialectical behaviour therapy (Chapter 12), psychodynamic psychotherapies (Chapter 13), and sex and couples therapy (Chapter 14).

The next two chapters look at two specific issues that form part of the mental health spectrum and whilst not the only two specific aspects we need to consider both are highly prevalent in LGBTQ people. Chapter 15 looks at substance abuse services and treatment, whilst Chapter 16 looks at the prevalence of suicide, offering different approaches for understanding the higher prevalence of suicide among the LGBTQ population, and among LGBTQ youth in particular. The chapter also outlines various suicide prevention practices.

In Chapter 17, the reader is offered a reflective approach to the consideration of sexual minority mental health through a public health lens. Written as an interview with the current President of the Association of Directors of Public Health, in this final chapter, sexual minority mental health is problematised as a public health issue with clear directives for interdisciplinary ways forward relevant to all professions working with this population.

The collection of chapters each highlight the heterogeneity of the sexual minority population, the complexity of issues and the various intersecting identities that need to be held in mind. The chapters outline the prevalence of historical and present pathologizing and prejudice and highlight this as a backdrop within which one must consider intervention, and the clinician's own positionings and biases. Inevitably, the various chapters touch on similar topic areas, and there are overlaps. While we have made attempts to avoid unnecessary repetition across the book, various key issues or theories (for example Minority Stress Theory) make several repeated appearances. We felt it important not to erase these overlaps and revisiting of key issues, as we wanted each chapter to be able to read on its own, as well as part of an edited volume. And, we feel that some points require emphasis!

Situating the Problem

In any publication that focuses on mental health in sexual minorities, it is an imperative to situate the problem both in terms of observed prevalence (which is detailed in Chapter 2), and also to present the population context, which we present here. That way the level of impact can be understood and throughout this book what will become evident, is that for sexual minorities, mental health is a significant and enduring health disparity.

UK Census Data: Sexual Orientation, 2021

Until UK Census 2021 data was released in 2023, we had only ever been able to estimate the number of sexual minorities in the UK population. In representative national health surveys, e.g. *Understanding Society*, with 100,000 participants (Institute for Social & Economic Research, 2022), approximately 3% select a sexual orientation identity other than heterosexual (Semlyen et al., 2016; Semlyen et al., 2020). In the 2009/2010 English General Practice Patient Survey (GPPS) (Ipsos-MORI, 2012) with 2,169,718 respondents, approximately 3.1% responded as gay, bisexual or 'other' male and 1.8% as lesbian, bisexual or 'other' female rising to 3.9% and 2.7% respectively in 2017 (Cross & Llewellyn, 2020).

On January 6th 2023, the very first data on sexual orientation collected by the UK Census in 2021, was released, revealing that 3.2% of the population identifies as LGBO,[1] this amounts to approximately 1.5 million people. Across the categories, 748,000 (1.54%) people aged 16 years and over described themselves as gay or lesbian, 624,000 (1.28%) described themselves as bisexual and 165,000 (0.3%) selected other sexual orientation. See Table 1.1.

This census data is important, but it must be noted that 7.5% (3.6 million people) did not answer this question, thus the figure of 3.2% may well be a significant underestimate. We know that disclosure carries

---

[1] *LGBO is the initialism that represents Lesbian, Gay, Bisexual or Other sexual orientation.*

Table 1.1 Sexual Orientation, 2021, England and Wales

Sexual Orientation	2021 (number)	2021 (%)
Straight or Heterosexual	43,403,110	89.37
Gay or Lesbian	747,805	1.54
Bisexual	623,504	1.28
Pansexual	112,386	0.23
Asexual	28,172	0.06
Queer	14,511	0.03
All other sexual orientations	10,236	0.02
Not answered	3,626,649	7.47

Source Office for National Statistics (ONS), released 6 January 2023, ONS website, statistical bulletin, Sexual orientation, England and Wales: Census 2021 (https://www.ons.gov.uk/peoplepopulationandcommunity/culturalidentity/sexuality/bulletins/sexualorientationenglandandwales/census2021)

a significant anxiety for many people and the Census is sent to households not individuals, so inaccurate data may have been recorded on behalf of someone. The question itself also was voluntary. Despite these caveats, it is worthy of note that 44.9 million people in the UK population aged 16 years and over (92.5% of those invited to respond) answered the question.

There is evidence that supports the notion of under reporting. There is an observed variation in sexual orientation identity which is directly determined by whether the question being asked refers to orientation, attraction or behaviour. The Census 2021 asked about identity but figures can be much higher when sexuality is measured by behaviour or attraction (Johnson et al., 2001). Indeed, recent modelled estimates suggest that LGB people form up to 11.5% of the UK population (Geary et al., 2018). This may be determined by the method by which the question is answered. An earlier, frequently cited estimate of 6%, came from the work by the Equalities Commission in 2009, finding that 5.7% of their online survey respondents identified as lesbian, gay or bisexual (LGB) (Ellison & Gunstone, 2009). This figure may reflect the open sampling mechanisms used in the study (i.e. online may reach a wider population) but may equally reflect increased confidence in self-identifying in an anonymous survey method.

The inclusion of sexual orientation in the Census was a long-fought battle. Indeed, a question designed to measure sexual orientation in the population was ready for inclusion in the 2011 Census, having been developed by the ONS in 2009 (Haseldon et al., 2009), but it was felt at the time that confidentiality and privacy could not be assured and it was withheld (ONS, 2006; Cabinet Office, 2008; ONS, 2010). The question was asked in the 2021 Census (HM Government, 2018) but was made voluntary to reflect sensitivities. To achieve this, the Census Act 1920 was amended with the Census (Return Particulars and Removal of Penalties) Act 2019 to remove penalties for non-completion of this question (ONS, 2020).

It is possible to assess the reported size of sexual orientation identity over time. Representative studies such as the Integrated Household Survey added a question on sexual orientation in 2010 and the Office for National Statistics have provided population statistics since then (ONS, 2011). Table 1.2 shows population data on sexual orientation in the UK from 2014 to 2020. Earlier data are still available in the National Archives.[2] These data show that identifying as heterosexual has declined since 2014. It is notable that rates of 'refuse/don't know' answers have remained stable whilst LGBO categories have all steadily increased. Detailed examination of the data by sex shows that more men identify as gay/lesbian than women and more women identify as bisexual than men. There are no differences in sex for other or refuse/don't know. Younger age groups are more highly reflected in this data, with one third being aged 16–24. This age group are more likely to identify as bisexual than gay/lesbian. There has been a large increase in young people identifying as LGBO; in 2018 it was 4.4%, in 2019 it was 6.6% and in 2020 was 8.0%.

Future Directions

With the very real and unavoidable population data, and the compelling disparities in mental health this population face, outlined in Chapter 2, there is an imperative to drive forward an intervention development and research agenda that seeks to understand and address the inequities we

---

[2] https://webarchive.nationalarchives.gov.uk

Table 1.2 Sexual Orientation, UK, 2014 to 2020 (%) Data from Annual Population Survey, ONS

Sexual orientation	2014	2015	2016	2017	2018	2019	2020
Heterosexual or straight	95.3	95.2	95.0	95.0	94.6	93.7	93.6
Gay or lesbian	1.1	1.2	1.2	1.3	1.4	1.6	1.8
Bisexual	0.5	0.7	0.8	0.8	0.9	1.1	1.3
Other	0.3	0.4	0.5	0.6	0.6	0.7	0.7
Do not know or refuse	2.8	2.6	2.5	2.3	2.5	3.0	2.6

observe. As the reader navigates the book, we hope they engage with some of the critical questions being posed whilst remaining aware that we consider this book just the very *start* of addressing mental health in this thus far under-served population.

References

Cabinet Office. (2008). Helping to shape tomorrow: The 2011 census of population and housing in England and Wales. *Cm 7513.*

Cross, H., & Llewellyn, C. D. (2020). A decline in patient disclosure of heterosexuality in the English general practice patient survey: A longitudinal analysis of cross-sectional data. *Family Practice, 37*(5), 661–667.

Ellison, G., & Gunstone, B. (2009). *Sexual orientation explored: A study of identity, attraction, behaviour and attitudes in 2009.* Equality and Human Rights Commission Manchester.

Geary, R. S., Tanton, C., Erens, B., Clifton, S., Prah, P., Wellings, K., … & Mercer, C. H. (2018). Sexual identity, attraction and behaviour in Britain: The implications of using different dimensions of sexual orientation to estimate the size of sexual minority populations and inform public health interventions. *PloS one, 13*(1), e0189607.

Haseldon, L., Joloza, T., & Household, L. M. (2009). *Measuring sexual identity: A guide for researchers.* Newport: Office for National Statistics.

HM Government. (2018). *Help shape our future. The 2021 census of population and housing in England and Wales.* HM Government.

Institute for Social and Economic Research. (2022). *Understanding society: Waves 1–12, 2009–2021 and Harmonised BHPS: Waves 1–18, 1991–2009.* University of Essex.

Ipsos-MORI, (2012). *Technical annex for the GP patient survey 2011–12.* Ipsos MORI.

Johnson, A. M., Mercer, C. H., Erens, B., Copas, A. J., McManus, S., Wellings, K., … & Field, J. (2001). Sexual behaviour in Britain: Partnerships, practices, and HIV risk behaviours. *The Lancet, 358*(9296), 1835–1842.

ONS. (2006). *Sexual orientation and the 2011 Census: background information,* Office for National Statistics.

ONS. (2010). *Measuring sexual identity: An evaluation report.* Office of National Statistics.

ONS, (2011). *Integrated household survey April 2010 to March 2011 : Experimental statistics,* Office for National Statistics.

ONS. (2020). *Sexual orientation question development for Census 2021,* Office for National Statistics.

Semlyen, J., King, M., Varney, J., & Hagger-Johnson, G. (2016). Sexual orientation and symptoms of common mental disorder or low wellbeing: Combined meta-analysis of 12 UK population health surveys. *BMC Psychiatry, 16*, 1–9.

Semlyen, J., Curtis, T. J., & Varney, J. (2020). Sexual orientation identity in relation to unhealthy body mass index: Individual participant data meta-analysis of 93 429 individuals from 12 UK health surveys. *Journal of Public Health, 42*(1), 98–106.

Part I

Issues

2

Sexual Minority Mental Health: Measurement, Prevalence, and Treatment

Joanna Semlyen

Introduction

This chapter will present an overview of mental health in sexual minorities with a particular focus on a UK context. Firstly, it will present prevalence of mental health in sexual minorities, and along with a brief consideration of causal pathways in an attempt to understand the context of this observed disparity, it will then go on to discuss data collection, sampling and research quality issues and will finish with providing some recommendations for interventions. In focusing on prevalence, it will start with a consideration of the complexities of sexual orientation identity (SOI) measurement, the categorising of sexual orientation identities and issues around sexual minority mental health (SMMH) data capture.

J. Semlyen (✉)
Norwich Medical School, UEA, Norwich, UK
e-mail: j.semlyen@uea.ac.uk

J. Semlyen and P. Rohleder (eds.), *Sexual Minorities and Mental Health*,
https://doi.org/10.1007/978-3-031-37438-8_2

Measuring Sexual Orientation Identity

We absolutely need to be measuring sexual orientation identity to allow us to capture information, health status, health outcomes and other crucial intelligence about this population. And meaningful, useful measurement allows meaningful data capture, which itself provides the compelling and unavoidable data (i.e., that which cannot be dismissed as estimates or low-quality evidence) that can change policy, funding and therefore impact of sexual minority peoples' lives. Capturing sexual orientation identity data is complex and challenging, in part because of sensitivities around disclosure but also in part because of capturing the complexity of the identity itself. It is beyond the scope of this chapter to address in full the issues around identity categories (such as limitations of LGB) but there currently are two, conflicting views that are in danger of becoming (unhelpfully) entrenched.

On the one hand, there is the view that it is crucial to capture sexual identity in all its variation, in its self-selected and potentially flux and fluid complexity, based on the well understood premise that not everyone identifies with the currently accepted, fixed (and limited) categories. This can be supported by the numbers of people selecting something 'other' rather than refusing to answer or choosing 'gay/lesbian', 'bisexual' or 'heterosexual' (Eliason & Streed, 2017; Eliason et al., 2016) in SOI questions. There is some, albeit minimal, research on what 'other' means/may consist of as a group (Betts, 2008, 2009) but the detailed exploration of this is beyond the scope of this chapter.

Conversely, the continued standardisation of sexual orientation identity into 'LGBO' (Lesbian, Gay, Bisexual, Other), as developed by the Office for National Statistics (ONS) and adopted in a wide range of national surveys, as well as the Census 2021, allows for meaningful epidemiological analysis across, within and between groups and over time, across surveys and among health outcomes. It permits the pooling of data where there are small samples (so very common in sexual orientation identity samples) and the greater statistical power pooling confers, permits disaggregated analyses across different identity categories (Semlyen, 2017) allowing us to understand the very different, nuanced experiences and health outcomes of, say, lesbians as distinct from bisexual women or gay men for example. Pooling allowed us to understand bisexual populations have poorer mental health than lesbian, gay and heterosexual populations (Semlyen et al., 2016). Whilst arguably there are disadvantages to both of these positions, the greatest disadvantage is that it is hard, perhaps impossible, to have both at the same time but that disagreeing about this may well lead us to a place where we have no data and nothing meaningful to say.

Researching Sexual Minority Mental Health

There is an abundance of research evidence now available on prevalence of mental health in sexual minorities but much of it has used study designs that lack rigour, often using unvalidated questionnaires and weak sampling, limiting usefulness. It is important before presenting prevalence date that level of evidence is understood to guide interpretation of findings and to understand the relationship between level of evidence and impact. There are numerous aspects to research design that could be drawn on to inform this point, I will illustrate this by focusing on sampling in sexual minority studies.

Sampling is a key component to research design, as poorly designed research with convenience samples leads to possible bias and it would be understandable (and right) for policy makers, practice leads and funders to mistrust those findings. For those research minded readers who might want a deep dive into sampling designs, I draw your attention to a super helpful paper by Ilan Meyer and Patrick Wilson who looked at this within LGB study designs (Meyer & Wilson, 2009).

When we are thinking about prevalence, the way you sample can have a direct effect on the prevalence you might 'find' in an analysis. For example, in their comparison between probability and nonprobability study designs, Hottes and colleagues found, compared to the heterosexual sample (4%), the prevalence of LGB suicide was much larger in the non-probability (20%) than probability sample (11%) (Hottes et al., 2016). One might argue that this (20%) is an important finding, but it is representative data we need for policy makers as this leads to the most accurate findings. Convenience sample studies, using venues or online resources are by design, *less* representative reflections of the LGB population attracting those who self-select by being at an LGB venue, or having demonstrable interest in the topic (Dodds et al., 2006; Evans et al., 2007). Higher levels of reported psychological distress or other mental health issues through selective recruitment may reflect nuances about those samples, such as higher willingness to disclose, or higher levels of community connection because of poorer mental health (Kuyper et al., 2016). Generalisability from these findings is limited, and provide impoverished evidence base upon which to determine resource, policy or political action.

Studies that collect representative data and also collect sexual orientation identity are few and far between, rendering quality evidence extremely elusive. Numbers of participants disclosing as sexual minority in these studies are usually small (around 3%, see Chapter 1) and techniques to combine through pooling to gain power are often necessary (Semlyen, 2017) so it would be useful, as has been done with ethnic minority sample, if efforts to oversample sexual minority populations in national health surveys are undertaken (King et al., 2007).

It is of course possible to record SOI by same sex *attraction* and same sex *behaviour* as well as sexual orientation *identity*; these three all forms different dimensions of sexual orientation, can lead to larger samples (Geary et al., 2018) and are differently linked to health outcomes (see Savin-Williams & Ream, 2007 for a comprehensive review). Recording sexual orientation through identity is accepted to be the most accurate dimension, overlapping closely with both other dimensions, is considered most closely related to discrimination and associated health outcomes.

Prevalence of Mental Health Disparities

There is now a clearly documented, significant and sustained mental health disparity observed in sexual minority individuals when compared to heterosexual counterparts. In a systematic review published in 2008 there was unarguable evidence demonstrated that lesbian, gay, and bisexual men and women have demonstrable higher levels of suicide ideation, suicide attempts, depression, anxiety, substance misuse and self-harm than the heterosexual population (King et al., 2008). The majority of the research studies included were drawn from USA samples, but representative data means that generalisability to a similar (Eurocentric, Western) context is possible. However a UK context is important to understand the specifics of that particlaur population. Significant available studies within a UK context are presented here. The evidence presented is drawn from a decade (2008–2018) of rapid legal, structural and social change and beginning at the end point from the first systematic review of lesbian, gay, bisexual mental health was published (King et al., 2008). A systematic approach to the search was adopted.

UK Mental Health Prevalence

The majority of studies with available data on LGB mental health in a UK setting have used non probability samples (Colledge et al., 2015; Hickson et al., 2017; Rimes et al., 2018b), or clinical samples (Rimes et al., 2018a) or were not UK wide (Calzo et al., 2018; Jones et al., 2017; McNamee et al., 2008; Pesola et al., 2014; Schubotz & O'Hara, 2011; Woodhead et al., 2016; Young et al., 2011).

Evidence drawn from studies with a comparative group, shows poorer mental health amongst LGB people (Chakraborty et al., 2011; McNamee et al., 2008; Semlyen et al., 2016; Woodhead et al., 2016) and higher rates of low well-being (Semlyen et al., 2016; Woodhead et al., 2016), substance misuse (Hagger-Johnson et al., 2013, Mercer et al., 2016; Pesola et al., 2014; Taibjee et al., 2013; Woodhead et al., 2016), eating disorders (Calzo et al., 2018), anxiety (Jones et al., 2017) and self-reported longstanding psychological or emotional problems (Elliott et al., 2015) than heterosexual people. One Scottish longitudinal study using a schools-based sample demonstrated a link between same-sex sexual behaviour and self-harm in young people (Young et al., 2011).

There are no UK health service records available on mental health prevalence in this population. Records held by NHS do not capture sexual orientation identities consistently, if at all, despite the development of a monitoring standard (see Chapter 17) (NHS England,

2017a), thus data on prevalence must be captured through secondary data analysis of national health surveys and other research studies. Until recently this has not been possible, as sexual orientation data was also not recorded and data on sexual minority mental health was limited to convenience sample studies. Since the emergence of health survey data sets that collect sexual orientation identity data (and sometimes behaviour and attraction) it has been possible more recently to locate and assess the prevalence of mental health outcomes in a representative sample within a UK context. Following agreement on a question on sexual orientation (Haseldon et al., 2009), the first health survey collected data on sexual orientation identity in 2008 (Scottish Health Survey) followed by Health Survey for England in 2011.

It must be noted, attempts to capture prevalence require sexual minority self-identification in surveys, sometimes interviewer-led, leading to disclosure-related anxiety regarding possible poor treatment, care or even harm (Aspinall, 2009). In surveys where sexual orientation identity is collected, this can have a direct impact on participant numbers. Where participant numbers are small, data analysis is difficult and frequently data is provided aggregated across sexual minority groups (e.g., grouping into non-heterosexual) key differences experienced by subgroups. Pooling data techniques can address this issue and it is this method that led to the first representative study of common mental disorder and UK sexual minorities.

Using pooled data from 12 UK national health surveys with a sample size of 94,818, Semlyen et al (2016) provide an analysis of a population-based, representative sample of lesbian, gay, bisexual and other-identified participants with data available on common mental disorder.[1] Common mental disorder was found to be twice as high for lesbian, bisexual, gay and 'other'-identified respondents in a representative sample, compared to heterosexual counterparts, with both younger people under 35, and

---

[1] Common mental disorder (CMD) is defined by the National Institute for Health and Clinical Excellence National Institute for Health and Clinical Excellence (2011). Common Mental Disorders: Full Guideline. London, NICE and is a technical classification for six common mental health diagnoses. These include Mixed Anxiety and Depression, Generalised Anxiety Disorder, Depression, Phobias, Obsessive Compulsive Disorder, and Panic Disorder.

those aged 55 and over having the highest levels of disparity (Semlyen et al., 2016).

There is minimal research in the UK looking directly at bisexual mental health (Barker, 2015), but from a self-selected sample of lesbian and bisexual women, (Colledge et al., 2015) found that bisexual women reported poorer mental health than lesbian respondents. A recent representative population study has found that levels of poorer mental health are higher for bisexual men and women (Semlyen et al., 2016).

Experiences of Mental Health Services

Little is known about sexual minority population levels of engagement with mental health services as most studies evaluating services provide no data on sexual orientation—not through accident but through omission. Typically, services and studies fail to record it in the first place (Heck et al., 2017). Despite the development of the monitoring standard in 2017 (NHS England, 2017b), there is little evidence of this being successfully implemented (Almack, 2023). Data on attendance at health services throughout the UK would offer helpful knowledge for service planning. Such data would also go some way to meet the requirements of equality legislation.

Research drawn from community samples and using qualitative methods shows clearly that LGB people often are not successful in getting the help they need (Guasp & Taylor, 2012; Rivers et al., 2018). Data from the UK Government LGBT survey reported that mental health services were accessed by 24% of the 108,000 respondents (Government Equalities Office, 2018a). Whilst not offering comparative data, and reflecting a self-selecting sample of LGBT respondents, this is still compelling statistics. We know from the survey that treatment for mental health conditions is accessed more frequently by people who identify with sexual orientations that are less common (such as pansexual-identified people) and that pansexual and queer identified people found accessing mental health services more difficult, in particular experiencing a long waiting time (Government Equalities Office, 2018a).

Causal Pathways to Mental Health

Throughout this book, it will be evident that structural, social and individual determinants can be drawn upon to explain observed mental health disparities in LGB populations. At minimum, growing up and navigating an identity that is marginal and stigmatised in a society with a strong social desirability bias i.e., heteronormativity, will bring challenges.

Studies examining causal pathways to this inequity lag far behind the inequalities data corpus. Evidence linking this disparity to epigenetic changes from stress exposure go some way to explain the wide range of physical *and* mental health inequalities experienced in sexual minorities (Flentje et al., 2020) but we still know relatively little as trials that consider pathways research questions invariably collect no sexual orientation data and almost no longitudinal studies in this population exist.

The minority stress theory (MST) offers an enduring, theoretical premise for understanding how stigma and stress are intertwined (Meyer, 1995, 2003), bringing together work from Goffman on stigma and Brooks' ground-breaking model of minority stress in lesbian women (Brooks, 1981; Goffman, 2009; Rich et al., 2020). The detail of the model is covered in detail throughout the book so will not be described here, but the dominant explanatory models of minority stress theory (Meyer, 1995, 2003) and its extensions, the psychological mediation framework (Hatzenbuehler, 2009) and Feinstein's rejection sensitivity model (2020), along with Diamond's very recent addition of social safety (Diamond and Alley, 2022), position the significance of discrimination, prejudice and stigma, and the psychological processes associated with their impact, as *fundamental* to our understanding of the pathway to poor mental health in this population. Psychological processes associated with this minority related stress include expectation of rejection, the need for concealment (of one's sexual identity) and internalisation of negative cognitions (Pachankis et al., 2020; Walch et al., 2016). Concealment, an active position, in contrast to absence of disclosure, (Pachankis et al., 2020), has been shown to be linked directly to sexual minority mental health likely through mechanisms such as reduced levels of perceived belonging, self esteem and social support (Le Forestier et al., 2023).

Mental Health Interventions for Sexual Minorities

Operationalising the minority stress model would allow consideration of routes to prevent and treat. At an individual level, tackling resilience, improving coping, increasing social support, reducing internalised homophobia and rejection sensitivity are all significantly useful targets for minority stress-based treatments for example (Meyer, 2003, 2015; Ngamake et al., 2016). However, as Meyer himself points out, the stressful event itself is an objective event and thus needs to be targeted with interventions too. Targeting interventions at societal level allows us to address structural stressors through, say, family or community level interventions or at policy level. Indeed, we know that structural stigma impacts significantly on this population (Hatzenbuehler and Link, 2014) with research illustrating that legal and policy protections along with cultural norms have been demonstrably linked to poor mental health (Hatzenbuehler et al., 2009) leading to increased levels of concealment in countries with high structural stigma (Pachankis et al., 2015).

Whilst societal change is the ultimate intervention, the necessary collective, systemic, structural, and ecological transformations, while possible in some UK contexts, are slow, subject to change and likely conditional on political whim. Instead, most efforts place the individual as the fundamental focus for treatment. Chapters in Part II of this book consider the usefulness of current existing approaches to addressing mental health in the general population for sexual minorities and explore current psychological provision in a UK context such as Dialectical Behaviour Therapy (Chapter 12) and Cognitive Behaviour Therapy (Chapter 11). It is crucial that these interventions, likely accessed with more frequency by this group, need to be equally beneficial, safe and affirming for sexual minority populations as others.

Affirmative Treatment

Affirmative treatment, that which is affirming of sexual minority identity and provides a supportive and safe space for individuals to explore mental distress, as distinct from their sexual identity, needs to be standard within any psychological treatment for sexual minorities. In interrogating psychological treatment for LGBT individuals, a British Association for Counselling and Psychotherapy commissioned systematic review demonstrated that from the literature (at that time in 2006) there were a number of difficulties being experienced by LGBT people with therapeutic provision at that time including: concerns about safety, therapy/therapists making heterosexual (heteronormative) assumptions and misattribution of problem to LGBT identity (King et al., 2007). Furthermore, LGBT individuals demonstrated concerns about lack of therapist knowledge of LGBT lives and expressed a preference for a LGBT therapist (King et al., 2007). Evidence shows that some health care professionals conflate LGBT identity with their mental health condition, such that for some LGBT people with schizophrenia their identity is seen as a symptom (Drinkwater & Semlyen, 2012).

Change to practice and training is slow; it is striking that the nine recommendations from that review remain just as relevant to practitioners now (King et al., 2007 - See Box 2.1).

Box 2.1: Recommendations for Practice and Practitioners (King et al., 2007)

1. All psychotherapy training institutes regard knowledge of LGBT development and lifestyles as part of core training.

   (a) Heteronormative bias must be recognised and avoided.
   (b) Therapists should increase their knowledge of LGBT issues and keep up to date.
   (c) Psychotherapeutic practice that pathologizes homosexuality, bisexuality and transgenderism should be replaced by more modern understandings of sexual identity.

(d) Therapists should become aware of internalised bias in the LGBT clients themselves.

(e) Therapists should receive training on the impact of self disclosure for all clients, including the sensitive issue of their own sexual orientation and gender identity.

2. All psychotherapy training institutes encourage greater numbers of LGBT people to train as therapists in order to improve knowledge in the professional therapeutic community and enable choice of therapists for clients where possible.

3. Psychotherapists consider very carefully the advantages and disadvantages of self-disclosure of their sexual identity, gender identity or lifestyle for each particular client and not expect to follow any general rules.

4. Psychotherapists take care to inform themselves about LGBT cultures and lifestyles through their personal or professional lives, rather than expecting their LGBT clients to educate them.

5. More services are provided for transgender people that focus on general psychotherapeutic issues rather than exclusively on the pathway to or from gender change.

6. Affirmative psychotherapy for LGBT people is operationalised in order for it to be evaluated.

7. Funding is made available for the evaluation of the effectiveness of LGBT-affirmative therapy in cohort studies and randomised controlled trials.

8. Prospective research should evaluate the degree to which our training recommendations are implemented and determine predictors of their implementation.

9. Mental health and psychotherapy services should routinely audit outcomes for LGBT people, including satisfaction, access, engagement, perceived homophobia, and mental health outcomes, including psychological and emotional wellbeing and functioning.

Future Directions

There has been and still is a proliferation of poorly designed studies 'measuring' sexual minority mental health being badged as LGB research. Frequent calls for 'opportunities' through social media invite the LGB population to partake in repetitive, poorly designed unnecessary studies of mental health prevalence. Ethically, repetition and poor design should be avoided at all costs. Yet when faced with the question of what to do about these observed disparities, the doing of research is often in and of itself the suggested solution to a problem! Indeed, the UK Government itself, in response to a seminar held in 2018 that presented health disparities in this population, was to carry out a convenience sample survey, albeit of 108,000 people, (Government Equalities Office, 2018a), which they used to develop their action plan (Government Equalities Office, 2018b). At time of writing most of these actions were paused and stalled.

Furthermore, research on sexual minority health is hugely under-funded, under-resourced and poorly disseminated. The endless misuse of mental health inequality as a justification for the "homosexuality is a mental illness" trope remains problematic especially within the influential sphere of religious and faith groups (APA, 2009; King, 2015) and there is a distinct lack of research activity focused on the necessary and urgent need to develop interventions (Semlyen & Meads, forthcoming).

In developing further research or interventions, approaches that remain committed to looking at and thinking about identities disaggregated across the subgroups, recognising that all have different and diverse mental health outcomes, needs and service use requirements are key. Studies that are properly funded, well-constructed with rigorous design, and with robust and useful data, that measure sexual orientation identity in ways that allow meaningful comparison with existing knowledge, that don't replicate what is known but bring something new to the table and that provide opportunity to change the landscape of knowledge through intervention development are what we need to focus on now.

Continued collection of data that allows monitoring of interventions and treatments (existing and new) is imperative and a continued recognition that sexual minority mental health must become a significant priority for health professionals cannot be overstated.

References

Almack, K. (2023). Monitoring patients' sexual orientation and gender identity: Can we ask? Should we ask? How do we ask? *BMJ Quality & Safety, 32*, 73–75.

APA. (2009). *Appropriate affirmative responses to sexual orientation distress and change efforts*. Retrieved February 10, 2013.

Aspinall, P. J. (2009). *Estimating the size and composition of the lesbian, gay and bisexual population in Britain* (Research Report 37). Equality and Human Rights Commission.

Barker, M.-J. (2015). Depression and/or oppression? Bisexuality and Mental Health. *Journal of Bisexuality, 15*(3): 369–384.

Betts, P. (2008). *Developing survey questions on sexual identity: UK experiences of administering survey questions on sexual identity/orientation*. SM Division. Office for National Statistics.

Betts, P. (2009). *ONS developing survey questions on sexual identity: Cognitive/in-depth interviews*. Office for National Statistics.

Brooks, V. R. (1981). *Minority stress and lesbian women*. Lexington Books.

Calzo, J. P., Austin, S. B., & Micali, N. (2018). Sexual orientation disparities in eating disorder symptoms among adolescent boys and girls in the UK. *European Child & Adolescent Psychiatry, 27*(11), 1483–1490.

Chakraborty, A., McManus, S., Brugha, T., Bebbington, P., & King, M. (2011). Mental health of the non-heterosexual population of England. *British Journal of Psychiatry, 198*(2), 143–148.

Colledge, L., Hickson, F., Reid, D., & Weatherburn, P. (2015). Poorer mental health in UK bisexual women than lesbians: Evidence from the UK 2007 Stonewall Women's Health Survey. *Journal of Public Health, 37*(3), 427.

Diamond, L. M., & Alley, J. (2022). Rethinking minority stress: A social safety perspective on the health effects of stigma in sexually-diverse and gender-diverse population. *Neuroscience & Biobehavioral Reviews, 138*, 104720.

Dodds, J. P., Mercer, C. H., Mercey, D., Copas, A., & Johnson, A. (2006). Men who have sex with men: A comparison of a probability sample survey and a community based study. *Sexually Transmitted Infections, 82*(1), 86–87.

Drinkwater, D., & Semlyen, J. (2012). Why sexuality and gender identity matter: A discourse analysis of LGBT mental health services user's talk of recovery. *Qualitative Methods in Mental Health*. University of Nottingham.

Eliason, M. J., Radix, A., McElroy, J. A., Garbers, S., & Haynes, S. G. (2016). The "something else" of sexual orientation: Measuring sexual identities of older lesbian and bisexual women using national health interview survey questions. *Women's Health Issues, 26*(Suppl 1), S71-80.

Eliason, M. J., & Streed, C. G., Jr. (2017). Choosing "SOMETHING ELSE" as a sexual identity: Evaluating response options on the national health interview survey. *LGBT Health, 4*(5), 376–379.

Elliott, M. N., Kanouse, D. E., Burkhart, Q., Abel, G. A., Lyratzopoulos, G., Beckett, M. K., Schuster, M. A., & Roland, M. (2015). Sexual minorities in England have poorer health and worse health care experiences: A national survey. *Journal of General Internal Medicine, 30*(1), 9–16.

Evans, A. R., Wiggins, R. D., Mercer, C. H., Bolding, G. J., & Elford, J. (2007). Men who have sex with men in Great Britain: Comparison of a self-selected internet sample with a national probability sample. *Sexually Transmitted Infections, 83*(3), 200–205.

Feinstein, B. A. (2020). The rejection sensitivity model as a framework for understanding sexual minority mental health. *Archives of Sexual Behavior, 49*(7), 2247–2258.

Flentje, A., Heck, N. C., Brennan, J. M., & Meyer, I. H. (2020). The relationship between minority stress and biological outcomes: A systematic review. *Journal of Behavioral Medicine, 43*, 673–694.

Geary, R. S., Tanton, C., Erens, B., Clifton, S., Prah, P., Wellings, K., Mitchell, K. R., Datta, J., Gravningen, K., Fuller, E., Johnson, A. M., Sonnenberg, P., & Mercer, C. H. (2018). Sexual identity, attraction and behaviour in Britain: The implications of using different dimensions of sexual orientation to estimate the size of sexual minority populations and inform public health interventions. *PLoS ONE, 13*(1), e0189607.

Goffman, E. (2009). *Stigma: Notes on the management of spoiled identity*. Simon and Schuster.

Government Equalities Office. (2018a). *National LGBT survey: Research report*.

Government Equalities Office. (2018b). *LGBT Action Plan*.

Guasp, A., & Taylor, J. (2012). *Experiences of healthcare: Stonewall health briefing*. Stonewall.

Hagger-Johnson, G., Taibjee, R., Semlyen, J., Fitchie, I., Fish, J., Meads, C., & Varney, J. (2013). Sexual orientation identity in relation to smoking history and alcohol use at age 18/19: Cross-sectional associations from the Longitudinal Study of Young People in England (LSYPE). *BMJ Open, 3*(8), e002810.

Haseldon, L., Joloza, T., & Household, L. M. (2009). *Measuring sexual identity: A guide for researchers*. Office for National Statistics.

Hatzenbuehler, M., Keyes, K., & Hasin, D. (2009). State-level policies and psychiatric morbidity in lesbian, gay, and bisexual populations. *American Journal of Public Health, 99*(12), 2275–2281.

Hatzenbuehler, M. L. (2009). How does sexual minority stigma "get under the skin"? A psychological mediation framework. *Psychological Bulletin, 135*(5), 707.

Hatzenbuehler, M. L., & Link, B. G. (2014). Introduction to the special issue on structural stigma and health. *Social Science & Medicine, 103*, 1–6.

Heck, N. C., Mirabito, L. A., LeMaire, K., Livingston, N. A., & Flentje, A. (2017). Omitted data in randomized controlled trials for anxiety and depression: A systematic review of the inclusion of sexual orientation and gender identity. *Journal of Consulting and Clinical Psychology, 85*(1), 72.

Hickson, F., Davey, C., Reid, D., Weatherburn, P., & Bourne, A. (2017). Mental health inequalities among gay and bisexual men in England, Scotland and Wales: A large community-based cross-sectional survey. *Journal of Public Health, 39*(3), 645.

Hottes, T. S., Bogaert, L., Rhodes, A. E., Brennan, D. J., & Gesink, D. (2016). Lifetime prevalence of suicide attempts among sexual minority adults by study sampling strategies: a systematic review and meta-analysis. *American Journal of Public Health 106* (5), e1–12.

Jones, A., Robinson, E., Oginni, O., Rahman, Q., & Rimes, K. A. (2017). Anxiety disorders, gender nonconformity, bullying and self-esteem in sexual minority adolescents: Prospective birth cohort study. *Journal of Child Psychology and Psychiatry, 58*(11), 1201–1209.

King, M. (2015). Attitudes of therapists and other health professionals towards their LGB patients. *International Review of Psychiatry, 27*(5), 396–404.

King, M., Semlyen, J., Killaspy, H., Nazareth, I., & Osborn, D. (2007). *A systematic review of research on counselling and psychotherapy for lesbian, gay, bisexual & transgender people*. British Association for Counselling and Psychotherapy.

King, M., Semlyen, J., Tai, S. S., Killaspy, H., Osborn, D., Popelyuk, D., & Nazareth, I. (2008). A systematic review of mental disorder, suicide, and deliberate self harm in lesbian, gay and bisexual people. *BMC Psychiatry*, 8(1), 70.

Kuyper, L., Fernee, H., & Keuzenkamp, S. (2016). A comparative analysis of a community and general sample of lesbian, gay, and bisexual individuals. *Archives of Sexual Behavior*, 45(3), 683–693.

Le Forestier, J. M., Chan, E. W., Shephard, R., Page-Gould, E., & Chasteen, A. L. (2023). *Why is Concealment Associated with Health and Wellbeing? An Investigation of Fifteen Potential Mechanisms*. PsyArXiv.

McNamee, H., Lloyd, K., & Schubotz, D. (2008). Same sex attraction, homophobic bullying and mental health of young people in Northern Ireland. *Journal of Youth Studies*, 11(1), 33–46.

Mercer, C. H., Prah, P., Field, N., Tanton, C., Macdowall, W., Clifton, S., Hughes, G., Nardone, A., Wellings, K., Johnson, A. M., & Sonnenberg, P. (2016). The health and well-being of men who have sex with men (MSM) in Britain: Evidence from the third National Survey of Sexual Attitudes and Lifestyles (Natsal-3). *BMC Public Health*, 16, 525.

Meyer, I. (2003). Prejudice, social stress, and mental health in lesbian, gay, and bisexual populations: Conceptual issues and research evidence. *Psychological Bulletin*, 129(5), 674–697.

Meyer, I. H. (1995). Minority stress and mental health in gay men. *Journal of Health and Social Behavior*, 36(1), 38–56.

Meyer, I. H. (2015). Resilience in the study of minority stress and health of sexual and gender minorities. *Psychology of Sexual Orientation and Gender Diversity*, 2(3), 209.

Meyer, I. H., & Wilson, P. A. (2009). Sampling lesbian, gay, and bisexual populations. *Journal of Counseling Psychology*, 56(1), 23.

National Institute for Health and Clinical Excellence. (2011). *Common mental disorders: Full guideline*. NICE.

Ngamake, S. T., Walch, S. E., & Raveepatarakul, J. (2016). Discrimination and sexual minority mental health: Mediation and moderation effects of coping. *Psychology of Sexual Orientation and Gender Diversity*, 3(2), 213–226.

NHS England. (2017a). *DCB2094: Sexual orientation monitoring standard*.

NHS England. (2017b). *Sexual orientation monitoring: Full specification*.

Pachankis, J. E., Hatzenbuehler, M. L., Hickson, F., Weatherburn, P., Berg, R. C., Marcus, U., & Schmidt, A. J. (2015). Hidden from health: Structural stigma, sexual orientation concealment, and HIV across 38 countries in the European MSM Internet Survey. *AIDS*, 29(10), 1239.

Pachankis, J. E., Mahon, C. P., Jackson, S. D., Fetzner, B. K., & Bränström, R. (2020). Sexual orientation concealment and mental health: A conceptual and meta-analytic review. *Psychological Bulletin, 146*(10), 831.

Pesola, F., Shelton, K. H., & van den Bree, M. B. (2014). Sexual orientation and alcohol problem use among UK adolescents: An indirect link through depressed mood. *Addiction, 109*(7), 1072–1080.

Rich, A. J., Salway, T., Scheim, A., & Poteat, T. (2020). Sexual minority stress theory: Remembering and honoring the work of Virginia Brooks. *LGBT Health, 7*(3), 124–127.

Rimes, K. A., Broadbent, M., Holden, R., Rahman, Q., Hambrook, D., Hatch, S. L., & Wingrove, J. (2018a). Comparison of treatment outcomes between lesbian, gay, bisexual and heterosexual individuals receiving a primary care psychological intervention. *Behavioural and Cognitive Psychotherapy, 46*(3), 332–349.

Rimes, K. A., Shivakumar, S., Ussher, G., Baker, D., Rahman, Q., & West, E. (2018b). Psychosocial factors associated with suicide attempts, ideation, and future risk in lesbian, gay, and bisexual youth. *Crisis, 40*(2), 83–92.

Rivers, I., Gonzalez, C., Nodin, N., Peel, E., & Tyler, A. (2018). LGBT people and suicidality in youth: A qualitative study of perceptions of risk and protective circumstances. *Social Science & Medicine, 212*, 1–8.

Savin-Williams, R. C., & Ream, G. L. (2007). Prevalence and stability of sexual orientation components during adolescence and young adulthood. *Archives of Sexual Behavior, 36*(3), 385–394.

Schubotz, D., & O'Hara, M. (2011). A shared future? Exclusion, stigmatization, and mental health of same-sex-attracted young people in Northern Ireland. *Youth & Society, 43*(2), 488–508.

Semlyen, J. (2017). Recording sexual orientation in the UK: Pooling data for statistical power. *American Journal of Public Health, 107*(8), 1215–1217.

Semlyen, J., King, M., Varney, J., & Hagger-Johnson, G. (2016). Sexual orientation and symptoms of common mental disorder or low wellbeing: Combined meta-analysis of 12 UK population health surveys. *BMC Psychiatry, 16*(1), 67.

Semlyen, J., & Meads, C. (Forthcoming). A systematic review of interventions addressing health disparities in LGBT popualtions in the UK.

Walch, S. E., Ngamake, S. T., Bovornusvakool, W., & Walker, S. V. (2016). Discrimination, internalized homophobia, and concealment in sexual minority physical and mental health. *Psychology of Sexual Orientation and Gender Diversity, 3*(1), 37.

Woodhead, C., Gazard, B., Hotopf, M., Rahman, Q., Rimes, K., & Hatch, S. (2016). Mental health among UK inner city non-heterosexuals: The role of risk factors, protective factors and place. *Epidemiology and Psychiatric Sciences, 25*(5), 450–461.

Young, R., Riordan, V., & Stark, C. (2011). Perinatal and psychosocial circumstances associated with risk of attempted suicide, non-suicidal self-injury and psychiatric service use. A longitudinal study of young people. *BMC Public Health, 11*(1), 875.

3

Social Prejudice

Sonja J. Ellis

Introduction

Internationally, over the last two decades there has been unprecedented positive social change around the inclusion of sexual minorities in society. As well as greater social inclusion in society more generally, in many places (primarily in Europe, North America, and Australasia) this has been accompanied by substantive advances including marriage equality, parenting rights, and protection from discrimination in the workplace. For example, in the UK, protection against discrimination on the grounds of 'sexual orientation' came into effect in 2003, same-sex couples have been able to 'marry' through a civil partnership since 2005, have been able to marry since 2014 (2020 in Northern Ireland), and since 2005 have been able to jointly adopt children (2009 in Scotland; 2013 in Northern Ireland).

S. J. Ellis (✉)
The University of Waikato, Hamilton, New Zealand
e-mail: sonja.ellis@waikato.ac.nz

© The Author(s), under exclusive license to Springer Nature
Switzerland AG 2023
J. Semlyen and P. Rohleder (eds.), *Sexual Minorities and Mental Health*,
https://doi.org/10.1007/978-3-031-37438-8_3

Although in many instances legal changes have brought with them increased social acceptance and inclusion, this is not universally true. In many countries in Asia, the Middle East, Africa, and the Pacific, homosexuality is illegal. While in a number of countries in Asia (for example, China, India, and Thailand) homosexuality is not criminalised, and in some instances certain legal protections are afforded, sexual minorities still experience widespread stigmatisation. Similarly, even in western contexts where social and legal inclusion are well established, those from minority ethnic and (in some cases) indigenous cultures experience stigmatisation in their own communities and are multiply marginalised due to the stigmatisation they also experience through systemic—and sometimes overt—racism within mainstream society (see Chapter 6).

Despite considerable progress in both the recognition and inclusion of sexual minorities within western society, social prejudice has never been eradicated. Recent years, particularly in Europe and North America, have seen the rise of populist politics and with it, a resurgence of anti-gay sentiment. For the first time in decades far right groups have been afforded a platform which has resulted in an increased prevalence of state sanctioned anti-gay rhetoric. For example, in the US the Trump administration initiated attacks on a range of LGBT protections including protections in healthcare, education, and employment (see Levin, 2019) while in an election campaign the President of Poland threatened to ban LGBTQ subject matter in schools and forbid same-sex marriage and adoption (see Porterfield, 2020). In tandem with this, there have been noticeable changes in the prevalence of anti-gay sentiment within wider society and also an increase in hostility towards sexual minorities. In the UK, one clear example is that sexual orientation motivated hate crimes reported to the police have doubled in the five years ending 2021 (Gov.uk, 2021). While some of the increase may be attributable to increases in rates of reporting and changes in methods of recording, the level of change would seem to indicate re a substantive increase in actual incidences of hate crime over this period even when these factors are accounted for.

Defining Social Prejudice Against Sexual Minorities

In the psychological literature there are a wide range of terms used to refer to social prejudice against sexual minorities. While terms such as 'homonegativity' and 'anti-gay prejudice' are widely used, the most commonly used term is 'homophobia'. The use of the term homophobia dates back to the early 1970s (Smith, 1971; Weinberg, 1972) and throughout the late twentieth century it was conceptualised as negative perceptions, attitudes, and behaviours towards lesbians and gay men. With the increased recognition of diversity, and substantive shifts in the way that sexuality is understood, today the term homophobia is often used as an umbrella term for negative perceptions, attitudes, and behaviours towards all sexual minorities, including those who identify as bisexual, pansexual, and other non-heterosexual identities. Sometimes the term 'biphobia' is used to refer to social prejudice that is specifically anti-bisexual; for example, perceptions of bisexuals as confused about their sexual identity, as really lesbians or gay men who refuse to come out, or as being promiscuous (Eliason, 2000; Hayfield, 2020). However, it is important to recognise that homophobia is not always perpetrated against sexual minorities but may also be used against heterosexual people, either as a way of socialising gender conformity (for example, see Poteat et al., 2012) or because they are *perceived* to be lesbian, gay, or bisexual.

Generally speaking, homophobia is manifested by individuals—typically against individuals—as symbolic representatives of sexual minorities as a group. It is usually framed as overt expressions of anti-LGB sentiments or specific acts of aggression or violence against sexual minorities. However, social prejudice is not necessarily overt. In many instances prejudice is systemic, and in the case of sexual minorities is manifested in societal customs and often institutionalised (embedded in the education and legal system) resulting in the erasure or marginalisation of sexual minorities and their culture (for example, customs and history); and by implication privileging heterosexuality and its culture. This type of prejudice is commonly referred to as heterosexism (Herek, 1990) and is made possible through the taken-for-granted normalisation of heterosexuality.

This phenomenon is often referred to as 'heteronormativity' (Warner, 1991).

Over the last few decades in western societies, it has become socially unacceptable to express overtly prejudiced views, and considerable sociolegal changes have meant that organisations are legally obligated to address institutionalised prejudice against sexual minorities. For example, in most western jurisdictions it is no longer legal to discriminate on the basis of 'sexual orientation' in relation to employment or the provision of goods and services. Despite this, both heterosexuality and heteronormativity are still deeply embedded in the fabric of society. So, while overt forms of homophobia and overt discrimination against sexual minorities in institutional settings are (arguably) less common today in a country like the UK, there is still much residual prejudice. The most common type of prejudice today is everyday incidences of heterosexism that are relatively unnoticed or unnoticeable; a phenomenon referred to as 'mundane heterosexism' (Peel, 2001). In the early 2000s, critical social psychologists (for example, Gough, 2002 and Kitzinger, 2005) explored the ways in which mundane heterosexism is conveyed in talk. For example, in group discussions with men Gough (2002) explored the way in which men's talk routinely reproduced heterosexual versions of masculinity through the mobilisation of homophobic talk. In the discussions, homosexuality was negatively framed in ways that devalued gay men while simultaneously positioning the male speakers as heterosexually masculine. The findings of this and other studies of mundane heterosexism show the way in which through talk sexual minorities are 'othered' in ways that are often subtle.

Drawing on work around racial prejudice, recent work has shifted the focus to microaggressions (Sue et al., 2007); a form of subtle prejudice. Microaggressions are "brief and commonplace daily verbal, behavioural, and environmental indignities, whether intentional or unintentional, that communicate hostile, derogatory, or negative…slights and insights to the target person or group" (Sue et al., 2007, p. 273). Examples of sexual minority microaggressions include things like 'that's so gay' (said as a putdown), 'not a real family' (implying that families can only be headed by heterosexual couples), and 'you don't look gay' (regarding 'gay' people as fitting a specific stereotype). So, in a sexual minority context microaggressions may comprise the use of 'gay' to mean uncool or stupid (Amodeo, Esposito, & Bacchini, 2020) or to discredit, minimise, or assess one's status as a sexual minority (Dimberg et al., 2021). Essentially microaggressions are a mundane form of prejudice in that they are typically subtle, often unconsciously delivered, and are not usually intended to be prejudiced (Sue et al., 2007).

Social Prejudice in Interpersonal Settings

The most overt forms of social prejudice are those that constitute some level of victimisation. While physical and sexual assaults occur, verbal abuse is the most common form of victimisation experienced by sexual minorities. Verbal victimisation typically includes aggressive, insulting, or stigmatising language; typically used interpersonally by individuals or groups to discriminate against, stereotype, or hurt sexual minority individuals or groups (El-Khoury et al., 2020). This type of social prejudice may comprise anything from legally defined hate crime, to homophobic bullying, through to mundane heterosexism and microaggressions.

Recent research around victimisation overwhelmingly suggests that sexual minorities are at considerably higher risk of victimisation than their heterosexual peers (Daigle & Hawk, 2022; Felix et al., 2021; Ray et al., 2021). For adults in the UK, statistics suggest that homophobic hate crime has increased considerably (GOV.UK, 2021), and a relatively recent YouGov survey indicated that one-in-six LGB people (and who are not trans) have experienced a hate crime or incident due to their sexual orientation in the 12 months prior to the survey (Bachman & Gooch, 2017). Homophobic hate crime may comprise verbal victimisation (for example, insults; intimidation; harassment), violence (for example, physical assault; use of force; threats), or damage to property that is perpetrated against sexual minorities; and can be clearly linked to them being, or being perceived to be, a sexual minority. Characteristically, hate crimes are not (usually) random or opportunistic attacks against individuals, but rather a deliberate targeting of members of a specific group as *symbols* of that group. Consequently, homophobic hate crimes are deliberately designed to send a message of intimidation to the wider community of sexual minorities. It is commonly reported that homophobic hate crimes (and related behaviours) are under-reported, but the extent of social prejudice lies much deeper than acts perpetrated against sexual minorities. What is less often articulated is the lengths that some sexual minorities go to in order to avoid victimisation. Even in societies where sexual minorities are more readily accepted many sexual minority people do not feel comfortable disclosing their identity at work or in other settings, or being seen as 'gay'. Furthermore, sexual minority individuals who are also culturally marginalised (such as, have ethnic minority backgrounds) may not find it feasible to disclose their sexual identity at home; while others may change their behaviour (for example, avoid known lesbian/gay venues, and monitor their appearance or behaviour) in order to pass as 'straight'.

Not all forms of social prejudice constitute victimisation. For example, sexual minorities commonly experience implicit discrimination both in access to, and the delivery of healthcare (Fish & Williamson, 2018). Commonly reported experiences include health professionals who appear ill-informed about sexual minorities, and systemic heteronormativity, resulting in often inadequate or inappropriate health advice/care (see McNeill et al., 2021). Both mundane and institutionalised forms of heterosexism lead many sexual minorities to not feel comfortable about being open about their sexuality in health care settings. This may result in disengagement from health care provision (for example, not participating in cervical screening) or the perpetuation of health disparities between sexual minorities and their heterosexual counterparts (see Zeeman et al., 2019). In the UK, the national LGBT action plan (Government Equalities Office, 2018) is designed to address these inequities; both in health, and in other institutional settings such as education.

Among young people, homophobic bullying is a common form of social prejudice. It is perpetrated against sexual minority youth as well as those who are perceived not to conform to norms around gender and sexuality. Sexual minority youth are at significantly higher risk of homophobic bullying—whether in person or via electronic means—than their heterosexual peers (Kahle, 2020). In the UK, the Stonewall School Report (Stonewall, 2017) indicates that although homophobic bullying had decreased in the period 2012–2017, around half of LGBT students are bullied, and a similar percentage have frequently experienced microaggressions (for example, heard homophobic slurs) at school.

An especially challenging form of social prejudice faced by sexual minority young people today is scepticism around their sexual minority identity (Dimberg et al., 2021). A prevalent culture of sexual fluidity among young women has seen engagement in public displays of suggestive lesbian acts (for example, intimately kissing other women at parties) to demonstrate bravado, or to attract male attention, become a normalised part of the heterosexual repertoire. Essentially this is an appropriation of lesbian sexuality for the heterosexual male consumer (Diamond, 2005; Gill, 2008) while non-heterosexually palatable expressions of lesbian desire are marginalised (Farhall, 2018; Gill, 2017). Compounded by the popularisation of the concept of the so-called 'girl crush', and perpetuation of heterosexist language (for example, 'girls' or 'babes') in commercialised gay spaces (Gill, 2017), this culture has made it much harder for sexual minority young women to be understood as authentically 'gay'. Furthermore, characterised by an intense non-sexual admiration of women, the girl crush conflates lesbian desire with platonic love. The problem with this is that it trivialises sincere same-sex attraction positioning it as akin to appreciation and aesthetic value, emotions commonly constructed as less important or meaningful than sexual desire and romantic love (Farhall, 2018).

Another subtle way in which social prejudice marginalises sexual minorities is the mainstreaming and popularisation of sexual minority culture. Born out of the fight for equality, the activist pride events of yesteryear have given way to highly commercialised events in which sexual minority culture has become just another themed party (Ammaturo, 2016). Coupled with this, every aspect of sexual minority culture from pride playlists on Spotify, to LGBTQ streaming services (for example, Dekkoo; Revry), and 'pink tourism' (for example, gay exclusive resorts, and marketing of mainstream venues as 'gay friendly') is seen as a way to make money, not just from sexual minorities but also through capitalising on the fashionableness of 'gay culture'. Similarly, in highly urbanised environments, gay neighbourhoods (for example, Soho in London or Canal Street in Manchester) that were once run-down central

city areas reclaimed by sexual minorities have increasingly become gentri-
fied; appealing to a more mainstream—and more affluent—audience
(Hess, 2019), and a social 'theme park' for heterosexuals (Casey, 2004;
Emig, 2018). While appearing to increase inclusivity for sexual minorities, these processes instead result in increased marginalisation through
the dilution of sexual minority culture and decreased opportunities for
sexual minority people to organise in meaningful ways (Ammaturo,
2016; Hess, 2019). Furthermore, increasing homonormativity (Duggan,
2002) has resulted in more heterosexually normative versions of sexual
minorities (for example, monogamous coupledom, or lesbian and gay
parenting) being more readily included in society and the simultaneous
marginalisation of sexual minorities who do not fit the heterosexual
norm.

Attitudes Towards Sexual Minorities

Until the mid-1990s, sexual minorities in the western world were subject
to a social climate in which they were not readily accepted and often
actively discriminated against. To varying degrees this social climate
was state-sanctioned due to the lack of socio-legal protections afforded
to sexual minorities, and the legal status of homosexuality itself. For
example, while homosexuality was legalised in England and Wales in
1967 it had a heavily circumscribed status through the institution of
an age of consent of 21 (for heterosexuality it was 16) and through
the policing of homosexuals in public places, including clubs and pubs.
In many other western jurisdictions homosexuality was not legalised
until much later. Before "homosexuality per se" was removed from the
DSM-II in 1973, it was classified as a 'sexual deviation' which was
also classified as a 'personality disorder' (Drescher, 2015) resulting not
only in the psychological and medical stigmatisation of many lesbians
and gay men, but in numerous instances their incarceration in psychiatric institutions where they were subjected to aversion therapy in an
attempt to 'cure' them. Aversion therapy was still widely used in the
1980s, and although purported to be 'successful' (Dickinson et al., 2012)
there is no scientific evidence that these therapies actually worked. The

stigmatisation of sexual minorities was further intensified by the AIDS epidemic of the 1980s. The prevalence of HIV transmission among gay men resulted in sexual minorities, and in particular gay men, being seen as undesirables. The social stigmatisation of gay men in this way is well captured in the recent British television series *It's a Sin* (Davies, 2021). Despite the last 25 years being (arguably) more enlightened times, negative attitudes towards sexual minorities have tended to surface in relation to major social change, notably where these changes intersect with heteronormative understandings of family.

Early work on lesbian and gay human rights indicated that while the overwhelming majority of people support personal rights and freedoms for sexual minorities, support for social rights (for example, the right to marry, freedom of expression in public, access to information in school) is considerably less well supported (Ellis, 2002). Consistent with this, recent debates around key equity issues for sexual minorities (for example, same-sex marriage; sexual minority inclusion in education) have invariably been seen as contentious, and at times resulted in moral panic. Broadly speaking, a moral panic refers to "the creation of a situation in which exaggerated fear is manufactured about topics that are seen (or claimed) to have a moral component" (Ben-Yehuda, 2009, p. 1). Often moral panic relating to sexual minorities centres on unsubstantiated claims that affording rights and social inclusion to sexual minorities presents a threat to the existing social order, and to childhood innocence. These claims are designed to be emotive and are therefore neither rational, nor (in this context) justified. Furthermore, these forms of social prejudice are mobilised through the elevation of democratic rights (such as, majority rules) over sexual minority rights to equality/equity (Ellis & Kitzinger, 2002). With reference to two recent examples—same-sex marriage and sexual minority inclusion in sexuality education—I will now outline the way in which social prejudice is manifested.

Same-Sex Marriage

For same-sex couples, marriage equality has been seen as an integral part of social inclusion (Badgett, 2011). However, almost universally 'marriage' has been conceptualised as inherently heterosexual; by definition and tradition a union between a man and a woman. This, together with the biological determinist construction of marriage as a framework designed for raising children, has been commonly used to argue against same-sex marriage (Jowett, 2014). While in some jurisdictions—notably Canada—the fact that the country's Constitution did not specifically state that marriage could only be between a man and a woman enabled a smoother transition to marriage equality; in others this was not necessarily the case. For example, in Australia, 2004 saw the Marriage Amendment Act introduced. This act saw for the first time the idea of marriage being specifically stated as 'the union of a man and a woman to the exclusion of all others' and explicitly banned the recognition of same-sex marriages entered into in other jurisdictions. The Act enabled this very argument to be mobilised resulting in marriage equality not being achieved in Australia until 2017. Today, there are around 30 countries where same-sex marriages are legal, among the most recent being the Republic of Ireland in 2015 (the first to legalise same-sex marriage through a referendum), Taiwan in 2017 (the first in Asia to legalise same-sex marriage), and Northern Ireland in 2019 (the last constituent country of the UK to do so).

Same-sex marriage has also been problematic historically in its formulation. In some countries, marriage equality was preceded by a marriage-like alternative. For example, in the UK the Civil Partnership Act 2004 made it possible for same-sex couples to obtain legal recognition of their relationships, and access to the rights and responsibilities afforded married couples from December 2005 (Harding & Peel, 2006; Wright, 2006). To most, civil partnerships were seen as 'marriage in all but name' due to there being very few discernible legal differences between (heterosexual) marriage and civil partnership. However, as many highlighted, the very use of alternative nomenclature and a two-tier system meant that same-sex couples were being treated differently from other-sex couples resulting in civil partnerships being seen as an inferior form of marriage. Essentially, civil partnerships extended rights to same-sex couples, but were designed to distinguish the formal recognition of same-sex relationships from the 'gold standard' of marriage afforded heterosexual couples (Wilkinson & Kitzinger, 2006). This was demonstrated by the

British High Court's judgement in 2006 that Celia Kitzinger and Sue Wilkinson's Canadian marriage could not be recognised in England and Wales in that 'marriage is by long standing definition and acceptance, a formal relationship between a man and a woman, primarily (though not exclusively) with the aim of producing and rearing children' (Para. 119) (see Harding, 2007). Furthermore, while the media commonly referred to civil partnerships using the terms 'marriage' and 'wedding' this was often using scare quotes, potentially signalling an issue or irregularity with these terms; while at other times constructing marriage as very much the sole domain of heterosexual couples (Jowett & Peel, 2010).

Like other sexual minority equality issues before it (for example, see Ellis & Kitzinger, 2002), the path to marriage equality has been marked by social prejudice. In the UK, marriage equality came about through a series of legal and political processes so in the main arguments against same-sex marriage were played out in political settings and in the media; notably the British press. There was relatively little visible public opposition to the legalisation of same-sex marriages through civil partnerships, and subsequently the institution of marriage equality. As with many other jurisdictions, conservative arguments about same-sex marriage being a threat to 'traditional' marriage, moral values, and family were common in political rhetoric (Clarke, 2003; Jowett, 2014). However, in the British Press, an argument around same-sex marriage being the 'thin end of the wedge' was also prevalent. As Jowett (2014) highlights, this type of argument claimed that allowing same-sex marriage would effectively set a precedent, enabling arguments around legalisation of polygamy and incestuous marriage to be proffered. The proposition of full marriage equality when civil partnerships were already in place saw a new argument emerge - that there was no need to legalise same-sex marriage as sexual minorities were already afforded through civil partnership (Jowett, 2014). The mobilisation of this argument demonstrates the lack of a clear understanding of the ways in which civil partnership marginalises same-sex couples, effectively treating same-sex relationships as 'less than' heterosexual ones.

In contrast to the UK, marriage equality in Australia was brought about by a plebiscite (public referendum) in which Australian citizens were given the opportunity to vote on whether or not same-sex marriages should become legal. The proposition of same-sex marriage there was marked by inherent, and in many cases explicit, homophobia. For example, 'vote no to faggots' was sighted on a Sydney train, and 'vote no' skywritten over Sydney harbour (Flaherty & Wilkinson, 2020); while organisations vehemently opposed to the idea of same-sex marriage launched a series of emotive television adverts, and leafleted house-holds with anti-gay propaganda (Thomas et al., 2020). Much of the campaigning was based on false claims that legalising same-sex marriage would result in the expansion of 'gay freedoms' and radical forms of sex education.

Sexual Minority Inclusion in Schools

The inclusion of sexual minority perspectives/culture within school settings has often been seen as contentious. Notably, in the UK from the late 1980s the legislative context was actively exclusionary with the introduction of Section 28 of the Local Government Act in 1988 prohibiting schools from 'teaching the acceptability of homosexuality as a pretended family relationship'. This legislation arose out of fears about children having access to books that normalise parenting by same-sex couples; in particular, the book *Jenny lives with Eric and Martin*. Although eventually repealed in the early 2000s, for a whole genera-tion Section 28 imbued a culture of silence around homosexuality and exacerbated the marginalisation of sexual minority youth growing up in the UK. Across much of the western world over the past decade there have been moves to ensure sexual minority inclusivity in education. Such initiatives are inevitably fraught in that 'childhood innocence' is invari-ably constructed to mean a life without sex and the knowledge of sex and sexuality (Thompson, 2020). Therefore, despite considerable posi-tive social change for sexual minorities, the inclusion of sexual minority content in schools is often seen as highly controversial; and many western jurisdictions have been reticent to include such content (Gegenfurtner & Gebhardt, 2017; Shannon & Smith, 2015). The Safe Schools initiative in Australia, and the implementation of new regulations for Relationships and Sexuality Education (RSE) in England are recent examples, and both have been met with considerable resistance (Formby & Donovan, 2020; Rawlings & Loveday, 2021).

The Safe Schools Coalition Australia (SSCA) was initially established in the Australian state of Victoria in 2010. The programme was designed to promote affirmation and inclusivity for sexual minorities (and around gender diversity) with the aim of creating a safe and supportive environment for LGBTI students and to tackle homophobic (and transphobic) bullying and harassment (Rawlings & Loveday, 2021); and for its first few years was seen as relatively uncontroversial (Thompson, 2020). As the programme was rolled out nationally, it was funded by the Australian Federal Government, but following considerable opposition from right-wing conservative MPs, The Australian Christian Lobby, and others it was defunded in 2017. Although some states (notably, Victoria) have provided state funding to continue the programme, retention is not widespread. Fuelled by mass media, opponents saw it as a form of social engineering, radical left-wing propaganda, sexualising children, and exposing them to inappropriate content (Zaglas, 2019). Overwhelmingly, representations of the SSCA were problematically framed through allusions to the promotion of paedophilia and grooming through to accusations of political correctness gone mad (see Rawlings & Loveday, 2021). Such protestations were specifically designed to invoke indignation and opposition from parents, the presumed reader of media reports (Thompson, 2020).

Similarly, in England, an overhaul of Sex and Relationships Education (SRE) has been undertaken making SRE in schools a statutory requirement from September 2020. The new regulations were released in 2019 and included a requirement that all primary schools teach Relationships Education; and that SRE, including relationships education in primary school, should include the integration of LGBT perspectives, introduced in a timely and age-appropriate way (Department for Education, 2019). In practice this means ensuring that at primary school, teaching about different types of families includes LGBT families; and that in secondary school 'sexual orientation' is included, explored in relation to stable and healthy relationships, and integrated into the programme rather than addressed separately (Lee, 2021). While there was considerable support for these changes, the release of these regulations sparked protests primarily from conservative Muslims, but also from Christian parents and organisations (for example, Christian Concern), opposing the inclusion of sexual minority perspectives. The protests initially began at Parkhill School, Birmingham in response to the *No Outsiders* lessons aimed at promoting inclusivity by helping children to "grow up with respectful and positive attitudes towards people who are different to them" (Lee, 2021, p. 2). Opposition was directed in particular at the use of two children's picture books '*Mommy, Mama, and Me*' and '*And Tango makes Three*' that feature families with same-sex parents (see Kotecha, 2019; Lightfoot, 2019). The protests quickly spread nationwide and centred on a range of claims including that such content would condition children to accept homosexuality as a normal way of life, convert them to homosexuality, and make them more promiscuous as they grow older (for example, see LGBT school lessons protests spread nationwide, BBC News, 2019). As Lee (2021) notes, this level of opposition is unprecedented and indicates a growing climate of moral panic in education around the inclusion of content relating to sexual minorities.

While problematic enough, social prejudice in relation to sexual minority inclusion in schools is by no means restricted to external opposition to taught content. Often, the documentation itself perpetuates the existence of prejudice against sexual minorities by enabling exclusion. For example, the recently implemented guidelines for SRE in both England and New Zealand include provision for parents to withdraw their children from lessons; and in the case of New Zealand, school Boards of Trustees are required to consult with their communities (such as, parents) and stakeholders (for example, proprietors of state integrated schools) about proposed content. These measures mean that sexual minority content can effectively be censored. However, as research (for example, Røthing & Svendsen, 2010; Svendsen, 2012) suggests, even in contexts where the inclusion of sexual minority content is encouraged this does not necessarily result in inclusive education provision. For example, despite the explicit inclusion of sexual minorities in the 2015 guidelines for sexuality education in New Zealand (Ministry of Education, 2015) a recent study of New Zealanders aged 16–19 (Ellis & Bentham, 2021) indicated that sexuality education at secondary school is still overwhelmingly heteronormative, and that content around sexual minority identities or relationships was, at best, only tokenistically included. Furthermore, guidelines for the teaching of SRE at secondary school commonly reproduce heteronormativity by framing heterosexuality as actively sexual (such as, in relation to sexual behaviours and outcomes) while framing sexual minorities solely in relation to 'identities' (Ellis & Bentham, 2021). Sexual minorities—in particular gay and bisexual men—are further marginalised by the framing of sexual health in male-to-male sex solely in connection with HIV/AIDS risk (for example, Hoefer & Hoefer, 2017; Lee & Carpenter, 2015).

Social Prejudice and Mental Health

As highlighted in Chapter 2, sexual minorities are at high risk of experiencing mental health issues such as anxiety, depression, self-harm, and suicidality (Pitman et al., 2021). While individual differences (for example, personality; resiliency) undoubtedly play a part, social prejudice is a key factor in the mental health of sexual minorities. Studies of both homophobic victimisation (for example, El-Khoury et al., 2020) and on implicit forms of prejudice such as microaggressions, perceived discrimination, and systemic prejudice (for example, Chan et al., 2020; Cronin et al., 2021) have consistently found that social prejudice against sexual minority people has a significant negative impact on psychological wellbeing. Amount of exposure to negative rhetoric is also a factor in the relationship between social prejudice and psychological wellbeing. For example, a study of 1305 sexual minority adults in Australia (Verrelli et al., 2019) found that during the campaign for marriage equality, frequent exposure to negative media messages about same-sex marriage was associated with greater psychological distress. However, it is not usually single instances of social prejudice that result in adverse effects on mental health, but the cumulative effect of day-to-day marginalisation resulting from social prejudice in its various forms.

Based on research with lesbians, Sophie (1987) developed the theory of 'internalised homophobia' to explain the psychological trauma experienced by sexual minorities as a result of negative views of homosexuality prevalent in society. As the name suggests, internalised homophobia (sometimes called 'internalised homonegativity') is characterised by personally taking on board anti-gay sentiment and stigma to the detriment of one's own sense of self-worth. Typically, the internalisation of homophobia is not conscious (see Chapter 13), but the experience of ongoing negativity (for example, criticism, judgement, and/or discrimination) and the perpetuation of stereotypes in society contributes to a negative perception that makes identifying as a sexual minority person difficult and sometimes confusing (Kanbur, 2020).

The relationship between internalised homophobia and markers of wellbeing (for example, self-esteem, depressive symptoms, anxiety, and suicidal ideation) and/or problematic behaviours (for example, substance use, sexual risk behaviour, etc.) amongst sexual minorities has been well researched. Over recent years, research of this kind has focused primarily on sexual minorities in non-western countries such as China (Sun et al., 2020), South Korea (Lee et al., 2019), and Russia (Yanykin & Nasledov, 2017) finding strong links between internalised homophobia—typically measured using psychometric scales—and adverse mental health outcomes (for example, higher levels of depression; increased suicidality) and relationship quality. While the construct 'internalised homophobia' is still widely used, particularly in counselling and psychotherapy contexts (see Chapter 13), it might be seen as simplistic, individualistic, and pathologising in that it focuses on personal rather than socio-cultural factors that result in the marginalisation of sexual minorities.

Minority Stress Theory (Meyer, 1995) offers a more nuanced explanation in suggesting that sexual minorities are subjected to chronic stress due to both internal and external factors (Meyer, 2003). In particular, based on a rigorous scientific study with gay men, Meyer (1995) demonstrated that three components—internalized homophobia, stigma (such as, expectations of rejection/discrimination), and prejudice (such as, actual events of discrimination and violence)—individually and in combination produce psychological distress. In his later work, Meyer (2003) extended his research to include lesbian, gay, and bisexual persons; additionally, focusing on the effects of concealing one's sexual orientation, and on the role of coping processes in mitigating against the effects of stress. The findings of this study suggested that due to social prejudice, sexual minorities were at 2–3 times greater risk of psychological distress than their heterosexual counterparts. While it might be expected that increased inclusion of sexual minorities in society would result in decreased exposure to minority stressors, this is not necessarily the case. For example, large scale research using a national (US) probability sample (Meyer et al., 2021) found no signs that an improved social environment reduced exposure to minority stressors. Furthermore, the study found that psychological distress was worse for those in younger cohorts than it was for those in older cohorts. Also contrary to what might be expected, other studies (for example, Douglass et al., 2020; Pepping et al., 2019) have found that minority stressors adversely affected couple relationship satisfaction, increased expectations of rejection, and heightened the motivation to conceal one's sexual minority identity.

One of the issues with minority stress theory though is the assumption that minority stress (brought about by social prejudice) directly impacts mental health. However, in the 'psychological mediation framework', Hatzenbuehler (2009) suggests that minority stress is a catalyst for triggering psychological processes around coping and affect which in turn impact mental health. In this conceptualization, personal factors (for example, coping; affect) are understood to mediate the relationship between social prejudice and mental health. Both conceptualisations offer a largely individualised analysis of the relationship between sexual minority status and mental health. Although the catalyst is social (such as, stigma; prejudice) the focus is on individual processes (such as internalized homophobia, concealment of identity, and coping skills) and the effect these have on the *individual* in impacting mental health. In this respect it does not account for the role of social norms in shaping how sexual minorities might be seen as legitimate targets of negative sentiments (Riggs & Treharne, 2017); and fails to explain the role that institutionalized, systematic oppression (for example, lack of legal recognition, insensitivity to and ignorance of sexual minority perspectives/experiences, and social exclusion) may have on wellbeing of sexual minority persons individually and collectively. So, even this more nuanced approach is limited in providing an understanding of the interface between social prejudice and psychological distress. To under-stand—and challenge—social prejudice, it needs to be addressed at a systemic rather than individual level (Rivas-Koehl et al., 2021).

One of the things which is often overlooked when considering social prejudice amongst sexual minorities is how to account for the way in which those within sexual minority communities are differentially impacted (Riggs & Treharne, 2017). Some sexual minority individuals are at greater risk of psychological distress than others, but the aggrega-tion of data *across* a diverse range of sexual minorities, serves to obscure important differences between constituent parts of the LGBTIQ+ popu-lation. For example, research (for example, Cyrus, 2017; Logie et al., 2017) seems to suggest that sexual minority women and those from ethnic minority backgrounds are at greater risk of psychological distress due to social prejudice. So, those who occupy multiple marginalised positions (for example, woman and sexual minority; gay and ethnic minority) are at much greater risk of psychological distress than those occupying just one marginalised subject position. However, there is very limited research exploring mental health in different subgroups of sexual minorities. Furthermore, collectively exploring social prejudice in LGBTIQ+ populations obscures important differences resulting from gender. For example, the impact of social prejudice on sexual minority women (marginalised as both women and sexual minorities) is likely to be different from the impact on trans and gender diverse people (marginalised by cisgenderism). Routinely researching social prejudice in sexual minorities as a collective assumes a homogeneity that prevents us gaining a better understanding of the way in which social preju-dice impacts mental health for constituent groups within the LGBTIQ+ umbrella (see Chapter 7 for an exploration of the intersections of sexual and gender diversity).

While research around the risks of social prejudice for the psycho-logical wellbeing of sexual minorities is well established, the factors mitigating these risks are much less well understood. The main factor that seems to have a positive effect is social support. While the specifics about how social support makes a difference are not well defined, there is a growing body of evidence suggesting that support from social networks (for example, family and peers) acts as a buffer between social prejudice and negative mental health outcomes (Russell & Fish, 2016; Ybarra et al., 2015). Another important source of social support is sexual minority communities. For example, in many instances there are social groups (for example, youth groups, LGBT choirs, online networks) that are an important source of social support and affirmation for sexual minority people. However, being able to connect in these ways often requires a certain level of outness which for some carries a risk of increased exposure to social prejudice (Begeny & Huo, 2017; Chang et al., 2021). For some sexual minority people, particularly those from ethnic minority groups (where being out is problematic for maintaining cultural connections) and those who work with children (where the prejudices of parents may impact them) accessing these networks is often problematic. Similarly, those who are older and those who live in less urbanised settings may also struggle to connect with these communities. Where they exist, LGB activities typically occur in spaces where alcohol consumption is prevalent (for example, pubs; clubs) and this in itself may impact mental health.

Conclusion

As outlined in this chapter, despite considerable social and legal change in relation to the inclusion of sexual minorities, social prejudice is still common. Social prejudice is manifest both in interpersonal settings and also through attitudes towards sexual minorities individually and collectively; often in subtle or implicit forms such as through microaggressions, the assimilation of sexual minority culture and spaces. As highlighted, attempts to effect greater inclusivity for sexual minorities have often resulted in increased resistance to inclusivity and the re-inscription of heterosexuality as the norm. This chapter has explored the way in which social prejudice negatively impacts the mental health of sexual minorities. It also highlights the need for research to use a disaggregated approach to the study of sexual minorities in order to gain a more nuanced understanding of the way in which the dynamics of social prejudice impact the mental health of different sexual minority groups.

References

Ammaturo, F. R. (2016). Spaces of pride: A visual ethnography of gay pride parades in Italy and the United Kingdom. *Social Movement Studies, 15*(1), 19–40. https://doi.org/10.1080/14742837.2015.1060156

Amodeo, A. L., Esposito, C., & Bacchini, D. (2020). Heterosexist microaggressions, student academic experience and perception of campus climate: Findings from an Italian higher education context. *PLoS ONE, 15*(4), Article e0231580. https://doi.org/10.1371/journal.pone.0231580

Bachman, C. L., & Gooch, B. (2017). *LGBT in Britain: Hate crime and discrimination*. YouGov/Stonewall. https://www.stonewall.org.uk/lgbt-britain-hate-crime-and-discrimination

Badgett, M. V. (2011). Social inclusion and the value of marriage equality in Massachusetts and the Netherlands. *Journal of Social Issues, 67*(2), 316–334. https://psycnet.apa.org/doi/10.1111/j.1540-4560.2011.01700.x

Begeny, C. T., & Huo, Y. J. (2017). When identity hurts: How positive intragroup experiences can yield negative mental health implications for ethnic and sexual minorities. *European Journal of Social Psychology, 47*(7), 803–817. https://doi.org/10.1002/ejsp.2292

Ben-Yehuda, N. (2009). Foreword: Moral panics—36 years on. *The British Journal of Criminology, 49*(1), 1–3. https://doi.org/10.1093/bjc/azn076

Casey, M. (2004). De-dyking queer space(s): Heterosexual female visibility in gay and lesbian spaces. *Sexualities, 7*(4), 446–461. https://doi.org/10.1177/1363460704047062

Chan, K. K. S., Yung, C. S. W., & Nie, G. M. (2020). Self-compassion buffers the negative psychological impact of stigma stress on sexual minorities. *Mindfulness, 11*(10), 2338–2348. https://psycnet.apa.org/doi/10.1007/s12671-020-01451-1

Chang, C. J., Kellerman, J. K., Fehling, K. B., Feinstein, B. A., & Selby, E. A. (2021). The roles of discrimination and social support in the associations between outness and mental health outcomes among sexual minorities. *American Journal of Orthopsychiatry, 91*(5), 607. https://doi.org/10.1037/ort0000562

Clarke, V. (2003). Lesbian and gay marriage: Transformation or normalization? *Feminism and Psychology, 13*(4), 519–529. https://doi.org/10.1177/09593535030134016

Cronin, T. J., Pepping, C. A., Halford, W. K., & Lyons, A. (2021). Minority stress and psychological outcomes in sexual minorities: The role of barriers to accessing services. *Journal of Homosexuality, 68*(14), 2417–2429. https://www.tandfonline.com/doi/full/10.1080/00918369.2020.1804264

Cyrus, K. (2017). Multiple minorities as multiply marginalized: Applying the minority stress theory to LGBTQ people of color. *Journal of Gay & Lesbian Mental Health, 21*(3), 194–202. https://doi.org/10.1080/19359705.2017.1320739

Daigle, L. E., & Hawk, S. R. (2022). Sexual Orientation, Revictimization, and Polyvictimization. *Sexuality Research and Social Policy, 19*, 308–320.

Davies, R. T. (Creator). (2021). *It's a sin* [TV series]. Red Production Company.

Department for Education. (2019). *Relationships education, relationships and sex education (RSE) and health education: Statutory guidance for governing bodies, proprietors, head teachers, principals, senior leadership teams, teachers.* https://www.gov.uk/government/publications/relationships-education-relationships-and-sex-educationrse-and-health-education

Diamond, L. M. (2005). 'I'm straight, but I kissed a girl': The trouble with American media representations of femalefemale sexuality. *Feminism & Psychology, 15*(1), 104–110. https://doi.org/10.1177/0959353505049712

Dickinson, T., Cook, M., Playle, J., & Hallett, C. (2012). Queer' treatments: Giving a voice to former patients who received treatments for their 'sexual deviations.' *Journal of Clinical Nursing, 21*(9–10), 1345–1354. https://doi.org/10.1111/j.1365-2702.2011.03965.x

Dimberg, S. K., Clark, D. A., Spanierman, L. B., & VanDaalen, R. A. (2021). "School shouldn't be something you have to survive": Queer women's experiences with microaggressions at a Canadian University. *Journal of Homosexuality, 68*(5), 709–732. https://doi.org/10.1080/00918369.2019.1661729

Douglass, R. P., Conlin, S. E., & Duffy, R. D. (2020). Beyond happiness: Minority stress and life meaning among LGB individuals. *Journal of Homosexuality, 67*(11), 1587–1602. https://psycnet.apa.org/doi/10.1080/00918369.2019.1600900

Drescher, J. (2015). Queer diagnoses revisited: The past and future of homosexuality and gender diagnoses in DSM and ICD. *International Review of Psychiatry, 27*(5), 386–395. https://doi.org/10.3109/09540261.2015.1053847

Duggan, L. (2002). The new homonormativity: The sexual politics of neoliberalism. In R. Castronovo & Nelson, D. D. (Eds.), *Materializing democracy: Toward a revitalized cultural politics* (pp. 175–194). Duke University Press.

El-Khoury, F., Heron, M., Van der Waerden, J., Leon, C., du Roscoat, E., Velter, A., Lydie, N., & Sitbon, A. (2020). Verbal victimisation, depressive symptoms, and suicide risk among sexual minority adults in France: Results from the nationally-representative 2017 Health Barometer survey. *Social Psychiatry and Psychiatric Epidemiology, 55*, 1073–1080. https://doi.org/10.1007/s00127-020-01848-2

Eliason, M. (2000). Bi-negativity: The stigma facing bisexual men. *Journal of Bisexuality, 1*(2–3), 137–154. https://doi.org/10.1300/J159v01n02_05

Ellis, S. J. (2002). Student support for lesbian and gay human rights: Findings from a large-scale questionnaire study. In A. Coyle & C. Kitzinger (Eds.), *Lesbian & gay psychology: new perspectives* (pp. 239–254). BPS Blackwell.

Ellis, S. J., & Bentham, R. M. (2021). Inclusion of LGBTIQ perspectives in school-based sexuality education in Aotearoa/New Zealand: An exploratory study. *Sex Education, 21*(6), 708–722. https://doi.org/10.1080/14681811.2020.1863776

Ellis, S. J., & Kitzinger, C. (2002). Denying equality: An analysis of arguments against lowering the age of consent for sex between men. *Journal of Community & Applied Social Psychology, 12*(3), 167–180. https://doi.org/10.1002/casp.670

Emig, R. (2018). Mainstreamed into oblivion? LGBTIQ+ cultures in the UK today. *Hard Times, 102*(2), 48–59.

Farhall, K. (2018). 'Girl-on-girl confessions!' Changing representations of female–female sexuality in two Australian women's magazines. *Sexualities, 21*(1–2), 212–232. https://doi.org/10.1177/1363460716679388

Felix, S. N., Daigle, L. E., Hawk, S. R., & Policastro, C. (2021). Lesbian, gay, and bisexual victims' reporting behaviors to informal and formal sources. *Sexuality Research and Social Policy, 18*, 281–289. https://doi.org/10.1007/s10896-022-00438-x

Fish, J., & Williamson, I. (2018). Exploring lesbian, gay and bisexual patients' accounts of their experiences of cancer care in the UK. *European Journal of Cancer Care, 27*(1), e12501. https://doi.org/10.1111/ecc.12501

Flaherty, I., & Wilkinson, J. (2020). Marriage equality in Australia: The 'no' vote and symbolic violence. *Journal of Sociology, 56*(4), 644–674. https://doi.org/10.1177/1440783320969882

Formby, E., & Donovan, C. (2020). Sex and relationships education for LGBT+ young people: Lessons from UK youth work. *Sexualities, 23*(7), 1155–1178. https://doi.org/10.1177/1363460719888432

Gegenfurtner, A., & Gebhardt, M. (2017). Sexuality education including lesbian, gay, bisexual, and transgender (LGBT) issues in schools. *Educational Research Review, 22*, 215–222. https://doi.org/10.1016/j.edurev.2017.10.002

Gill, R. (2008). Empowerment/sexism: Figuring female sexual agency in contemporary advertising. *Feminism & Psychology, 18*(1), 35–60. https://doi.org/10.1177/0959353507084950

Gill, R. (2017). The affective, cultural and psychic life of postfeminism: A postfeminist sensibility 10 years on. *European Journal of Cultural Studies, 20*(6), 606–626. https://doi.org/10.1177/1367549417733003

Gough, B. (2002). 'I've always tolerated it but…': Heterosexual masculinity and the discursive reproduction of homophobia. In A. Coyle & C. Kitzinger (Eds.), *Lesbian & gay psychology: New perspectives* (pp. 219–238). BPS Blackwell.

Government Equalities Office. (2018). *LGBT action plan: Improving the lives of lesbian, gay, bisexual and transgender people.* https://www.gov.uk/government/organisations/government-equalities-office

GOV.UK. (2021). *Hate crime, England and Wales, 2020 to 2021.* https://www.gov.uk/government/statistics/hate-crime-england-and-wales-2020-to-2021/hate-crimeengland-and-wales-2020-to-2021

Harding, R. (2007). Sir Mark Potter and the protection of the traditional family: Why samesex marriage is (still) a feminist issue. *Feminist Legal Studies, 15*(2), 223–234. https://philpapers.org/go.pl?id=HARSMP&proxyId=&u=https%3A%2F%2Fdx.doi.org%2F10.1007%2Fs10691-007-9057-y

Harding, R., & Peel, E. (2006). We do? International perspectives on equality, legality and same-sex relationships. *Lesbian & Gay Psychology Review, 7*(2), 123–140.

Hatzenbuehler, M. L. (2009). How does sexual minority stigma "get under the skin"? A psychological mediation framework. *Psychological Bulletin, 135*(5), 707–730. https://doi.org/10.1037/a0016441

Hayfield, N. (2020). The invisibility of bisexual and pansexual bodies: Sexuality, appearance norms, and visual identities. In E. Maliepaard & R. Baumgartner (Eds.), *Bisexuality in Europe: Sexual citizenship, romantic relationships, and Bi+ identities* (pp. 178–191). Routledge.

Herek, G. M. (1990). The context of anti-gay violence: Notes on cultural and psychological heterosexism. *Journal of Interpersonal Violence, 5*(3), 316–333. https://doi.org/10.1177/088626090005003006

Hess, D. B. (2019). Effects of gentrification and real-estate market escalation on gay neighbourhoods. *The Town Planning Review, 90*(3), 229–237. https://doi.org/10.3828/tpr.2019.16

Hoefer, S. E., & Hoefer, R. (2017). Worth the wait? The consequences of abstinence-only sex education for marginalized students. *American Journal of Sexuality Education, 12*(3), 257–276. https://doi.org/10.1080/15546128.2017.1359802

Jowett, A., & Peel, E. (2010). Seismic culture change?' Media representations of same-sex 'marriage. *Women's Studies International Forum, 33*(3), 206–214. https://doi.org/10.1016/j.wsif.2009.12.009

Jowett, A. (2014). 'But if you legalise same-sex marriage…': Arguments against marriage equality in the British press. *Feminism & Psychology, 24*(1), 37–55. https://doi.org/10.1177/0959353513510655

Kahle, L. (2020). Are sexual minorities more at risk? Bullying victimization among lesbian, gay, bisexual, and queer youth. *Journal of Interpersonal Violence, 35*(21–22), 4960–4978. https://doi.org/10.1177/0886260517718830

Kanbur, N. (2020). Internalized Homophobia in Adolescents: Is it really about Culture or Religion? *Journal of the Canadian Academy of Child and Adolescent Psychiatry, 29*(2), 124–126. https://www.ncbi.nlm.nih.gov/pmc/articles/PMC7213920/

Kitzinger, C. (2005). Heteronormativity in action: Reproducing the heterosexual nuclear family in after-hours medical calls. *Social Problems, 52*(4), 477–498. https://doi.org/10.1525/sp.2005.52.4.477

Kotecha, S. (2019, 26 July). *LGBT teaching row: DfE 'pressured school' to Halt Lessons.* https://www.bbc.co.uk/news/uk-england-birmingham-49110151

Lee, C. (2021). Inclusive relationships, sex and health education: Why the moral panic? *Management in Education.* Advance online publication. https://doi.org/10.1177/08920206211016453

Lee, D., & Carpenter, V. M. (2015). "What would you like me to do? Lie to you?" Teacher education responsibilities to LGBTI students. *Asia-Pacific Journal of Teacher Education, 43*(2), 169–180. https://doi.org/10.1177/016146812012200704

Lee, H., Operario, D., Yi, H., Choo, S., & Kim, S. S. (2019). Internalized homophobia, depressive symptoms, and suicidal ideation among lesbian, gay, and bisexual adults in South Korea: An age-stratified analysis. *LGBT Health, 6*(8), 393–399. https://doi.org/10.1089/lgbt.2019.0108

Levin, S. (2019, September 3). 'A critical point un history': How Trump's attack on LGBT rights is escalating. *The Guardian.* https://www.theguardian.com/world/2019/sep/03/trump-attack-lgbt-rights-supreme-court

BBC News. (2019, May 16). *LGBT school lessons protests spread nationwide.* https://www.bbc.com/news/uk-england-48294017

Lightfoot, L. (2019, April 2). *Parkfield LGBT protest: Why has the school's Top Teacher Been Silenced?* https://www.theguardian.com/education/2019/apr/02/parkfield-school-protest-teacher-silenced

Logie, C. H., Lacombe-Duncan, A., Poteat, T., & Wagner, A. C. (2017). Syndemic factors mediate the relationship between sexual stigma and depression among sexual minority women and gender minorities. *Women's Health Issues, 27*(5), 592–599. https://doi.org/10.1016/j.whi.2017.05.003

McNeill, S. G., McAteer, J., & Jepson, R. (2021). Interactions between health professionals and lesbian, gay and bisexual patients in healthcare settings: a systematic review. *Journal of Homosexuality.* Advance online publication. https://doi.org/10.1080/00918369.2021.1945338

Meyer, I. H. (1995). Minority stress and mental health in gay men. *Journal of Health and Social Behavior, 36*(1), 38–56. https://doi.org/10.2307/2137286

Meyer, I. H. (2003). Prejudice, social stress, and mental health in lesbian, gay, and bisexual populations: Conceptual issues and research evidence. *Psychological Bulletin, 129*(5), 674–697. https://doi.org/10.1037/0033-2909.129.5.674

Meyer, I. H., Russell, S. T., Hammack, P. L., Frost, D. M., & Wilson, B. D. (2021). Minority stress, distress, and suicide attempts in three cohorts of sexual minority adults: A US probability sample. *PLoS ONE, 16*(3), Article e0246827. https://doi.org/10.1371/journal.pone.0246827

Ministry of Education. (2015). *Sexuality education: A guide for principals, boards of trustees, and teachers.* Ministry of Education, NZ.

Peel, E. (2001). Mundane heterosexism: Understanding incidents of the everyday. *Women's Studies International Forum, 24*(5), 541–554. https://psycnet.apa.org/doi/10.1016/S0277-5395(01)00194-7

Pepping, C. A., Cronin, T. J., Halford, W. K., & Lyons, A. (2019). Minority stress and same-sex relationship satisfaction: The role of concealment motivation. *Family Process, 58*(2), 496–508. https://doi.org/10.1111/famp.12365

Pitman, A., Marston, L., Lewis, G., Semlyen, J., McManus, S., & King, M. (2021). The mental health of lesbian, gay, and bisexual adults compared with heterosexual adults: Results of two nationally representative English household probability samples. *Psychological Medicine*. Advance online publication. https://doi.org/10.1017/S0033291721000052

Porterfield, C. (2020, June 10). Anti-LGBTQ rhetoric is ramping up in Eastern Europe, human rights advocates say. *Forbes*. https://www.forbes.com/sites/carlieporterfield/2020/06/10/anti-lgbtq-rhetoric-is-ramping-up-in-eastern-europe-human-rights-advocates-say/?sh=3f8cf3cf231e

Poteat, V. P., O'Dwyer, L. M., & Mereish, E. H. (2012). Changes in how students use and are called homophobic epithets over time: Patterns predicted by gender, bullying, and victimization status. *Journal of Educational Psychology, 104*(2), 393–406. https://psycnet.apa.org/doi/10.1037/a0026437

Rawlings, V., & Loveday, J. (2021). 'A threat to the social order': A 'problem frame' analysis of the Safe Schools Coalition Australia programme within print media. *Discourse: Studies in the Cultural Politics of Education*. Advance online publication. https://www.tandfonline.com/doi/full/10.1080/01596306.2021.1918060

Ray, T. N., Lanni, D. J., Parkhill, M. R., Duong, T. V., Pickett, S. M., & Burgess-Proctor, A. K. (2021). Interpersonal violence victimization among youth entering college: A preliminary analysis examining the differences between LGBTQ and non-LGBTQ youth. *Violence and Gender, 8*(2), 67–73. https://doi.org/10.1089/vio.2020.0076

Russell, S. T., & Fish, J. N. (2016). Mental health in lesbian, gay, bisexual, and transgender (LGBT) youth. *Annual Review of Clinical Psychology, 12*, 465–487. https://doi.org/10.1146/annurev-clinpsy-021815-093153

Riggs, D. W., & Treharne, G. J. (2017). Decompensation: A novel approach to accounting for stress arising from the effects of ideology and social norms. *Journal of Homosexuality, 64*(5), 592–605. https://psycnet.apa.org/doi/10.1080/00918369.2016.1194116

Røthing, Å., & Svendsen, S. (2010). Homotolerance and heterosexuality as Norwegian values. *Journal of LGBT Youth, 7*(2), 147–166. https://doi.org/10.1080/19361651003799932

Rivas-Koehl, M., Valido, A., Espelage, D. L., Robinson, L. E., Hong, J. S., Kuehl, T., et al. (2021). Understanding protective factors for suicidality and depression among US sexual and gender minority adolescents: Implications for school psychologists. *School Psychology Review, 51*, 290–303. https://www.tandfonline.com/doi/abs/10.1080/2372966X.2021.1881411

Shannon, B., & Smith, S. (2015). 'A lot more to learn than where babies come from': Controversy, language and agenda setting in the framing of school-based sexuality education curricula in Australia. *Sex Education, 15*(6), 641–654. https://doi.org/10.1080/14681811.2015.1055721

Smith, K. T. (1971). Homophobia: A tentative personality profile. *Psychological Reports, 29*(3_Suppl.), 1091–1094. https://doi.org/10.2466/pr0.1971.29.3f.1091

Sophie, J. (1987). Internalized homophobia and lesbian identity. *Journal of Homosexuality, 14*(1–2), 53–65. https://doi.org/10.1300/J082v14n01_05

Stonewall. (2017). *School report: The experiences of lesbian, gay, bi, and trans young people in Britain's schools in 2017*. https://www.stonewall.org.uk/system/files/the_school_report_2017.pdf

Sue, D. W., Capodilupo, C. M., Torino, G. C., Bucceri, J. M., Holder, A., Nadal, K. L., & Esquilin, M. (2007). Racial microaggressions in everyday life: implications for clinical practice. *American Psychologist, 62*(4), 271–286. https://psycnet.apa.org/doi/10.1037/0003-066X.62.4.271

Sun, S., Pachankis, J. E., Li, X., & Operario, D. (2020). Addressing minority stress and mental health among men who have sex with men (MSM) in China. *Current HIV/AIDS Reports, 17*(1), 35–62. https://doi.org/10.1007/s11904-019-00479-w

Svendsen, S. (2012). Elusive sex acts: Pleasure and politics in Norwegian sex education. *Sex Education, 12*(4), 397–410. https://doi.org/10.1080/14681811.2012.677209

Thomas, A., McCann, H., & Fela, G. (2020). 'In this house we believe in fairness and kindness': Post-liberation politics in Australia's same-sex marriage postal survey. *Sexualities, 23*(4), 475–496. https://doi.org/10.1177/1363460719830347

Thompson, J. D. (2020). Your parents will read this: Reading (as) parents in journalistic coverage of the Safe Schools Coalition Australia controversy. *Journalism, 21*(12), 1951–1964. https://doi.org/10.1177/1464884918755638

Verrelli, S., White, F. A., Harvey, L. J., & Pulciani, M. R. (2019). Minority stress, social support, and the mental health of lesbian, gay, and bisexual Australians during the Australian Marriage Law Postal Survey. *Australian Psychologist, 54*(4), 336–346. https://psycnet.apa.org/doi/10.1111/ap.12380

Warner, M. (1991). Introduction: Fear of a queer planet. *Social Text, 9*(4), 3–17. https://www.jstor.org/stable/466295

Weinberg, G. (1972). *Society and the healthy homosexual*. St Martins Press.

Wilkinson, S., & Kitzinger, C. (2006). In support of equal marriage: Why civil partnership is not enough. *Psychology of Women Review, 8*(1), 54–57.

Wright, W. K. (2006). The tide in favour of equality: Same-sex marriage in Canada and England and Wales. *International Journal of Law, Policy and the Family, 20*(3), 249–285. https://doi.org/10.1093/lawfam/edl008

Yanykin, A. A., & Nasledov, A. D. (2017). Internalized homophobia in Russia. *Psychology in Russia, 10*(2), 103–116. https://psycnet.apa.org/doi/10.11621/pir.2017.0207

Ybarra, M. L., Mitchell, K. J., Palmer, N. A., & Reisner, S. L. (2015). Online social support as a buffer against online and offline peer and sexual victimization among U.S. LGBT and non-LGBT youth. *Child Abuse and Neglect, 39*, 123–136. https://doi.org/10.1016/j.chiabu.2014.08.006

Zaglas, W. (2019, May 24). Looking back at safe schools. *Education Review.* https://www.educationreview.com.au/2019/05/looking-back-at-safe-schools/

Zeeman, L., Sherriff, N., Browne, K., McGlynn, N., Mirandola, M., Gios, L., et al. (2019). A review of lesbian, gay, bisexual, trans and intersex (LGBTI) health and healthcare inequalities. *European Journal of Public Health, 29*(5), 974–980. https://doi.org/10.1093/eurpub/cky226

4

Coming Out: Conceptualising a Reflexive Model of Disclosure and Non-disclosure

Joshua K. Simpson and Ian Rivers

Introduction

'Coming out' has been described as the process through which individuals come to recognise their non-heterosexual or alternate gender identities and subsequently disclose or share those identities with others through, "an unambiguous and public declaration" (Jagose, 1996, p. 38). It represents an internal—almost existential—acceptance of self that requires the individual to redefine the 'self' and, for others, their relationship to that 'self' (Hill, 2009; Troiden, 1989). It has also been described as a process of identity-centred development, emphasising self-recognition and an internal sense of identity rather one based specifically

J. K. Simpson
University of Worcester, Worcester, UK
e-mail: jk.simpson@icloud.com

I. Rivers (✉)
University of Strathclyde, Glasgow, Scotland, UK
e-mail: ian.rivers@strath.ac.uk

© The Author(s), under exclusive license to Springer Nature
Switzerland AG 2023
J. Semlyen and P. Rohleder (eds.), *Sexual Minorities and Mental Health*,
https://doi.org/10.1007/978-3-031-37438-8_4

on sexual acts (Dubé, 2000). Coming out is not, as we will see, "a static action, but a range of various motivations, goals, and strategies that people wrap up in a single term, a catch-all for this complex identity management system" (Orne, 2011, p. 699).

In this chapter we explore the intricacies of disclosure and its relationship to mental health and well-being. We propose a model to better reflect the varied relevance of coming out for some today. In line with other chapters in the book, we focus primarily upon lesbian, gay, and bisexual (LGB) populations but acknowledge that there are commonalities in experience for those who are trans, queer, intersex or asexual.

Understanding the Coming Out Process

Coming out is complex and the research has, historically, tended to focus on the reactions of immediate others (family and friends) to disclosure and, of course, the social, cultural, political, and religious contexts that surround individuals at the time (D'Augelli, 1994). Coming out has often been characterised as a singular occurrence. For example, Savin-Williams (2001) presented it as a "critical milestone" where emotional, practical, and economic factors come into play as part of identity formation. However, in a society underpinned by assumptions of heterosexuality and cisgender status, LGB, trans, queer, intersex and asexual people regularly find themselves in the position of having to come out to others to correct those underpinning assumptions (Manning, 2015a) and many have come to accept this as a "fundamental feature" of their lives (Knoble & Linville, 2012, p. 330). Furthermore, lived experience shows that not only is coming out actually an ongoing process where there is a constant need to define oneself and correct assumptions, in a society that shows ongoing prejudice, it is also a risky one (Ragins, 2008; see also Pachankis, 2007). We explore this further later in this chapter.

Being out is also not a process that is entirely within an individual's control; information is shared across networking groups, and that information (i.e., disclosure of another's actual or perceived sexual orientation, gender identity or status) can be passed on. This sometimes occurs without malice (e.g., Cho, 2018), and may even be preferred by some individuals as an "easier" means of disclosure. As one participant in Orne's (2011) study shared, "Some of my family has found out through means such as MySpace or Facebook, which I almost prefer" (p. 690).

Numerous stage theories and models of identity formation have sought to explain 'coming out' (e.g. Cass, 1979; D'Augelli, 1994; Troiden, 1989). As we have noted above, such theories and models tend to characterise disclosure as moving from a personal position of identity confusion to a position of commitment to an LGB identity, acknowledging wider contexts and prohibitions. Perhaps one of the most fundamental models has been that posited by Cass (1979), which includes six stages of progressive LGBT identity formation: confusion, which includes first becoming aware of one's attraction; comparison, in which the implications of a particular identity are considered; tolerance, which includes acknowledgement of one's likely identity and outreach toward or interaction with others; acceptance, in which a positive tolerance is attached to the identity; pride, which includes disclosure; and synthesis, in which identity is integrated with other aspects of the self.

However, models such as Cass', have been criticised for their over-generalizations in terms of sexual identity (usually limited to lesbian and gay, excluding other sexual identities) and, latterly, gender identity development and their emphasis on linear progression (Diamond, 2006). For example, the assumption that bisexual people go through a similar pattern of disclosure has been contested by Manning (2015b), who argued that models of identity development tended to ignore bisexuality and failed to engage with cultural differences.

The Coming Out Process and Intersectional Perspectives

It has been argued that the concept of coming out has undergone significant change. For example, Kaufman and Johnson (2004) argued that, over the decades, both 'the closet' and coming out have altered in meaning, with the process of disclosure being described as one of a "situated negotiation of stigma management" (p. 821). Here disclosure is characterised in terms of "a revolving door" of being "in the closet" or "out" that depends much more upon individual circumstances than self-acceptance (p. 822). Indeed, according to Rivers (1997) the continuous process of disclosing to others means that LGB people have to navigate a complex decision-making process at different stages in their lives, judging the personal, social, political, cultural and economic implications in which they find themselves.

For example, the disclosure process may vary for LGB individuals who also identify as trans or non-binary and may therefore face different challenges and find themselves making repeated disclosures of both sexuality and gender (Matsuno, 2019). As Sansfaçon et al. (2020) described it, coming out and identity formation for trans (including non-binary) youth is a process of "pauses, advances and retreats" (p. 317). One participant in Sansfacon et al.'s study, for example, reported going through "many coming outs" as they explored different labels, while another participant described how, at one point, she "revoked" her coming out but then subsequently decided to continue her transition:

> It just came back as a feeling, and then I was like, "No. I don't want to stay how I was born." And then it just came back stronger than ever and then it [my transition] finally started. (Sansfaçon et al., 2020, p. 313)

Other factors that may affect the process of disclosure include differences in ability, age and generations. For disabled LGB people, disclosure can be complicated not only by heterosexism but also ableism (Toft, 2020, p. 1894). While disclosure may help one become part of a larger LGB community, some LGB disabled people may be more hesitant out of concern of potentially being excluded from non-heterosexual spaces for not being the 'right kind' of (i.e., non-disabled) LGB person (Toft, 2020, p. 1907), impacting the decision of whether or not to disclose.

Older LGB populations may also experience greater stressors that impact the coming out process (see also Chapter 5). Such stressors stem from the "hostile historical context in which they grew up" and by ageism or "negative attitudes toward aging" (Rosati et al., 2020, n.p.). Challenges for those who are older may also include requiring care from others or being unable to maintain their independence (Ward et al.,

2012) (acknowledging, of course, that such care and reduced levels of independence may also reflect the experiences of younger populations who still live at home and are dependent on their families).

Meanwhile, many sexuality and gender labels, and the differences which define them, have less resonance among younger people today who question the centrality of labelling desires to their core identities or sense of self (Allen et al., 2021; Coleman-Fountain, 2014; Savin-Williams, 2005). In other words, the process of disclosure may be less meaningful to younger people's sense of self and identity when compared to those form whom labels may still hold some essential meaning.

Further complexities may also be found at intersections of race and ethnicity. In the study by Bishop et al. (2020), for example, it was found that "Black and Latinx participants reported younger ages of same-sex attraction and self-realization, respectively, than White participants" (p. 16). The age at which the coming out process is first initiated (i.e., self-realisation or recognition of one's non-heterosexual identity) may therefore differ depending on one's race or ethnicity.

Similarly, religion too can impact the process of disclosure, as one's religious beliefs or the religious beliefs of one's family or community may compound the stressors associated with disclosure. As Rosati et al. (2020) argued, LGB people "may feel (or be) rejected by their religious community, or stop practicing a religion altogether, due to a perceived conflict with their sexual minority status" (n.p.). It should be recognised that, as with age, religion is not necessarily a negative factor and can indeed be a positive one in the lives of LGB people (e.g., Skidmore et al., 2022). Experiences of disclosure can further differ for those who experience multiple intersectional identities, include race, ethnicity, and religion. Consider also Jaspal's (2021) study of British South Asian gay men, which highlighted the experiences of participants who, upon returning to their family homes during the COVID-19 lockdowns imposed in the UK, found themselves having to choose between, or at least compartmentalise, their sexual and family identities. Political, cultural, and economic implications in which they find themselves.

Forms of Disclosure

Of course, many of the models of coming out have focused on face-to-face interactions, and the potential emotional consequences of acceptance or rejection by significant others (family, friends, opposite-sex partners and work colleagues). We know that, in the past, many LGB youth have tended to disclose their sexual orientation to a friend before disclosing to a parent (Savin-Williams, 2001; Wells & Kline, 1987), and this is particularly the case where those parents have strong traditional values encompassing marriage and, as discussed above, religious beliefs and the family (Newman & Muzzonigro, 1993).

However, such disclosures have not always involved face-to-face conversations, they have been made in writing or by the sharing of clues. One such example comes from Orne's (2011) study of gay men's processes of disclosure where one participant described his strategy for coming out at work as follows:

> At work, I make no secret of my sexuality, but rarely talk about it … I did put all my gay-complishments on my resume, so they knew I was gay since I started. (p. 690)

In other words, he came out in writing, via his resumé.

Online spaces also offer a means for coming out and exploring identities virtually without necessarily having to verbalise one's experiences. However, the digital world presents new opportunities (and challenges) for those wishing to come out and find communities of similar others. Today, many young people report that they choose to come out online in what they perceive to be a safe space (Alexander & Losh, 2010; Bond et al., 2009; Pascoe, 2011). While the anonymous nature of online spaces means that reactions are not always positive and can, of course, be very destructive (Bauman & Rivers, 2015), it nonetheless offers those who access such spaces opportunities for exploring identities before coming out offline and empowers them to make changes in the 'real' world (Alonzo & Buttitta, 2019; Cabiria, 2008). Coming out virtually, then, can have many benefits (see Craig & McInroy, 2014) by enabling audience separation, wherein identity formation and expression can be managed through partial disclosure (Duguay, 2016). For example, audience separation provides the opportunity to curate and negotiate content and interactions in some spaces and to some people, but not others. Through an exploration of their own identities, those wishing to come out not only connect with others who share similar experiences, but they also access relevant advice, resources, and information that may not be available at the beginning of their journey (Buss et al., 2021).

Lived Experiences of Coming Out

So, what do we know about the lived experience of those who have or are thinking about coming out? Firstly, many of the older studies of disclosure have involved young people who were members of community groups, gender-sexuality alliances (GSAs), or those who accessed services because they experienced negative reactions from others (Savin-Williams, 2005). In the absence of any other means of collecting data, the assumption was that their experiences were representative of the everyday rather than exceptional. Politically, these young people had also been seen as vulnerable rather than being self-actualised and able to make decisions for themselves. This construction of youth was particularly evident, for example, in the case of Section 28 of the Local Government Act 1988, a UK law that prohibited local authorities from, "promoting…homosexuality as a pretended family relationship" (s. 2A) Parliamentary debates surrounding Section 28 not only characterised children and young people as innocent and vulnerable, they also characterised them as requiring protection both from themselves—often being described in terms that inferred innate or latent homosexuality—and any materials (book and other resources) that might awaken that latent identity (Simpson, 2021).

Section 28 was the culmination of political attempts to select and organise the 'right' kind of knowledge to which children and young people should have access, and the rejection that children and young people possess capacities for agency and self-determination. These protectionist politics are more recently evidenced in the case of *Bell v. Tavistock*, where a UK court was asked to decide whether young people under the age of 18, seeking gender reassignment, could give informed consent to puberty blockers. In determining that it is "highly unlikely" or "doubtful", the court's decision echoed Section 28 in ruling that trans young people are not the experts in their own lives, they cannot know their own best interests, and must, therefore, be protected from themselves.

Positive Effects on Mental Health by Coming Out

Research has shown that coming out can have positive effects on mental health and wellbeing, and it is these benefits (as well as potential costs) that have to be considered when deciding whether or not to disclose to others (Waldner & Magrader, 1999). We know that coming out can reduce psychological distress and suicidality (Solomon et al., 2015), as well as aid resiliency, counteract stress, and present opportunities for growth (Meyer, 2003). It has also been correlated with increased satisfaction in same-sex relationships (Knoble & Linville, 2012). Where families are accepting, LGB people are likely to experience greater mental and physical health (Ryan et al., 2010). Evidence also indicates that disclosure can also be of benefit to those with mental illness, promoting acceptance, comfort, and happiness (Corrigan et al., 2009).

Coming out can also be a source of strength, particularly where it is, "associated with opportunities for affiliation, social support, and coping that can ameliorate the impact of stress" (Meyer, 2003, p. 679). Additionally, it has been beneficial in terms of furthering political activism. It has, for example, been used as a strategy to protest laws that force individuals to conceal their sexuality or gender identities (Cisneros & Bracho, 2019). Politically, then, disclosure can aid the achievement of legal reforms, raising awareness of sexual and gender minorities in broader society (Orne, 2011), and fostering greater acceptance by and within that society. Indeed, some same-sex couples have linked their level of 'outness' to their desire to be visible and serve as role models for others (Knoble & Linville, 2012) and encourage more positive attitudes towards non-heterosexual people more generally (Klein et al., 2015, p. 299).

Thus, coming out can be beneficial both to the individual and the wider community, in a reciprocal or mutually constitutive process.

Homonormativity

However, it should be noted too that coming out in order to achieve greater visibility may ultimately act to marginalise those who do not 'fit the mould' of what is deemed to be acceptable by the majority—whatever that majority is (cisgender, heterosexual or LGB). For example, one couple in Knoble and Linville's (2012) study said:

> We tell our son it's his responsibility to be well-behaved and to be a good representation of a lesbian-headed family. (p. 334)

Linking outness to notions of being "well-behaved" and being a "good representation" to achieve acceptance is problematic. In addition to subjecting non-heterosexuality to the heterosexual gaze, it risks reifying or bolstering the notion of the so-called 'good homosexual', in which the majority deem only certain sexual minorities to be worthy of respect because those individuals replicate heteronormative ideals. From within LGB communities we can see similar expression of what can be described as 'homonormativity'. For example, we regularly hear debates surrounding the acceptability or appropriateness of demonstrations of 'kink' at Pride events (Pohtinen, 2019). However, it can be argued that, if no other ways of being are modelled for LGB people, they cannot embrace the range of queer possibilities and expressions of gender and sexuality that exist and, thus, may therefore find it more difficult to come out if they do not see themselves reflected in LGB communities.

Potential Negative Effects of Coming Out

While coming out is seen as a healthy sign of maturation and identity integration, it also carries risks, including victimisation, stigmatisation, prejudice, and sexual violence (Bogaert & Hafer, 2009). Other negative outcomes can include becoming the target of prejudice, disruption of relationships with friends and family, and developing depression, suicidality, substance abuse, or low self-esteem (Solomon et al., 2015). These impacts are often compounded for those with intersectional identities or multiple minority status, resulting in multiple forms of oppression. They may experience, for example, both heterosexism and racism within and outside LGB communities (Balsam et al., 2011), or have to navigate an undocumented immigration status while facing both anti-LGB and anti-immigrant attitudes (Cisneros & Bracho, 2019). Disclosure in these contexts has been linked to negative outcomes in terms of mental health and wellbeing (Rivers et al., 2018). This has been explored in more detail in various other chapters in this book.

Coming out can also impact personal relationships, most obviously in the case of families, but friendships too. While several studies have documented the invaluable sources of support friendship networks bring, they have shown that disclosure often-times results in the loss of those networks (see Hershberger & D'Augelli, 1995; Pilkington & D'Augelli, 1995; Rivers, 2001; Rivers & Carragher, 2003). Physical, verbal, emotional and even sexual abuse have been reported and this can result in friends taking fright and disowning LGB peers means of self-preservation (O'Shaughnessy et al., 2004; Rivers, 2002; Saewyc et al., 2006).

These reasons demonstrate why many may remain in the closet, concealing their identities in order to avoid the anticipated risks and consequences associated with coming out, although this in turn may give rise to other risks.

We must acknowledge that there is a general consensus that remaining in 'the closet' can itself have negative outcomes (for those who desire to come out but are prevented from doing so). For example, early research by Weinberg and Williams (1974) indicated that staying 'in the closet' could lead to psychological stress in the anticipation of being exposed or involuntarily outed and, thus, subjected to discrimination (which, in turn, leads to strain in managing one's behaviours and expressions). Additionally, the negative impacts of not coming out may be compounded by well-meaning individuals who encourage disclosure or well-meaning workplace policies or practices.

Is Being Out Meaningful Still?

In the opening of this chapter, we discussed research on, and theorisations of, 'coming out', in which disclosure is emphasised as a necessary pathway or process for LGB people's self-acceptance and identity formation. However, we want to interrogate the perceived link between health development and the disclosure of one's identities, and in particular the assumption that 'coming out' is universally relevant to LGB people or indeed trans, queer, intersex or asexual people. This particular conception of disclosure of the idea that (repeated) declarations signal positive wellbeing—suggests that the process represents a form of liberation that allows individuals to be 'authentic' (and, conversely, those who remain in the closet, sometimes by choice, as 'inauthentic'). This assumption infers that identities are not yet fully legitimate or valid unless and until disclosed publicly. Indeed, as Snider (1996) noted, there is a presumption in 'coming out' discourses that being out is beneficial, which itself is underpinned by a perception that a dichotomy exists between the true self and the repressed self. Yet this line of thinking recalls and calcifies essentialist conceptions of sexuality, sexual orientation and gender whereby the discovery *and expression* of a person's identity reveals some inherent truth about that person. If that is the case, then post-structural views of sexuality, sexual-orientation and gender, in which identity is an ongoing social or relational process, are called into question.

Furthermore, we have to question where disclosure is important or relevant for some people, and this suggests that there is a need for a new way of thinking about the disclosure process in a way that does not elide or erase the experiences of those individuals, who may be marginalised even within their communities. While the experiences of those who desire but are unable to 'come out' are, of course, valid and worthy of investigation and understanding (see Clarke, 2002) there are also those who resist 'coming out' in ways that assign labels relating to sexuality, sexual orientation and gender altogether. As discussed earlier, for example, many labels, and the differences which define them, have less resonance among young people today who question the centrality of labelling desires to their core identities or sense of self (Allen et al., 2021; Coleman-Fountain, 2014; Savin-Williams, 2005). As Dilley (2010) argued, while there is the desire amongst some young people to, "recognize and acknowledge their non-heterosexual feelings, experiences, and social connections as not heterosexual", there is also the wish to "consciously refute [...] the primacy of those aspects of their identity in their overall sense of self" (p. 191).

Indeed, research conducted with young people who identify as being solely or primarily attracted to members of the same sex, but have not come out, indicates that while they have concerns about hostility from others, fear experiencing loneliness, and have a propensity for risk-taking behaviour, their psychological profile is not noticeably different from peers solely or primarily attracted to members of the opposite sex (see Rivers & Noret, 2008). Thus, if divisions based on desire are not significant to defining oneself and one's community, or to understanding psychological well-being, the question arises as to the continued importance of communities defined by sexual desire to the social identities adopted by young people today (which may not be based on sexual desire at all).

The continued emphasis we place on disclosure has the potential to exclude or erase those with 'other' experiences within 'other' populations as well as those who identify as asexual and do not experience sexual attraction or the desire to seek out romantic partners. For some, there may be little value placed in 'coming out' (Robbins et al., 2016). Indeed, some desire to live without having to disclose or explain their trans identity, for example (Klein et al., 2015). In these contexts, choosing not to 'come out' is not the result of shame or secrecy, as the notion of the closet implies, but a reflection of their sense of self which is not tied to public disclosure in the first place. Thus, while concealment can have detrimental effects (Pachankis, 2007) for some, for others, there may simply be a lack of desire to either conceal *or* disclose.

If we can disentangle the historical narratives surrounding disclosure and recognise that 'coming out' is not the goal for everyone from LGB, trans, queer, intersex or asexual communities, 'the closet' can be reconceptualised as a space of safekeeping for different people at the different stages in their lives. For some it is a place of safety early in their identity development, for others it is a refuge (either temporary or long-term). Privacy can also be essential for young people whose families are less accepting; for example, in families that emphasise certain traditional or religious values, as discussed above. Yet for others still, the act of keeping a 'secret' may be an erotic experience that enhances pleasure.

These arguments do not suggest that 'coming out' is a meaningless or arbitrary process, or that disclosure is a non-issue. Indeed, the research we have cited shows that this clearly is not the case, for it can be a transformative experience, just as it can be a dangerous one in certain contexts such as those discussed above and including social, religious, or familial. But what is key here is the recognition that, for some individuals, disclosure and the categorisations required to make disclosure possible—may constrain rather than liberate, and thus becomes a compulsory rather than emancipatory act—one that essentially creates a hierarchy of sexual identities in which one is either out and proud or closeted and shamed. The perpetuation of an in/out binary reinforces the experience of sexuality, sexual orientation and even gender-identity as fixed rather than fluid. Indeed, if we accept that they can be fluid, then can it be said that there is ever an end to the 'coming out' process?

A Reflexive Model of 'Coming Out'

Given this discussion, how can the process of 'coming out' be represented by a model that accounts for varied and individual experiences rather than a universal or singular process of identity development? To visualise disclosure as informed by the research discussed in this chapter—and, in particular, to represent the process of disclosure as non-linear and as person specific, recognising that healthy development and disclosure may not necessarily be linked—we propose the model in Fig. 4.1.

The process of conceptualising this model involved first familiarising ourselves with the research to identify the domains in which disclosure can take place and understand how those domains relate to the process of disclosure and how it may vary for individuals. This structure of the model is not intended to reflect a "spectrum of visibility" (Cisneros & Bracho, 2019, p. 717)—in which each domain or dimension is another level of increased or cumulative public awareness—that would imply that those who are not increasingly out are somehow less legible than those

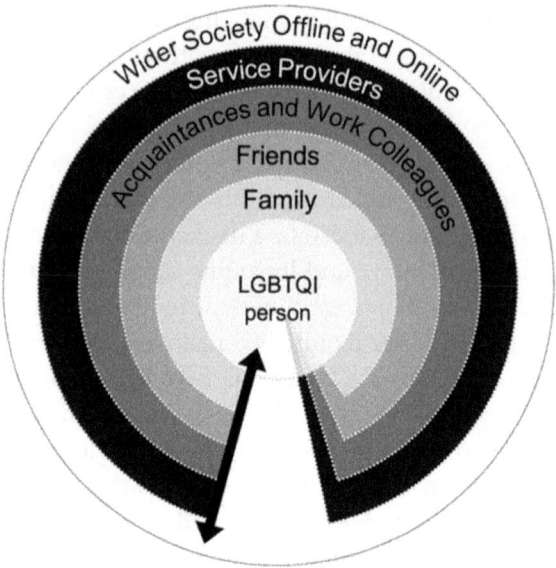

Fig. 4.1 A reflexive model of coming out

who are. Nor do the domains (represented by circles) infer that there is a natural progression to 'coming out'. As we have argued, private subjectivity and non-disclosure are as valid as public disclosure. Rather, the domains are intended to represent patterns of disclosure, should individuals so choose, while also recognising that sometimes there is not a choice (i.e., where one is involuntarily outed). By not tying disclosure to developmental stages, the model further reflects that, while the 'coming out' may or may not have value or relevance to wellbeing, the process is inherently a social one. It does not deny that 'coming out' can result in experiences of growth and healthy development, nor does it assume a link between the two or that the process is a universal one.

In the model, each domain visibly flows from the central LGBTQI person or self domain, indicating that a person can come out in any of these contexts at any time. Although there may be socially imposed expectations of an order or pathway (referencing a form of social ecology), there is no particular order or pathway, and some or all of these may be 'skipped' or 'jumped'. The pathways can also be read as flowing *into* the self, reflecting the socially constructed nature of sexual and gender identities. It also reflects the experience of being involuntary outed by others (see Jaspal, 2021). Finally, the arrow indicates the fluid and non-linear nature of coming out, including its often context-specific nature, wherein the individual may navigate and re-navigate different domains at different times and in different locations (such as in the workplace or when negotiating family relationships). In other words, the model's structure reflects disclosure as an ongoing, rather than static or one-time, process, which in turn may also provide sharper reflection of LGB people who experience fluid sexuality.

While further research on this model is needed, our hope is that it will serve as a tool or reference point for discussion and analysis in relation to the varied and contextual lived experiences and mental health and wellbeing of LGB people.

Conclusion

In addition to summarising much of the research that has gone before on the topic of disclosure, we have chosen to challenge some of the assumptions that have been made about the being 'out' recognising that past research does not always reflect the diversity that now exists in terms of sexualities, sexual orientations and gender identities. For many LGB people, as it is for those who are trans, queer and intersex, initial disclosure of sexual orientation or gender-identity is a pivotal milestone in the development of self and to mental health and wellbeing. It has both its personal benefits and its contextual risks. However, for some, 'coming out' may be seen as unnecessary or even limiting—casting off one inflexible identity for another for the sake of 'development'. Disclosure is a personal choice (or should be one) but so, too, is the decision not to disclose. It is important that we move away from linear models of 'coming out' in relation to development and wellbeing and reflect upon the inevitability that the lives and mental health of young people cannot be understood in terms of a simple binary—in or out—but involve degrees of 'outness' that reflect both context and personal choice.

References

Alexander, J., & Losh, E. (2010). 'A YouTube of one's own?': 'Coming out' videos as rhetorical action. In C. Pullen & M. Cooper (Eds.), *LGBT identity and online new media* (pp. 37–50). Routledge.

Allen, K., Cuthbert, K., Hall, J. J., Hines, S., & Elley, S. (2021). Trailblazing the gender revolution? Young people's understandings of gender diversity through generation and social change. *Journal of Youth Studies, 25*(5), 650–666. https://doi.org/10.1080/13676261.2021.1923674

Alonzo, D. J., & Buttitta, D. (2019). Is 'coming out' still relevant? Social justice implications for LGB-membered families. *Journal of Family Theory & Review, 11*(3), 354–366. https://doi.org/10.1111/jftr.12333

Balsam, K. F., Molina, Y., Beadnell, B., Simoni, J., & Walters, K. (2011). Measuring multiple minority stress: ILGBT people of color microaggressions scale. *Cultural Diversity and Ethnic Minority Psychology, 17*(2), 163–174. https://doi.org/10.1037/a0023244

Bauman, S., & Rivers, I. (2015). *Mental health in the digital age.* Palgrave Macmillan.

Bell and Another v. Tavistock and Portman NHS Foundation Trust (University College London Hospitals NHS Foundation Trust and others intervening), EHWC 3274 (admin). (2020). www.judiciary.uk/wp-content/uploads/2020/12/Bell-v-Tavistock-Judgment.pdf

Bishop, M. D., Fish, J. N., Hammack, P. L., & Russell, S. T. (2020). Sexual identity development milestones in three generations of sexual minority people: A national probability sample. *Developmental Psychology, 56*(11), 2177–2193. https://doi.org/10.1037/dev0001105

Bogaert, A. F., & Hafer, C. L. (2009). Predicting the timing of coming out in gay and bisexual men from world beliefs, physical attractiveness, and childhood gender identity/role. *Journal of Applied Social Psychology, 39*(8), 1991–2019. https://doi.org/10.1111/j.1559-1816.2009.00513.x

Bond, B. J., Hefner, V., & Drogos, K. L. (2009). Information-seeking practices during the sexual development of lesbian, gay, and bisexual individuals: The influence and effects of coming out in a mediated environment. *Sexuality & Culture: An Interdisciplinary Quarterly, 13*(1), 32–50. https://doi.org/10.1007/s12119-008-9041-y

Buss, J., Le, H., & Haimson, O. L. (2021). Transgender identity management across social media platforms. *Media, Culture & Society, 44*(1), 22–38. https://doi.org/10.1177/01634437211027106

Cabiria, J. (2008). Benefits of virtual world engagement: Implications for marginalized gay and lesbian people. *Media Psychology Review, 1*(1). http://mprcenter.org/review/cabiria-virtual-world/

Cass, V. C. (1979). Homosexual identity formation: A theoretical model. *Journal of Homosexuality, 4*(3), 219–235. https://doi.org/10.1300/J082v04n03_01

Cho, A. (2018). Default publicness: Queer youth of color, social media, and being outed by the machine. *New Media & Society, 20*(9), 3183–3200. https://doi.org/.o0r.g1/107.171/1774/61144614448418717744784

Cisneros, J., & Bracho, C. (2019). Coming out of the shadows and the closet: Visibility schemas among undocuqueer immigrants. *Journal of Homosexuality, 66*(6), 715–734. https://doi.org/10.1080/00918369.2017.1423221

Clarke, G. (2002). Outlaws in sport and education? Exploring the sporting and education experiences of lesbian physical education teachers. In S. Scraton & A. Flintoff (Eds.), *Gender and sport: A reader* (pp. 209–221). Routledge.

Coleman-Fountain, E. (2014). Lesbian and gay youth and the question of labels. *Sexualities, 17*(7), 802–817. https://doi.org/10.1177/1363460714534 1432

Corrigan, P. W., Larson, J. E., Hautamaki, J., Matthews, A., Kuwabara, S., Rafacz, J., Walton, J., Wassel, A., & O'Shaughnessy, J. (2009). What lessons do coming out as gay men or lesbians have for people stigmatized by mental illness? *Community Mental Health Journal, 45*(5), 366–374. https://doi.org/10.1007/s10597-009-9187-6

Craig, S. L., & McInroy, L. (2014). You can form a part of yourself online: The influence of new media on identity development and coming out for LGBTQ Youth. *Journal of Gay & Lesbian Mental Health, 18*(1), 95–109. https://doi.org/10.1080/19359705.2013.777007

D'Augelli, A. R. (1994). Identity development and sexual orientation: Toward a model of lesbian, gay and bisexual development. In E. J. Trickett, R. J. Watts, & D. Birman (Eds.), *Human diversity: Perspectives on people in context* (pp. 312–333). Jossey-Bass.

Diamond, L. M. (2006). What we got wrong about sexual identity development: Unexpected findings from a longitudinal study of young women. In A. M. Omoto & H. S. Kurtzman (Eds.), *Sexual orientation and mental health: Examining identity and development in lesbian, gay, and bisexual people* (pp. 73–94). American Psychological Association.

Dilley, P. (2010). New century, new identities: Building on a typology of nonheterosexual college men. *Journal of LGBT Youth, 7*, 186—199. https://doi.org/10.1080/19361653.2010.488565

Dubé, E. M. (2000). The role of sexual behavior in the identification process of gay and bisexual males. *The Journal of Sex Research, 37*(2), 123–132. https://doi.org/10.1080/00224490009552029

Duguay, S. (2016). 'He has a way gayer Facebook than I do': Investigating sexual identity disclosure and context collapse on a social networking site. *New Media & Society, 18*(6), 891–907. https://doi.org/10.1177/146144481 4549930

Hershberger, S. L., & D'Augelli, A. R. (1995). The impact of victimization on the mental health and suicidality of lesbian, gay, and bisexual youths. *Developmental Psychology, 31*(1), 65–74. https://doi.org/10.1037/0012-1649.31. 1.65

Hill, N. L. (2009). Affirmative practice and alternative sexual orientations: Helping clients navigate the coming out process. *Clinical Social Work Journal, 37*(4), 346–356. https://doi.org/10.1007/s10615-009-0240-2

Jagose, A. (1996). *Queer theory: An introduction.* New York University Press.

Jaspal, R. (2021). Identity threat and coping among British South Asian gay men during the COVID-19 lockdown. *Sexuality & Culture, 25*(5), 1428–1446. https://doi.org/10.1007/s12119-021-09817-w

Kaufman, J. M., & Johnson, C. (2004). Stigmatized individuals and the process of identity. *The Sociological Quarterly, 45*(4), 807–833. https://doi.org/10.1111/j.1533-8525.2004.tb02315.x

Klein, K., Holtby, A., Cook, K., & Travers, R. (2015). Complicating the coming out narrative: Becoming oneself in a heterosexist and cissexist world. *Journal of Homosexuality, 62*(3), 297–326. https://doi.org/10.1080/00918369.2014.970829

Knoble, N. B., & Linville, D. (2012). Outness and relationship satisfaction in same-gender couples. *Journal of Marital and Family Therapy, 38*(2), 330–339. https://doi.org/10.1111/j.1752-0606.2010.00206.x

Manning, J. (2015a). Communicating sexual identities: A typology of coming out. *Sexuality & Culture, 19*(1), 122–138. https://doi.org/10.1007/s12119-014-9251-4

Manning, J. (2015b). Identity, relationships, and culture: A constitutive model of coming out. In J. Manning & C. M. Noland (Eds.), *Contemporary studies of sexuality & communication: Theoretical and applied perspectives* (pp. 93–108). Kendall Hunt Publishing Company.

Matsuno, E. (2019). Nonbinary-affirming psychological interventions. *Cognitive and Behavioral Practice, 26*(4), 617–628. https://doi.org/10.1016/j.cbpra.2018.09.003

Meyer, I. H. (2003). Prejudice, social stress, and mental health in lesbian, gay, and bisexual populations: Conceptual issues and research evidence. *Psychological Bulletin, 129*(5), 674–697. https://doi.org/10.1037/0033-2909.129.5.674

Newman, B. S., & Muzzonigro, P. G. (1993). The effects of traditional family values on the coming out process of gay male adolescents. *Adolescence, 28*(109), 213–226.

Orne, J. (2011). 'You will always have to "out" yourself': Reconsidering coming out through strategic outness. *Sexualities, 14*(6), 681–703. https://doi.org/10.1177/1363460711420462

O'Shaughnessy, M., Russell, S. T., Heck, K., Calhoun, C., & Laub, C. (2004). *Safe place to learn: Consequences of harassment based on actual or perceived sexual orientation and gender non-conformity and steps for making schools safer.* California Safe Schools Coalition.

Pachankis, J. E. (2007). The psychological implications of concealing a stigma: A cognitive-affective-behavioral model. *Psychological Bulletin, 133*(2), 328–345. https://doi.org/10.1037/0033-2909.133.2.328

Pascoe, C. J. (2011). Resource and risk: Youth sexuality and new media use. *Sexuality Research & Social Policy: A Journal of the NSRC, 8*(1), 5–17. https://doi.org/10.1007/s13178-011-0042-5

Pilkington, N. W., & D'Augelli, A. R. (1995). Victimization of lesbian, gay, and bisexual youth in community settings. *Journal of Community Psychology, 23*(1), 33–55. https://doi.org/10.1002/1520-6629(199501)23:1%3C34::AID-JCOP2290230105%3E3.0.CO;2-N

Pohtinen, J. (2019). From secrecy to pride: Negotiating the kink identity, normativity, and stigma. *Ethnologia Fennica, 46*(1), 84–108. https://doi.org/10.23991/ef.v46i0.74306

Ragins, B. R. (2008). Disclosure disconnects: Antecedents and consequences of disclosing invisible stigmas across life domains. *The Academy of Management Review, 33*(1), 194–215. https://doi.org/10.2307/20159383

Rivers, I. (1997). Lesbian, gay and bisexual development: Theory, research and social issues. *Journal of Community and Applied Social Psychology, 7,* 329–343. https://doi.org/10.1002/(SICI)1099-1298(199712)7:5%3C329::AID-CASP432%3E3.0.CO;2-E

Rivers, I. (2001). The bullying of sexual minorities at school: Its nature and long-term correlates. *Educational and Child Psychology, 18*(1), 33–46.

Rivers, I. (2002). Developmental issues for lesbian and gay youth. In A. Coyle & C. C. Kitzinger (Eds.), *Lesbian and gay psychology: New perspectives* (pp. 30–44). Blackwell/BPS Books.

Rivers, I., & Carragher, D. J. (2003). Social-developmental factors affecting lesbian and gay youth: A review of cross-national research findings. *Children and Society, 17*(5), 374–385. https://doi.org/10.1002/CHI.771

Rivers, I., Gonzalez, C., Nodin, N., Peel, E., & Tyler, A. (2018). LGBT people and suicidality in youth: A qualitative study of perceptions of risk and protective circumstances. *Social Science and Medicine, 212*(September), 1–8. https://doi.org/10.1016/j.socscimed.2018.06.040

Rivers, I., & Noret, N. (2008). Well-being among same-sex and opposite sex attracted youth at school. *School Psychology Review, 37*(2), 174–187. https://doi.org/10.1080/02796015.2008.12087892

Robbins, N. K., Low, K. G., & Query, A. N. (2016). A qualitative exploration of the 'coming out' process for asexual individuals. *Archives of Sexual Behavior, 45*(3), 751–760. https://doi.org/10.1007/s10508-015-0561-x

Rosati, F., Pistella, J., Nappa, M. R., & Baiocco, R. (2020). The coming-out process in family, social, and religious contexts among young, middle, and older Italian LGBQ+ adults. *Frontiers in Psychology, 11*, 617217. https://doi.org/10.3389/fpsyg.2020.617217

Ryan, C., Russell, S. T., Huebner, D., Diaz, R., & Sanchez, J. (2010). Family acceptance in adolescence and the health of LGBT young adults. *Journal of Child and Adolescent Psychiatric Nursing, 23*(4), 205–213. https://doi.org/10.1111/j.1744-6171.2010.00246.x

Saewyc, E. M., Skay, C. L., Reis, E., Pettingell, S. E., Bearinger, L. H., Resnick, M. D., Murphy, A., & Combs, L. (2006). Hazards of stigma: The sexual and physical abuse of gay, lesbian, and bisexual adolescents in the US and Canada. *Child Welfare, 85*(2), 195–213.

Sansfaçon, A. P., Medico, D., Suerich-Gulick, F., & Temple, J. (2020). "I knew that I wasn't cis, I knew that, but I didn't know exactly": Gender identity development, expression and affirmation in youth who access gender affirming medical care. *International Journal of Transgender Health, 21*(3), 307–320. https://doi.org/10.1080/26895269.2020.1756551

Savin-Williams, R. C. (2001). *Mom, dad. I'm gay. How families negotiate coming out*. American Psychological Association.

Savin-Williams, R. C. (2005). *The new gay teenager*. Harvard University Press.

Simpson, J. K. (2021). *Section 28 then and now: A tripartite investigation into narratives of sexuality, gender, and the role of fiction for children and young people in shaping LGBT+ exclusion and inclusion* (Unpublished doctoral dissertation). University of Strathclyde.

Skidmore, S. J., Lefevor, G. T., & Perez-Figueroa, A. M. (2022). "I come out because I love you": Positive coming out experiences among Latter-day Saint sexual and gender minorities. *Review of Religious Research, 64*, 539–559. https://doi.org/10.1007/s13644-022-00501-5

Snider, K. (1996). Race and sexual orientation: The (im)possibility of these intersections in educational policy. *Harvard Educational Review, 66*(2), 294–302.

Solomon, D., McAbee, J., Åsberg, K., & McGee, A. (2015). Coming out and the potential for growth in sexual minorities: The role of social reactions and internalized homonegativity. *Journal of Homosexuality, 62*(11), 1512–1538. https://doi.org/10.1080/00918369.2015.1073032

Toft, A. (2020). Identity management and community belonging: The coming out careers of young disabled LGBT+ persons. *Sexuality & Culture, 24*, 1893–1912. https://doi.org/10.1007/s12119-020-09726-4

Troiden, R. R. (1989). The formation of homosexual identities. *Journal of Homosexuality, 17*(1–2), 43–74. https://doi.org/10.1300/J082v17n01_02

Waldner, L. K., & Magrader, B. (1999). Coming out to parents: Perceptions of family relations, perceived resources, and identity expression as predictors of identity disclosure for gay and lesbian adolescents. *Journal of Homosexuality, 37*(2), 83–100. https://doi.org/10.1300/J082v37n02_05

Ward, R., Rivers, I., & Sutherland, M. (Eds.). (2012). *Lesbian, gay, bisexual and transgender ageing: Providing effective support through biographical practice.* Jessica Kingsley Press.

Weinberg, M. S., & Williams, C. J. (1974). *Male homosexuals: Their problems and adaptations.* Oxford University Press.

Wells, J. W., & Kline, W. B. (1987). Self-disclosure of homosexual orientation. *Journal of Social Psychology, 127*(2), 191–197. https://doi.org/10.1080/00224545.1987.9713679

5

Mental Health and Sexual Orientation Across the Life Course

Paul Willis and Sue Westwood

Introduction

This chapter considers mental health and wellbeing at two ends of the age spectrum, comparing current cohorts of young and older LGBTQ[1] people. We first consider temporal contexts and the themes of minority

[1] Throughout this chapter we use the abbreviation 'LGBTQ' to encompass those identifying as lesbian, gay, bisexual, trans and queer. When using this acronym we are mindful of the generational differences that accompany these identity makers, including recognition that many older people will not affiliate themselves with the expression 'queer' because of its historical homophobic connotations.

P. Willis (✉)
Cardiff University, Cardiff, UK
e-mail: paul.willis@bristol.ac.uk

S. Westwood
University of York, York, UK
e-mail: sue.westwood@york.ac.uk

J. Semlyen and P. Rohleder (eds.), *Sexual Minorities and Mental Health*, https://doi.org/10.1007/978-3-031-37438-8_5

stress and intersectionality before then summarising the relevant literature. This is followed by a discussion comparing and contrasting the two
sets of experiences, with concluding key messages being drawn from this
analysis.

Temporal Contexts

Chronological age is a crude construct for taking into account changes
in sexual and gender identities, and associated changes in mental health,
over the life course. The categories of 'younger' and 'older' encompass
multiple cohorts and generations who are experiencing different social
transitions across diverse social circumstances. For example, older people
belonging to the 'third age' may be experiencing transitions from paid
employment to retirement while older adults in the 'fourth age' may
be experiencing transitions into supported living and long-term care,
dependent on their needs and circumstances. For younger adults, the
transitions adolescents experience as they move between primary and
secondary school, and associated changes in psychological development
and identity, will dramatically differ from the experiences of older teens
taking up paid employment for the first time or relocating to further
education and university.

These transitions are also taking place against wide-ranging social,
legal and cultural reforms between the 1960s and the present day. The
world young people are growing up in now is a very different one
from when older LGBTQ people were young adults. Within the UK,
older gay men grew up during a time when sex between men was
unlawful, then witnessed a period of decriminalisation commencing with
the Sexual Offences Act 1967 in England and Wales (men over 21 years)
through to the equal age of consent for all (Sexual Offences (Amendment) Act 2000). In some nations homosexuality is still criminalised.[2]
Homosexuality was declassified as a mental illness in the Diagnostic
Statistical Manual III in 1973 and in the International Classification of

---

[2] ILGA reports that in 2020 67 UN member states had in place legal provisions criminalising
consensual same-sex activity.

Diseases (ICD-10) in 1990. In the UK significant advances have been made in granting equal recognition of rights to LGBTQ people across child and family policy (including equal adoption rights), social security, employment law and the expansion of marriage to include recognition of same-sex relationships. Discrimination, harassment and victimisation on the basis of age and sexual orientation have been recognised and outlawed in the last twenty years, with current anti-discrimination provisions enshrined in the Equality Act 2010.

For trans people in the UK, 'gender reassignment' is also a protected characteristic under the Equality Act, determined by case law to encompass all trans identities, not only those of trans women and men who have transitioned. Prior to the Gender Recognition Act 2004, trans individuals were not permitted to legally change their gender, now they can. However, for many this legal improvement has not gone far enough. The Act require a medical assessment and diagnosis of 'gender dysphoria' as grounds for legal change. Many trans groups and organisations have campaigned for a removal of this medical requirement in favour of an alternative model based on principles of self-determination and self-identification.

The world of young LGBTQ adults today is, then, very different from the world experienced by now-ageing older LGBTQ adults when they were young, with the law, even so, still playing catch-up with increasing social inclusion and acceptance, particularly in relation to trans issues. However, that is not to say that prejudices towards LGBTQ individuals do not continue to prevail (see Chapter 3) and that some religious views still regard homosexuality as problematic (see Chapter 6).

Key Concepts

To understand these changes and their significance for LGBTQ mental health and wellbeing, we draw here on two key conceptual frameworks: minority stress and intersectionality. As outlined in previous chapters, minority stress is excess stress to which individuals from marginalised and stigmatized social categories are routinely exposed, and which has a detrimental effect on mental and physical wellbeing (Meyer, 2003, 2015). For

LGBTQ people in particular, it can occur through one or more of four processes: objective stressful events such as the experience of hostility and discrimination (for example, homophobia, biphobia and transphobia); the expectation of this and the associated perceived need to be vigilant; the internalising of homonegative and trans-negative beliefs; and hiding one's sexual orientation and/or gender identity.

Authors engaged in LGBTQ youth research have adopted an ecological model for strengthening understanding of the ways in which young people experience different and overlapping stressors across interpersonal, social and cultural contexts, including the family home and settings where they interact with peers (Russell & Fish, 2016). In relation to later life, researchers have increasingly focussed on a life course approach to understanding the accumulation of minority stress over time among older LGBTQ people (Fredriksen-Goldsen et al., 2014). The impact on the cognitive health of older LGBTQ people is a topic of increasing importance (see Correro & Nielson, 2020).

A central theme throughout this chapter is the ways in which being LGBTQ *and* younger *or* older impact the lived experience and mental wellbeing of both cohorts. Here, an intersectional perspective is needed. Intersectionality, first discussed by Crenshaw (1991), provides a sociological lens for understanding the complex ways in which social identity categories coalesce and compound experiences of social disadvantage and inequality. In the context of ageing, gender and sexuality, it has been discussed notably by Witten (2016), Averett et al. (2011), Traies (2016), Hulko (2016), Westwood (2016a), and King et al. (2019). Crucially, it is the intersection of age, gender and sexuality within specific temporal sociolegal contexts which shapes how minority stress is experienced.

Young LGBTQ People and Mental Health

Mental health disparities among LGBTQ young people in comparison to heterosexual peers has been a growing area of international research over the last two decades. Two parallel trends have been the increasing levels of social acceptability of non-heterosexual identities and amplified concerns for LGBTQ young people's mental wellbeing (Fish, 2020). Arguably the increasing visibility of LGBTQ youth, including 'coming out' at much earlier ages in comparison to older LGBTQ generations (Bishop et al., 2020), has heightened awareness of young people's mental wellbeing and welfare. The pressures of living in heteronormative and cisnormative cultures and homonegative and trans-negative environments generate stressors for young LGBTQ people's mental wellbeing (see also Chapter 7 for exploration of intersecting sexual and gender diverse identities). Reported outcomes include lowered self-esteem, higher levels of depression, heightened psychological distress, including PTSD and increased risk of self-harm and suicide (Baker et al., 2016; Hill et al., 2021; McDermott et al., 2018b; Mereish, 2019; Mustanski et al., 2016; Russell & Fish, 2016).

An overarching narrative within this body of research is the location of young LGBTQ people as more at risk of mental health problems and suicidality in comparison to heterosexual and cisgender peers (Rivers et al., 2018). A closer examination of mental health outcomes on the basis of gender *and* sexuality highlights important differences. From Shearer et al.'s (2016) survey of LGBTQ and heterosexual youth, young bisexual and questioning women were more at risk of mental health problems compared to young heterosexual women, with young bisexual women exhibiting the highest scores for suicidality. A similar finding is echoed in Ream's secondary analysis of youth suicide data—bisexual women had higher prevalence for mental health problems and suicidal thoughts compared to other groups (LGBT+ and heterosexual). Trans men had the highest prevalence for prior suicide attempt compared to other trans and cis groups (Ream, 2019). The marginalisation of young bisexual people is more complex as they encounter exclusion and stigmatisation from lesbian and gay groups and communities and across heteronormative contexts (e.g. the negative stereotyping of bisexual youth as promiscuous or merely going through a phase) (Shearer et al., 2016). Rivers et al. (2018) qualitative research with LGBT people in the UK suggest that young people are mindful of and seek to distance themselves from the stereotypical trope of 'depressed gay teenager' and resist disease connotations attached to LGBTQ identities and stigmas.

Researchers within this field are quick to locate the mental health stressors young people experience within the wider hetero- and cisnormative environments in which young people are situated and through which they build LGBTQ identities. McDermott et al. (2018a) point to five interconnected social determinants of suicidality (suicidal thoughts, planning and attempting suicide) amongst this group: (1) experiences of homophobia, biphobia and transphobia, (2) pressures of sexual and gender norms, (3) stressors of managing minority identities across different life domains, including home and school, (4) experiencing difficulties in discussing emotional responses, and (5) other life crises, for example financial pressures in the family home. In England, young LGBTQ people indicate common experiences of verbal abuse, including name calling, harassment and threats and intimidation, and physical assault across school and home life (Baker et al., 2016). Homophobic discourses are conveyed through verbal and physical abuse to evoke shame and position young LGBTQ people as "abnormal, dirty and disgusting" (McDermott et al., 2008, p. 821). Despite these oppressive discourses young LGBTQ people continue to construct identities of pride and affirmation (Willis, 2012). However, pride identities are difficult to sustain, and young people may not always have the resources available to them to construct such identities. Secondary schools remain prevalent sites of exposure to homonegative and trans-negative views and attitudes (Hill et al., 2021), with some longitudinal evidence indicating that experiences of victimisation decline as young people transition out of them (Mustanski et al., 2016).

The primacy of risk discourse within this body of literature is unsurprising given that "LGBTQ+ young people mental health research is overwhelmingly conducted within a biomedical psychiatric paradigm that tends to pathologize young people's emotions" (Gabb et al., 2020, pp. 536–537). Adolescence for LGBTQ people is framed as a 'time of mental health risk' (McConnell et al., 2016) with a dominant focus on the struggles and life-challenges of growing up queer. Problem-saturated accounts of young LGBTQ people's lives convey totalising stories of distress, damage and injury, and do not reflect the diversity of young people's wellbeing and resilience. Talburt (2004, p. 118) has argued that the representation of young LGBTQ people 'at risk' contributes to their life-stories as 'suffering, isolated and suicidal' subjects. Similarly, Harwood (2004) articulates how a 'discourse of woundedness' transmits a conservative understanding of young LGBTQ people's sexual lives and discursively regulates what kinds of sexual experiences, pleasures and relationships are spoken about within social settings such as schools. These critiques raise a fundamental question of how researchers approach the mental wellbeing of young LGBTQ people in a holistic and enabling manner beyond pathological discourses of risk and harm.

Another stream within this body of literature focuses on increasing knowledge of access to services and support-seeking. Barriers to accessing mental health services include the unique pressures LGBTQ youth experience in having to conceal their sexual and gender identities from parents and caregivers versus the requirement for parental consent to access such services. At a systemic level the lack of 'LGBTQ competent' services in mental health support and gaps in professional knowledge are two interconnected barriers to receiving good support (Higgins et al., 2021). Young LGBTQ people may wait until they reach crisis point before seeking help and their attempts at help-seeking may be hindered by pressures to conceal LGBTQ identities, worries about adverse responses from caregivers and professionals, difficulties in articulating emotional distress, and perceptions of help-seeking as a sign of weakness and losing control (McDermott et al., 2018b). The double stigma of mental health problems and identifying as LGBTQ impede help-seeking with mixed-methods research in the UK suggesting that young LGBTQ people normalise their emotional distress and only seek help at crisis point (McDermott et al., 2018b).

Supportive families have been highlighted as an important factor for ameliorating levels of psychological distress—young people lacking family support report higher levels of distress (McConnell et al., 2016). Having supportive parents is also correlated with lower depression for young LGB people and higher self-esteem amongst gay and bisexual youth (Watson et al., 2019). Seeking family support may be complicated by ethnic differences across family groupings. A recent Australian study reports that young LGBTQ people from Anglo-Celtic backgrounds report supportive family in greater numbers than those from multicultural backgrounds. Multicultural young people in the same study also report higher levels of physical, verbal and sexual abuse compared to Anglo-Celtic respondents, highlighting the greater safety concerns for young LGBTQ people from ethnically diverse backgrounds (Hill et al., 2021). Gabb et al. (2020) discuss the notion of 'paradoxical families' to capture the ways in which UK-based families seek to exercise care and support for LGBTQ children while young people continue to negate hetero- and cisnormative assumptions and beliefs present within family interactions. Peers are an equally important source of support. Young LGBTQ Australians report higher levels of disclosure to friends compared to family, and friends as the most likely to be supportive with family and classmates ranked as the least supportive (Hill et al., 2021). This is supported by US research indicating that LGBTQ youth rate friendship support as more important than support from family and school (Watson et al., 2019).

Australian survey research has highlighted higher levels of psychological distress and increased concealment of sexual minority identities for young gay men in rural contexts in comparison to those in urban settings (Lyons et al., 2015). During COVID19-related lockdowns in 2020 young LGBTQ people reported frustrations about lack of access to LGBTQ spaces outside of school and being stuck at home with unsupportive parents (for example, religious parents). The shift from in-person LGBTQ services and groups also raises privacy concerns about parents overhearing online conversations in the family home (Fish et al., 2020). US research conducted during the pandemic suggests that trans young people are experiencing greater mental health deterioration than cis peers and experiencing more disruptions in accessing mental health services (Hawke et al., 2021).

After two decades of scholarship on LGBTQ youth, research on resilience and strengths-based perspectives continues to be limited in scope (Fish, 2020). Alongside this, more attention needs to be given to intersectional perspectives to understand more fully how other social identities, including religious, ethnic minority and disabled identities, shape youth mental health and wellbeing. Another key area for investigation is how community contexts and resources promote better mental health for LGBTQ young people, including LGBTQ and non-LGBTQ community spaces and services (Fish, 2020).

Older LGBTQ People and Mental Health

Older LGBTQ people share the same concerns as the ageing majority population (increasing physical and mental decline into older old age, bereavement, potential loneliness and isolation, heightened care needs and questionable care quality) but this is nuanced by LGBTQ issues (Fish & Weis, 2019; Fredriksen-Goldsen et al., 2014, 2017a, 2017b; Hash & Rogers, 2013; Kim et al., 2017; Lyons et al., 2021; Smith et al., 2019; Yarns et al., 2016). Older LGBTQ people are differentiated by those who exhibit enduring resilience across their lives, which assists them in coping with the ageing process, compared with those who have found dealing with their circumstances more difficult, in ways which are then compounded in older age (Allen & Lavender-Stott, 2020; Bower et al., 2021; Fredriksen-Goldsen et al., 2013). Many older LGBTQ people have 'emotional, social and economic resources' (Kneale et al., 2021) which buffer them from life's stresses and the challenges of ageing. Some include family of origin, some include 'families of choice', and some include organised networks, either organised within particular communities, or arranged and coordinated by lesbian/gay/bisexual/trans and/or LGBTQ groups and organisations. Where older LGBTQ people do not have access to these resources, they are more likely to experience heightened loneliness and isolation, with associated risks to their mental health and wellbeing.

Older LGBTQ people generally report poorer mental health than the majority population (Fredriksen-Goldsen et al., 2013, 2017a, 2017b; Kneale et al., 2021; Semlyen et al., 2016; Tinney et al., 2015; Westwood et al., 2020; Yarns et al., 2016). A UK study which conducted a survey of 1,000 older lesbian, gay and bisexual (LGB) people and 1,000 heterosexual people (Guasp, 2011) reported that older LGB people, compared with older heterosexual people, drink alcohol more often (45% compared with 31%); are more likely to take drugs (1 in 11 compared with 1 in 50); and are more likely to be concerned about their mental health (49% compared with 37%). The study identified two key differentiators among LGB older people in relation to mental health and wellbeing: relationship status, with single LGB older people being three times as likely as LGB older people in a relationship to rate their mental health as 'poor'; and socioeconomic status, with individuals in lower socioeconomic categories being more than twice as likely as those in higher socioeconomic categories to rate their mental health as 'poor' (14% compared with 6%). Despite its important insights, the data from this study need to be approached with caution, as there were several methodological flaws (Westwood, 2020), and lesbians, especially older lesbians, were significantly under-represented (Traies, 2016).

Comparatively poorer health among older LGBTQ people is attributable to (Fredriksen-Goldsen et al., 2017a; Kneale et al., 2021; Westwood, 2020) the accumulated impact of minority stress, i.e. the physical and psychological effects of stigma and marginalisation, and health risk behaviours linked to that stress (e.g., smoking, excessive drug/alcohol use, obesity). Having strong identity-validating personal support networks, and "a strong sense of agency, and emotional control" (King & Richardson, 2017, p. 62) can act as buffers to the worst effects of minority stress.

Westwood (2020) has commented on the need to differentiate between issues affecting LGBTQ sub-populations and their intersection with other social locations (for example ethnicity, socioeconomic status) in order to better appreciate specific needs. For example, older cis gay men are at high risk of loneliness and isolation than both older cis lesbians (Guasp, 2011) and older cis heterosexual men (Willis et al., 2022). This is for several reasons: ageism within the gay commercial scene and the invisibility of older gay men (Brennan-Ing et al., 2021; Simpson, 2013; Willis et al., 2022); diminished ageing cohorts due to so many gay men dying young during the HIV/AIDs crisis in the 1980s and 1990s; being less likely to be in a couple and less likely to have children (Guasp, 2011; Westwood, 2016a); and gendered social networking styles (Toze et al., 2023; Willis et al., 2022). Older lesbians and gay men tend to use formal support groups in gendered ways (Knocker et al., 2012): firstly, preferring gender-specific support; and secondly in how they use that support, with the gay men using the groups as their social networks, while older lesbians use them to 'top up' their existing social networks.

Accounts in the literature about the mental health of older trans people suggest that they are at higher risk of mental health problems compared with the non-trans population, including non-trans LGBQ people (Bailey et al., 2018; Fabbre & Gaveras, 2020; Fredriksen-Goldsen et al., 2014; Hoy-Ellis & Fredriksen-Goldsen, 2017), attributable to the accumulated effects of 'multi-level stigma' (Fabbre et al., 2020). Findings from research conducted by Jones et al. (2019) suggest that the mental health of non-binary trans adults its better than that of binary trans adults. For many trans women and trans men, transitioning in later life can dramatically improve their health and wellbeing (Bailey et al., 2018). However, this may put them out of temporal sync with their cis peers (Pearce, 2018; Toze, 2019) and while newly transitioned older individuals may experience a 'new lease of life' (Willis et al., 2021, p. 1), they may also experience associated family rejections (Riggs & Kentlyn, 2014) at a time in life when it can be difficult to compensate socially and personally, making formally organised networks more important for wellbeing.

Older bisexual people's lives in general, and more specifically their mental health, are not yet well-understood (Fredriksen-Goldsen et al., 2017b; Jen, 2018; Jones, 2018; Scherrer, 2017; Witten, 2016). A recent review of the UK and US literature has suggested that older bisexual people have poorer mental health than both older heterosexual people and older lesbians and gay men (Jen & Jones, 2019). However, older bisexual people are often under-represented in mixed LGBTQ studies, and it is not yet clear how robust and/or reliable these findings are. A UK based study with 12 bisexual people aged over 50 (Jones et al., 2018) suggests that while lifelong experiences of biphobia may affect health and wellbeing in later life, older bisexual people may also have developed a range of resiliencies which better-prepare them to deal with the challenges of ageing.

The extent to which older LGBTQ people are living in inclusive environments as they age impacts their mental health. Heaphy (2009) observed that greater access to material resources gave older LGB greater choice about where and how they lived in later life. For older LGB people ageing in rural environments, whose social connections are further afield, i.e. in cities, having the funds to use costly public transport when no longer able to drive, can make all the difference between remaining connected to social networks and becoming disconnected from them. Access to material resources can also determine what type and quality of housing is lived in (including retirement housing and housing with care), in what neighbourhoods, and to what extent they are inclusive of people from diverse background, including older LGBTQ people (Westwood, 2016b).

Older LGBTQ people are very worried about needing care in later life, and about care providers not being equipped to understand or meet their needs. There is a growing body of UK-based evidence which suggests older age care providers are ill-equipped to meet the diverse needs of older LGBTQ people (Almack, 2018; Hafford-Letchfield et al., 2018; Simpson et al., 2018; Willis et al., 2016, Willis et al., 2018). This in turn will have a detrimental effect on their mental health and wellbeing (Smith et al., 2019). Dementia is a particular concern for older LGBTQ people (Westwood & Price, 2016) who are worried about prejudice and discrimination, at a time when they may be especially vulnerable. Older trans people who have transitioned fear that with memory loss they may forget that they have done so and/or that their now aligned gender identity will not be respected in care contexts (Willis et al., 2021). Those whose bodies may not be congruent with their gender identity fear staff providing personal care will not be respectful or understanding towards them (Baril & Silverman, 2019). They may find themselves "reluctant educators and self-advocates" (Willis et al., 2020, p. 1231) with care providers at times and under circumstances when they would be better placed being supported in attending to their health and wellbeing.

COVID-19 has had a significant impact on the mental health of many older people in general, and LGBTQ older people in particular. In a recent UK survey of almost 400 older LGBTQ people, worsening mental health during the pandemic was reported by 54% of older lesbians/gay women (cis and trans), 45% of older gay men (cis and trans), 33% of bisexual individuals (cis and trans) and 53% or trans respondents (Westwood et al., 2021). Self-reported factors which informed declining mental health included being unable to physically connect with friends and loved ones, loneliness and isolation (especially among single individuals) and an inability to engage in normal leisure activities. Many survey respondents indicated that the constraints upon their social connections with L/G/B/T and/or LGBTQ networks—considered important for mitigating the impact of wider social exclusions—compounded the negative impact of social isolation on their mental health.

Comparing Younger and Older LGBT+ Mental Health Issues

Here we articulate some wider points of differentiation and commonality while recognising that these represent partial reflections that cannot capture all LGBTQ people's lived experiences of mental health and wellbeing. First, we discuss some points of differentiation.

For older people, LGBTQ discrimination and exclusion is magnified by their intersection with older age. While LGBTQ people of all ages can experience prejudice and discrimination, its impact on older people and their mental health is different from that of younger people in several ways (Lyons et al., 2021). Older LGBTQ people have experienced *more extreme* systemic discrimination than younger people, and complex trauma histories (Westwood, 2020) as they lived their earlier adult lives during times of far greater legal and social prohibition and thus greater and more protracted minority stress. Unlike younger cohorts of LGBTQ people, current cohorts of older LGBTQ people are ageing against the shadow of historical criminalisation, pathologisation, being regarded as sinful, and workplace and family exclusions. This was further compounded by the deaths of so many young gay men during the HIV/AIDs crisis and by the cruelties of Section 28, which banned the 'promotion' of homosexuality for over a decade. Many, especially older gay men, experienced the loss of close friends and loved ones, while some are ageing with HIV from that era, living their lives against a backcloth of additional stigma, and associated health issues (Rosenfeld et al., 2012). Put simply, older LGBTQ people, have not only experienced more extreme systematic discrimination, they have also experienced it for longer, compounding their experiences of cumulative disadvantage (Dannefer, 2003).

For trans people, the intersection with age also adds nuance to wellbeing. Forty years ago, trans adults in mid to later life in the UK did not have affirming language and reliable information about trans identities and social and medical transitioning available to them, along-side a legal process for changing gender status (Willis et al., 2021). Commencing transitioning (socially and/or medically) in mid to later life also generates unique stressors in having to renegotiate existing long-term relationships with spouses and partners and children (Willis et al., 2021). Unlike young people, older trans adults are more likely to be financially and socially independent. Young trans people are highly restricted with access to financial and material resources; their dependency on parent caregivers can amplify risks of exclusion or the removal of access to trans-affirming resources and services. Older and younger trans adults may experience family exclusions, especially those who transition, but for older adults this can be compounded by the greater challenges of developing alternative sources of support in later life.

In terms of commonalities, loneliness and social isolation are key factors informing the mental wellbeing of LGBTQ individuals, although the research evidence available suggest more nuanced differences on the basis of age and gender. There are particular life stage and spatial issues which intersect with and add nuance to LGBTQ people's experiences of loneliness and social isolation in younger and older age. In the UK loneliness amongst young people has been flagged as a growing phenomenon—younger people 16–24 years who are renting and single are more likely to report feeling often lonely than older age groups. Similarly geographical areas with a higher concentration of young people report higher levels of 'often or always lonely' (ONS, 2021). A recent charity report in Wales suggests that LGBTQ young people are twice as likely to feel lonely compared to their heterosexual, cis peers and that levels of loneliness have been exacerbated during the pandemic lockdowns (Just Like Us, 2021). Higher levels of reporting may also reflect young people's increased familiarity with loneliness and mental health discourse compared to older age groups. For young LGBTQ people who look more to their peers for support, peer-exclusions can be particularly challenging especially if family support is not available. For older people, loneliness and isolation may be more associated with restricted mobility and decreased opportunities for connecting with members of social networks outside of the home, such as LGBTQ friends, or with being located in older age housing and long-term care spaces where they are surrounded by non-LGBTQ people.

Technology also intersects with LGBTQ lives to inform the quality of those lives, especially in terms of social networking. The ubiquity of the Internet and social media for young people as important platforms for performing LGBTQ identities online and connecting with virtual groups may be less readily accessible and familiar to older generations. National UK statistics continue to show older adults (75+ years) as the group least likely to be accessing the Internet compared to younger age groups, however this digital divide is shrinking (ONS, 2021). For young LGBTQ people the Internet serves as an important source of information, support and social connection (Lucassen et al., 2018). However young people in the UK have identified concerns about cyberbullying, personal safety and potential for sexual exploitation online which compromise the effectiveness of the Internet for expanding social support networks and gaining access to helpful information and potential e-therapies. Lucassen et al. (2018) advocate for the online availability of mental health resources targeted at LGBTQ youth and the development and testing of e-therapies that are LGBTQ-specific. Similar technologies and applications may equally be beneficial for older LGBTQ adults. However, we have little evidence or information about their Internet use or levels of digital literacy.

As noted earlier, the personal, social and legal contexts have changed significantly over the last twenty years for younger and older LGBTQ people alike. There is a common sense that 'things are better' for LGBTQ citizens across the lifespan. There are many more social spaces where it is safe to be openly LGBTQ (while acknowledging not all of these are accessible to young people under eighteen, for example commercial bars and clubs) and there has been an easing of some of the psychosocial pressures of minority stress experienced by older LGBTQ people. However, many older people are still living with its aftereffects, captured in the notion of cumulative stress. For young LGBTQ people there are many more pathways for individual expression, collectivised group identities and social inclusion and approval. They are not experiencing the same legal oppression of older generations, and there are greater social and cultural representations of LGBTQ people for them to see and identify with.

Although younger LGBTQ people have many visible pathways to take, and many visible role models to follow, that itself can generate new stressors by having to construct sexual and gender identities in a social milieu of diversified and sometimes competing messages (online and off-line) about non-normative relationships, identities and gender expressions. Moreover, with the shifting UK demographic, there are more younger people from minoritised ethnic groups, who are navigating an LGBTQ identity at the intersection with issues of minority cultures, ethnicities and religions, which adds to the complexities of constructing an affirming identity while maintaining established cultural and religious affiliations. As noted by Rehman et al. (2020, p. 15) the 'intersections of sexual orientation, gender, and religion can increase the risk of psychological stress' for LGBTQ people from these groups. These authors note the continued familial and community pressures to enter heterosexual marriages, to single out one stressor that remains a reality for some young LGBTQ people. Chapter 6 explores this intersection in more detail.

This brings us to a final point of commonality—both cohorts continue to experience psychosocial stressors across social relationships and contexts, which negatively impacts their health and wellbeing. Certain social environments and settings continue to be problematic for LGBTQ people, younger and older. While some of them are different spaces, some are shared. Families, especially religious families, can still hold and express heteronormative and cisnormative expectations. LGBTQ young people are disproportionately represented among homeless young people (Norris & Quilty, 2020). Schools, colleges and universities are still often sites of LGBTQ oppression. For older LGBTQ people, they face new spatial challenges associated with finding and having access to appropriate age-related housing and care and support services. They are potentially relocated into new hetero- and cisnormative spaces where they face new sources of stigma and oppression at times in their lives when they may be more vulnerable due to older age dependencies (Westwood, 2016b; Willis et al., 2022). Crucially, age-related care needs may mean that they cannot—literally sometimes—walk away from people and spaces where they feel marginalised. In some ways, there are similarities for younger people here too. They cannot walk away from schools either, unless they risk being excluded.

It is not safe for any of us—younger or older—to openly express non-normative desires, attractions, relationships and love in many contexts (Hubbard, 2013). Showing affection to same-gender partners in public settings continues to be a vivid example of this—from the UK Government's (Government Equalities Office, 2018) national survey of 108 000+ LGBTQ respondents (16+ years), 68% with a minority sexual orientation report they avoid holding hands with a same-gender partner in public. From the same survey, 70% of cis respondents report avoiding being open about their sexuality with 67% trans respondents avoiding being open about their gender identity. Public transport and workplaces are identified as places of high safety risk and surveillance—spaces that younger and older LGBTQ+ adults negotiate daily. Specific to mental health, older cis respondents were more likely to have been offered or undergone conversion therapy (psychological and religious therapies aimed at changing people's sexual orientation and gender identity) than those in younger age groups, however experiences of conversion therapy were reported by respondents *across age groups* (Government Equalities Office, 2018).

Conclusion

This chapter has highlighted sites of commonality and difference between younger and older LGBTQ people. Both have higher rates of mental health problems than their majority peers, attributable to minority stress. Older LGBTQ people grew up in times of greater government sanctioned/legal oppression, and legitimised social oppression than younger LGBTQ people and have experienced minority stressors for longer than young LGBTQ people. However, they have also had more time to develop adaptive responses which act as buffers to that minority stress. Younger LGBTQ people have greater opportunities to live their lives openly and while this can be potentially liberating, it can also be potentially very stressful, in terms of navigating choices and risks with open self-identification and also challenges about how to self-identify, in ways which were not experienced by older LGBTQ people. Young LGBTQ people face the challenges of too many choices. Older LGBTQ people, when they were younger, faced the challenges of too few choices.

All LGBTQ people, young and old, still navigate a lack of social safety across social contexts. For older LGBTQ people this is compounded by age-related care and support needs and the potential total institutions of domiciliary, residential and/or nursing home care. For younger LGBTQ people this is compounded by the compulsory institutions of school and family life under parental control. For each cohort, it is the quality of inclusion and acceptance by others that will have a major impact on their mental health and wellbeing. Promoting intergenerational communication and support between younger and older LGBTQ people could potentially benefit the mental health of young and old alike: younger LGBTQ people would benefit from the mentorship and guidance of older LGBTQ people, while older LGBTQ people would benefit from sharing their experiences and insights with future generations.

Across the research literature is a clear message for more attention to be given to sources of social support for younger and older LGBTQ people and to accumulate more evidence of what factors (social, individual, cultural) support good mental wellbeing. Common to both groups is a predominant focus on social disadvantage and marginalisation and the adverse physical, mental and social outcomes that arise. More attention must be given to the factors that boost the mental wellbeing of younger and older individuals—their strengths and coping practices and the community and social resources they have access to—as they navigate heterocentric and cisgendered social norms and environments.

References

Allen, K. R., & Lavender-Stott, E. S. (2020). The families of LGBTQ older adults: Theoretical approaches to creative family connections in the context of marginalization, social-historical change, and resilience. *Journal of Family Theory and Review, 12*(2), 200–219.

Almack, K. (2018). 'I didn't come out to go back in the closet': Ageing and end of life care for older LGBT people. In A. King, K. Almack, S. Westwood, & Y. T. Sung (Eds.), *Older lesbian, gay, bisexual and trans people: Minding the knowledge gaps* (pp. 151–171). Routledge.

Averett, P., Yoon, I., & Jenkins, C. L. (2011). Older lesbians: Experiences of aging, discrimination and resilience. *Journal of Women and Aging, 23*(3), 216–232.

Bailey, L., McNeil, J., & Ellis, S. J. (2018). Mental health and well-being among older trans people. In A. King, K. Almack, Y. T. Suen, & S. Westwood (Eds.), *Older lesbian, gay, bisexual and trans people: Minding the knowledge gaps* (pp. 44–60). Routledge.

Baker, D., Durr, P., & Scott, P. (2016). *Youth chances: Integrated report.* Metro Charity. Accessed 30th July 2021, from https://metrocharity.org.uk/research/2016/nov/10/national-youth-chances

Baril, A., & Silverman, M. (2019). Forgotten lives: Trans older adults living with dementia at the intersection of cisgenderism, ableism/cogniticism and ageism. *Sexualities,* 1363460719876835.

Bishop, M. D., Fish, J. N., Hammack, P. L., & Russell, S. T. (2020). Sexual identity development milestones in three generations of sexual minority people: A national probability sample. *Developmental Psychology.* Advance online publication. https://doi.org/10.1037/dev0001105

Bower, K. L., Lewis, D. C., Bermúdez, J. M., & Singh, A. A. (2021). Narratives of generativity and resilience among LGBT older adults: Leaving positive legacies despite social stigma and collective trauma. *Journal of Homosexuality, 68*(2), 230–251.

Brennan-Ing, M., Haberlen, S., Ware, D., Egan, J. E., Brown, A. L., Meanley, S., Palella, F. J., Bolan, R., Cook, J. A., Okafor, C. N., & Friedman, M. R. (2021). Psychological connection to the gay community and negative self-appraisals in middle-aged and older men who have sex with men: The mediating effects of fitness engagement. *The Journals of Gerontology: Series B.* gbab076. https://doi.org/10.1093/geronb/gbab076

Correro, A. N., & Nielson, K. A. (2020). A review of minority stress as a risk factor for cognitive decline in lesbian, gay, bisexual, and transgender (LGBT) elders. *Journal of Gay and Lesbian Mental Health, 24*(1), 2–19.

Crenshaw, K. (1991). Mapping the margins: Intersectionality, identity politics, and violence against women of color. *Standford Law Review, 43*, 1241–1299.

Dannefer, D. (2003). Cumulative advantage/disadvantage and the life course: Cross-fertilizing age and social science theory. *The Journals of Gerontology Series B: Psychological Sciences and Social Sciences, 58*(6), S327–S337.

Fabbre, V. D., & Gaveras, E. (2020). The manifestation of multilevel stigma in the lived experiences of transgender and gender nonconforming older adults. *American Journal of Orthopsychiatry, 90*(3), 350.

Fish, J. N. (2020). Future directions in understanding and addressing mental health among LGBTQ youth. *Journal of Child and Adolescent Psychology, 49*(6), 943–956.

Fish, J. N., McInroy, L. B., Paceley, M. S., Williams, N. D., Henderson, S., Levine, D. S., & Edsall, R. N. (2020). "I'm kinda stuck at home with unsupportive parents right now": LGBTQ youths' experiences with COVID-19 and the importance of online support. *Journal of Adolescent Health, 67*(3), 450–452.

Fish, J. N., & Weis, C. (2019). All the lonely people, where do they all belong? An interpretive synthesis of loneliness and social support in older lesbian, gay and bisexual communities. *Quality in Ageing and Older Adults, 20*(3), 130–142.

Fredriksen-Goldsen, K. I., Cook-Daniels, L., Kim, H. J., Erosheva, E. A., Emlet, C. A., Hoy-Ellis, C. P., Goldsen, J., & Muraco, A. (2014). Physical and mental health of transgender older adults: An at-risk and underserved population. *The Gerontologist, 54*(3), 488–500.

Fredriksen-Goldsen, K. I., Emlet, C. A., Kim, H. J., Muraco, A., Erosheva, E. A., Goldsen, J., & Hoy-Ellis, C. P. (2013). The physical and mental health of lesbian, gay male, and bisexual (LGB) older adults: The role of key health indicators and risk and protective factors. *The Gerontologist, 53*(4), 664–675.

Fredriksen-Goldsen, K. I., Kim, H. J., Bryan, A. E., Shiu, C., & Emlet, C. A. (2017a). The cascading effects of marginalization and pathways of resilience in attaining good health among LGBT older adults. *The Gerontologist, 57*(suppl_1), S72–S83.

Fredriksen-Goldsen, K. I., Shiu, C., Bryan, A. E., Goldsen, J., & Kim, H. J. (2017b). Health equity and aging of bisexual older adults: Pathways of risk and resilience. *Journals of Gerontology Series B: Psychological Sciences and Social Sciences, 72*(3), 468–478.

Gabb, J., McDermott, E., Eastham, R., & Hanbury, A. (2020). Paradoxical family practices: LGBTQ+ young people, mental health and wellbeing. *Journal of Sociology, 56*(4), 535–553.

Government Equalities Office. (2018). *National LGBT survey: Research report*. Department for Education. Accessed 1 July 2021, from https://www.gov.uk/government/publications/national-lgbt-survey-summary-report

Guasp, A. (2011). *Lesbian, gay and bisexual people in later life*. Stonewall.

Hafford-Letchfield, T., Simpson, P., Willis, P. B., & Almack, K. (2018). Developing inclusive residential care for older lesbian, gay, bisexual and trans (LGBT) people: An evaluation of the care home challenge action research project. *Health and Social Care in the Community, 26*(2), e312–e320.

Harwood, V. (2004). Telling truths: Wounded truths and the activity of truth telling. *Discourse—Studies in the Cultural Politics of Education, 25*(4), 467–476.

Hash, K. M., & Rogers, A. (2013). Clinical practice with older LGBT clients: Overcoming lifelong stigma through strength and resilience. *Clinical Social Work Journal, 41*(3), 249–257.

Hawke, L. D., Hayes, E., Darnay, K., & Henderson, J. (2021). Mental health among transgender and gender diverse youth: An exploration of effects during the COVID-19 pandemic. *Psychology of Sexual Orientation and Gender Diversity*. Advance online publication. http://dx.doi.org/10.1037/sgd0000467

Heaphy, B. (2009). Choice and its limits in older lesbian and gay narratives of relational life. *Journal of GLBT Family Studies, 5*(1–2), 119–138.

Higgins, A., Downes, C., Murphy, R., Sharek, D., Begley, T., McCann, E., Sheerin, F., Smyth, S., De Vries, J., & Doyle, L. (2021). LGBT+ young people's perceptions of barriers to accessing mental health services in Ireland. *Journal of Nurse Management, 29*(1), 58–67.

Hill, A. O., Lyons, A., Jones, J., McGowan, I., Carman, M., Parsons, M., Power, J., & Bourne, A. (2021). *Writing themselves in 4: The health and wellbeing of LGBTQA+ young people in Australia. National report, monograph series number 124*. Australian Research Centre in Sex, Health and Society, La Trobe University. Accessed from http://www.latrobe.edu.au/arcshs

Hoy-Ellis, C. P., & Fredriksen-Goldsen, K. I. (2017). Depression among transgender older adults: General and minority stress. *American Journal of Community Psychology, 59*(3–4), 295–305.

Hubbard, P. (2013). Kissing is not a universal right: Sexuality, law and the scales of citizenship. *Geoforum, 49*, 224–232.

Hulko, W. (2016). LGBT* individuals and dementia: An intersectional approach. In S. Westwood & E. Price (Eds.), *Lesbian, gay, bisexual and trans* individuals living with dementia: Concepts, practice and rights* (pp. 35–50). Routledge.

ILGA. (2020). *State-sponsored homophobia: Global legislation overview update.* ILGA, Geneva. Accessed 20 July 2022 from https://ilga.org/state-sponsored-homophobia-report

Jen, S. (2018). Bisexual and aging: Striving for social justice. In S. Westwood (Ed.), *Ageing, diversity, and inequality: Social justice perspectives* (pp. 131–146). Routledge.

Jen, S., & Jones, R. L. (2019). Bisexual lives and aging in context: A cross-national comparison of the United Kingdom and the United States. *The International Journal of Aging and Human Development, 89*(1), 22–38.

Jones, B. A., Pierre Bouman, W., Haycraft, E., & Arcelus, J. (2019). Mental health and quality of life in non-binary transgender adults: A case control study. *International Journal of Transgenderism, 20*(2–3), 251–262.

Jones, R. L. (2018). Bisexual ageing: What do we know and why should we care? In A. King, K. Almack, Y. Suen, & S. Westwood (Eds.), *Older lesbian, gay, bisexual and trans people: Minding the knowledge gaps.* Routledge.

Jones, R. L., Almack, K., & Scicluna, R. (2018). Older bisexual people: Implications for social work from the 'Looking both ways' study. *Journal of Gerontological Social Work, 61*(3), 334–347.

Just Like Us. (2021). *'Growing up LGBT+' report.* Accessed 14 July 2021, from https://www.justlikeus.org/single-post/growing-up-lgbt-just-like-us-research-report

Kim, H. J., Fredriksen-Goldsen, K. I., Bryan, A. E., & Muraco, A. (2017). Social network types and mental health among LGBT older adults. *The Gerontologist, 57*(suppl_1), S84–S94.

King, A., Almack, K., & Jones, R. L. (Eds.). (2019). *Intersections of ageing, gender and sexualities: Multidisciplinary international perspectives.* Policy Press.

King, S. D., & Richardson, V. E. (2017). Mental health for older LGBT adults. *Annual Review of Gerontology and Geriatrics, 37*(1), 59–75.

Kneale, D., Henley, J., Thomas, J., & French, R. (2021). Inequalities in older LGBT people's health and care needs in the United Kingdom: A systematic scoping review. *Ageing and Society, 41*(3), 493–515.

Knocker, S., Maxwell, N., Phillips, M., & Halls, S. (2012). Opening doors and opening minds: Sharing one project's experience of successful community engagement. In R. Ward, I. Rivers, & M. Sutherland (Eds.), *Lesbian, gay, bisexual and transgender ageing: Biographical approaches for inclusive care and support* (pp. 150–164). Jessica Kingsley.

Lucassen, M., Samra, R., Iacovides, I., Fleming, T., Shepherd, M., Stasiak, K., & Wallace, L. (2018). How LGBT+ young people use the internet in relation to their mental health and envisage the use of e-therapy: Exploratory study. *JMIR Serious Games, 6*(4), e11249.

Lyons, A., Alba, B., Waling, A., Minichiello, V., Hughes, M., Barrett, C., Fredriksen-Goldsen, K., Edmonds, S., & Blanchard, M. (2021). Recent versus lifetime experiences of discrimination and the mental and physical health of older lesbian women and gay men. *Ageing and Society, 41*(5), 1072–1093.

Lyons, A., Hosking, W., & Rozbroj, T. (2015). Rural-urban differences in mental health, resilience, stigma, and social support among young Australian gay men. *Journal of Rural Health, 31*(1), 89–97.

McConnell, E. A., Birkett, M., & Mustanski, B. (2016). Families matter: Social support and mental health trajectories among lesbian, gay, bisexual, and transgender youth. *Journal of Adolescent Health, 59*(6), 674–680.

McDermott, E., Hughes, E., & Rawlings, V. (2018a). Norms and normalisation: Understanding lesbian, gay, bisexual, transgender and queer youth, suicidality and help-seeking. *Culture, Health and Sexuality, 20*(2), 156–172.

McDermott, E., Hughes, E., & Rawlings, V. (2018b). The social determinants of lesbian, gay, bisexual and transgender youth suicidality in England: A mixed methods study. *Journal of Public Health, 40*(3), e244–e251.

McDermott, E., Roen, K., & Scourfield, J. (2008). Avoiding shame: Young LGBT people, homophobia and self-destructive behaviours. *Culture, Health and Sexuality, 10*(8), 815–829.

Mereish, E. H. (2019). Substance use and misuse among sexual and gender minority youth. *Current Opinion in Psychology, 30*, 123–127.

Meyer, I. H. (2003). Prejudice, social stress, and mental health in lesbian, gay, and bisexual populations: Conceptual issues and research evidence. *Psychological Bulletin, 129*, 674–697.

Meyer, I. H. (2015). Resilience in the study of minority stress and health of sexual and gender minorities. *Psychology of Sexual Orientation and Gender Diversity, 2*(3), 209.

Mustanski, B., Andrews, R., & Puckett, J. A. (2016). The effects of cumulative victimization on mental health among lesbian, gay, bisexual, and transgender adolescents and young adults. *American Journal of Public Health, 106*(3), 527–533.

Norris, M., & Quilty, A. (2020). Unreal, unsheltered, unseen, unrecorded: The multiple invisibilities of LGBTQI homeless youth. *Critical Social Policy*. First published 8th October 2020. https://doi.org/10.1177/026101832095 3328

ONS. (2021). *Internet users, UK: 2020.* Released 6th April 2021. Accessed from https://www.ons.gov.uk/businessindustryandtrade/itandinternetindustry/bulletins/internetusers/2020

Pearce, R. (2018). Trans temporalities and non-linear ageing. In A. King, K. Almack, Y. T. Suen, & S. Westwood (Eds.), *Older lesbian, gay, bisexual and trans people: Minding the knowledge gaps* (pp. 1–9). Routledge.

Ream, G. L. (2019). What's unique about lesbian, gay, bisexual, and transgender (LGBT) youth and young adult suicides? Findings from the national violent death reporting system. *Journal of Adolescent Health, 64*(5), 602–607.

Rehman, Z., Jaspal, R., & Fish, F. (2020). 'Service provider perspectives of minority stress among Black, Asian and minority ethnic lesbian, gay and bisexual people in the UK. *Journal of Homosexuality.* Published online. 14 September 2020. https://doi.org/10.1080/00918369.2020.1804256

Riggs, D. W., & Kentlyn, S. (2014). Transgender women, parenting, and experiences of ageing. In M. F. Gibson (Ed.), *Queering motherhood: Narrative and theoretical perspectives* (pp. 219–230). Demeter Press.

Rivers, I., Gonzalez, C., Nodin, N., Peel, E., & Tyler, A. (2018). LGBT people and suicidality in youth: A qualitative study of perceptions of risk and protective circumstances. *Social Science & Medicine, 212*, 1–8.

Rosenfeld, D., Bartlam, B., & Smith, R. D. (2012). Out of the closet and into the trenches: Gay male baby boomers, aging, and HIV/AIDS. *The Gerontologist, 52*(2), 255–264.

Russell, S. T., & Fish, J. N. (2016). Mental health in lesbian, gay, bisexual, and transgender (LGBT) youth. *Annual Review of Clinical Psychology, 12*, 465–487.

Scherrer, K. S. (2017). Stigma and special issues for bisexual older adults. *Annual Review of Gerontology and Geriatrics, 37*(1), 43–57.

Semlyen, J., King, M., Varney, J., & Hagger-Johnson, G. (2016). Sexual orientation and symptoms of common mental disorder or low wellbeing: Combined meta-analysis of 12 UK population health surveys. *BMC Psychiatry, 16*(1), 1–9.

Shearer, A., Herres, J., Kodish, T., Squitieri, H., James, K., Russon, J., Atte, T., & Diamond, G. S. (2016). Differences in mental health symptoms across lesbian, gay, bisexual, and questioning youth in primary care settings. *Journal of Adolescent Health, 59*(1), 38–43.

Simpson, P. (2013). Alienation, ambivalence, agency: Middle-aged gay men and ageism in Manchester's gay village. *Sexualities, 16*(3–4), 283–299.

Simpson, P., Almack, K., & Walthery, P. (2018). 'We treat them all the same': The attitudes, knowledge and practices of staff concerning old/er lesbian, gay, bisexual and trans residents in care homes. *Ageing and Society, 38*(5), 869–899.

Smith, R. W., Altman, J. K., Meeks, S., & Hinrichs, K. L. (2019). Mental health care for LGBT older adults in long-term care settings: Competency, training, and barriers for mental health providers. *Clinical Gerontologist, 42*(2), 198–203.

Talburt, S. (2004). Constructions of LGBT youth: Opening up subject positions. *Theory into Practice, 42*(2), 116–121.

Tinney, J., Dow, B., Maude, P., Purchase, R., Whyte, C., & Barrett, C. (2015). Mental health issues and discrimination among older LGBTI people. *International Psychogeriatrics, 27*(9), 1411–1416. https://doi.org/10.1017/S10 41610214002671

Toze, M. (2019). Developing a critical trans gerontology. *The British Journal of Sociology, 70*(4), 1490–1509.

Toze, M., Westwood, S., & Hafford-Letchfield, T. (2023). Social support and unmet needs among older trans and gender non-conforming people during the COVID-19 'lockdown' in the UK. *International Journal of Transgender Health, 24*(3). 305–319. https://doi.org/10.1080/26895269.2021.1977210

Traies, J. (2016). *The lives of older lesbians: Sexuality, identity and the life course.* Springer.

Watson, R. J., Grossman, A. H., & Russell, S. T. (2019). Sources of social support and mental health among LGB Youth. *Youth and Society, 51*(1), 30–48.

Westwood, S. (2016a). *Ageing, gender and sexuality: Equality in later life.* Routledge.

Westwood, S. (2016b). 'We see it as being heterosexualised, being put into a care home': Gender, sexuality and housing/care preferences among older LGB individuals in the UK. *Health and Social Care in the Community, 24*(6), e155–e163.

Westwood, S. (2020). The myth of 'older LGBT+' people: Research shortcomings and policy/practice implications for health/care provision. *Journal of Aging Studies, 55*, 100880.

Westwood, S., Hafford-Letchfield, T., & Toze, M. (2021) *The impact of COVID-19 on the lives of older LGBT+ people in the UK.* https://covid1 9olderlgbt.wordpress.com/

Westwood, S., & Price, E. (Eds.). (2016). *Lesbian, gay, bisexual and trans* individuals living with dementia: Concepts, practice and rights.* Routledge.

Westwood, S., Willis, P., Fish, J., Hafford-Letchfield, T., Semlyen, J., King, A., Beach, B., Almack, K., Kneale, D., Toze, M., & Becares, L. (2020). Older LGBT+ health inequalities in the UK: Setting a research agenda. *Journal of Epidemiology and Community Health, 74*(5), 408–411.

Willis, P. (2012). Constructions of lesbian, gay, bisexual and queer identities among young people in contemporary Australia. *Culture, Health and Sexuality, 14*(9/10), 1213–1227.

Willis, P., Almack, K., Hafford-Letchfield, T., Simpson, P., Billings, B., & Mall, N. (2018). Turning the co-production corner: Methodological reflections from an action research project to promote LGBT inclusion in care homes for older people. *International Journal of Environmental Research and Public Health, 15*(4), 695.

Willis, P., Dobbs, C., Evans, E., Raithby, M., & Bishop, J. A. (2020). Reluctant educators and self-advocates: Older trans adults' experiences of health-care services and practitioners in seeking gender-affirming services. *Health Expectations, 23*(5), 1231–1240.

Willis, P., Maegusuku-Hewett, T., Raithby, M., & Miles, P. (2016). Swimming upstream: The provision of inclusive care to older lesbian, gay and bisexual (LGB) adults in residential and nursing environments in Wales. *Ageing and Society, 36*(2), 282–306.

Willis, P., Raithby, M., Dobbs, C., Evans, E., & Bishop, J. A. (2021). 'I'm going to live my life for me': Trans ageing, care, and older trans and gender non-conforming adults' expectations of and concerns for later life. *Ageing and Society, 41*(12), 2792–2813.

Willis, P., Vickery, A., & Jessiman, T. (2022). Loneliness, social dislocation and invisibility experienced by older men who are single or living alone: Accounting for differences across sexual identity and social context. *Ageing and Society, 42*(2), 409–431.

Witten, T. M. (2016). Aging and transgender bisexuals: Exploring the intersection of age, bisexual sexual identity, and transgender identity. *Journal of Bisexuality, 16*(1), 58–80.

Yarns, B. C., Abrams, J. M., Meeks, T. W., & Sewell, D. D. (2016). The mental health of older LGBT adults. *Current Psychiatry Reports, 18*(6), 60.

6

Identity Processes, Stressors and Mental Health in Black, Asian and Minority Ethnic Sexual Minorities

Rusi Jaspal ⓘ and Claire Bloxsom

Introduction

There has been much progress in establishing equal rights for lesbian, gay, and bisexual people (henceforth, sexual minorities) in the United Kingdom (UK). The Equality Act 2010, for instance, provides protection against discrimination on the basis of sexual orientation as well as seven other 'protected characteristics' in employment settings. Despite this progress, research shows that sexual minorities continue to report relatively high levels of prejudice due to their sexual orientation and that they are also at higher risk of poor mental health outcomes than the general population (Semlyen et al., 2016). As outlined in Chapter 3,

R. Jaspal (✉)
University of Brighton, Brighton, UK
e-mail: rusi.jaspal@cantab.net

C. Bloxsom
University of Warwick, Coventry, UK
e-mail: claire.bloxsom@warwick.ac.uk

© The Author(s), under exclusive license to Springer Nature
Switzerland AG 2023
J. Semlyen and P. Rohleder (eds.), *Sexual Minorities and Mental Health*,
https://doi.org/10.1007/978-3-031-37438-8_6

107

prejudice has many manifestations, ranging from overt denigration and rejection to more subtle 'microaggressions'. Given that overt prejudice on the basis of sexual orientation is increasingly stigmatised and, in employment settings, prohibited by law, it tends to be manifested more subtly. However, it is no less psychologically aversive.

There is evidence that sexual minorities from Black, Asian and Minority Ethnic (BAME) backgrounds face multiple forms of discrimination and emerging evidence that they may be at higher risk of poor mental health than White British people (Jaspal et al., 2021b). Many of the risk factors for poor mental health are preventable social and psychological stressors, such as homonegativity, racism, and internalised homonegativity. These appear to be rooted in experiences across the life course. Various theoretical frameworks have been proposed to shed light on the mechanisms of 'minority stress' among BAME sexual minorities, such as minority stress theory (Meyer, 2003) and the concept of intersectionality (Crenshaw, 1991).

This chapter provides a brief overview of these theoretical perspectives in relation to identity, stressors, and mental health in BAME sexual minorities and argues that identity process theory (Breakwell, 2015) provides an integrative framework within which the risk factors for poor mental health in this population can be examined, understood and addressed. The chapter concludes with reflections on counselling and social psychological interventions that may reduce the risk of poor mental health in BAME sexual minorities.

BAME Sexual Minorities: An Overview

The term Black, Asian, and Minority Ethnic (or BAME) is generally used as 'collective terminology' to describe (generally non-White) minority ethnic groups as a whole (Aspinall, 2002). It is acknowledged that this category is very diverse and broad in terms of ethnicity, culture, language, religion, and history (Jaspal et al., 2021a) and therefore does not fully encompass the complexity and multiplicity of individual experience and identity. For example, 'Asia' includes South Asia, East Asia, and Southeast Asia, and 'minority ethnic' may include anybody who does not see themselves as having an ethnicity rooted in one of the four nations of the United Kingdom.

However, in this chapter, BAME is used hereafter as a way to capture the potential commonality of experience among minority ethnic groups in the UK vis-à-vis the White British majority. Indeed, research into sexual identity, health, and wellbeing tends to show that BAME sexual minorities face higher levels of exposure to stressors associated with their sexuality which can result in poor health and wellbeing outcomes. As the most populous constituent ethnic groups within the BAME category, Indian, Pakistani, Black African, and Black Caribbean sexual minorities constitute the focus of the research outlined in this chapter. However, it is acknowledged that future research must attempt to capture the experiences of other minority ethnic groups, such as those of mixed heritage and Roma people. Nevertheless, a key aim is to highlight the gaps in knowledge concerning particular constituent groups within the BAME category to set an agenda for future research in this important area.

In 2011, the total population of England and Wales was 56.1 million and 14% reported a non-White ethnicity (ONS, 2012). People from Asian and Black ethnic groups make up the largest percentage of the BAME population. According to the ONS (2018), in 2018, a smaller proportion of BAME groups described their sexuality as lesbian, gay, bisexual, or 'other' and a large proportion of these groups either did not know, or refused to acknowledge, their sexuality. This observation could be attributed to at least two factors. First, it could be that fewer people in BAME communities are willing to acknowledge their sexuality due to social stigma which appears to be prevalent in these communities as well as the internalisation of this stigma at an individual level. Second, it is possible that these sexual identity labels are not deemed to be appropriate by some individuals from BAME communities because they may associate these labels with Western culture. This observation may say more about sexual identity, rather than sexual orientation (see Jaspal, 2019). As highlighted in this chapter, the recruitment of adequate samples of BAME sexual minority individuals can be challenging and may be one of the reasons that there is limited research focusing on these groups.

Theoretical Frameworks for Understanding Identity

Understanding mental health among BAME sexual minorities requires some insight into the potential stressors to which individuals within this community may be exposed as well as the ways in which their identities are constructed and managed. Accordingly, three significant frameworks are briefly outlined: minority stress theory, intersectionality and identity process theory.

Minority Stress Theory

Minority stress theory (Meyer, 2003), has become an important theoretical framework for examining the impact of 'stressors' associated with one's minority identity. Stressors refer to events, situations, and widespread societal perceptions that might lead to psychological stress. Despite the considerable diversity that characterises sexual minorities, experiences of stigma, prejudice, and discrimination are remarkably common in this broad community.

It is thus argued in minority stress theory that sexual minorities face stress that is *unique* to them and *additive* (over and above the habitual stressors that people from the general population face); *chronic* as it is rooted in long-standing and relatively stable social and cultural structures; and *socially based* because it arises from social processes, institutions, and representations rather than individual characteristics. The theory identifies three processes of minority stress, namely external events and conditions that cause stress; the expectation of such events and conditions, and the vigilance that this can create in the minority individual; and the internalisation of stigma directed towards sexual minorities (Meyer, 1995).

Minority stress theory refers to distal and proximal stressors and notes their differential impact on the psychological health of the sexual minority individual. Distal stressors are prejudice events that are external to the individual, such as the experience of 'microaggressions' or exclusion due to one's sexual orientation. Proximal stressors are the individual's internal response to these events, such as internalised homonegativity, that is, the acceptance of negative social representations of their sexual orientation. It has been found that these distinct types of stressors may contribute differently to depressive and anxious symptomatology in sexual minorities from BAME backgrounds (Jaspal et al., 2022; Ramirez & Paz-Galupo, 2019). In order to understand how and why particular types of stressors affect mental health, it is important to understand the individual's sense of identity. This has been one of the foci of the concept of intersectionality.

Intersectionality

The concept of intersectionality crosses the boundaries of the binary and the categorical and focuses on the dynamic interplay between and within aspects of difference and privilege. Intersectionality is thought to provide the "critical insight that race, class, gender, sexuality, ethnicity, nation, ability, and age operate not as unitary, mutually exclusive entities, but rather as reciprocally constructing phenomena" (Collins, 2015, p. 1). More recently, Turner (2021) has discussed in skilful depth the importance of understanding and engaging with "varying layers of oppression" (p. 18) that are present in many spheres, including in counselling and psychotherapy.

Intersectionality is associated with the work of Crenshaw (1991), which problematised the "single axis" approach to disadvantage. Focusing on gender and race in women of colour, Crenshaw (1991) emphasised that marginalisation could occur at the intersection of these group memberships and thus advocated an intersectional lens to uncover the complex interplay of multiple types and levels of oppression. In her work, she noted that Black women might be compared (unfavourably) to either Black men or White women. Furthermore, she highlighted that it is limiting to focus on marginalisation because of one's identity as either 'Black' or a 'woman', rather than the unique type of marginalisation that being a 'Black woman' might bring about. Likewise, individuals may be members of other oppressed groups, such as being a lesbian woman of colour. As Crenshaw (1991) describes—a Black woman and a White woman would differ in their experience of systemic racism, though they may have a shared experience of gender inequality. The intersectional approach emphasises that a simple combination of "double (or multiple) oppression" is not adequate to appreciate the individual lived experience of what it is like to be both Black and a woman. Indeed, Hancock (2007) notes "multiple marginalizations of race, class, gender, or sexual orientation at the individual and institutional levels create social and political stratification, requiring policy solutions that are attuned to the interaction of these categories" and that they are "more than the sum of mutually exclusive parts" (p. 65).

A deeper multidisciplinary assessment of the impact of intersectional oppression may therefore facilitate a richer and more accurate understanding of BAME sexual minorities' lived experience. This enhanced understanding may in turn inform and evolve research methodologies and subsequent policy recommendations as well as both practitioner professional development and therapeutic practice. A single axis framework for what it might mean for an individual to identify as a sexual minority *or* as a BAME individual cannot accurately encapsulate the potential experience of those individuals whose identities include both of these categories, where membership of these categories may expose them to threat, fear of threat, and stigma. For instance, as outlined in this chapter, being BAME may expose an individual to racism and being a sexual minority may expose them to homonegativity. Both categories are associated with the experience of marginalisation though the lived experience of this marginalisation may differ both individually and in combination. It must not be forgotten that the BAME sexual minority individual may also face homonegativity from within their ethnic ingroup or perhaps hostility towards their ethnicity and/ or religion from their sexual ingroup (i.e., other gay, bisexual, and/or lesbian people).

Identity Process Theory

Identity process theory (IPT) (Breakwell, 2015) has been proposed as a framework for understanding the diverse components that comprise identity. It enables researchers to explore the structure and content of intersectional identities because it focuses not on single identity characteristics (e.g., specific group memberships, personality traits, cognitive styles) but rather the interactions between them that produce a sense of identity. IPT also mirrors key tenets of minority stress theory given its focus on the experience of, and reaction to, identity threat (Jaspal et al., 2022). A key tenet of the theory is that individuals construct their identities by engaging in two processes:

- *assimilation-accommodation* refers to the incorporation of novel elements into the contents of identity and the changes that are subsequently made to identity content. For instance, when an individual accepts that they are gay, this novel identity element comes to form a part of the identity structure. This is assimilation. However, pre-existing elements, such as one's religion, may come to be attenuated or even removed from the contents of identity during accommodation. This example demonstrates how one characteristic may have implications for others in the overall identity structure.
- *Evaluation* refers to the allocation of meaning and value to the novel and existing elements of identity. Although the individual accepts that they are gay, they may initially believe that this is a flaw in their identity and feel ashamed of this, often because this is the dominant view of their sexual orientation in their particular societal context. In the case of BAME sexual minorities, this response may result from the perceived representations of sexuality within the relevant ethnic and/or religious group. This example of the evaluation of identity aspects demonstrates how one characteristic may acquire a specific meaning and value due to the presence of another characteristic that consciously exists in the identity structure.

IPT originally posited that individuals strive to construct an identity that is characterised by self-esteem, continuity, distinctiveness, and self-efficacy. Jaspal and Cinnirella (2010) have noted that, in some contexts, two or more identity elements may become 'inter-connected', that is, they may be perceived to be relevant to, and impacting upon, one another. In response to two or more inter-connected identity elements, the psychological coherence principle is activated, prompting the individual to seek compatibility and coherence between the elements (see Amiot & Jaspal, 2014). This motivation to integrate aspects of the identity structure may lead people to derive a particular perception of their level of self-esteem, continuity, and so on.

Both the four prime principles and the secondary principle of psychological coherence are essentially the desirable end-states of identity. Therefore, individuals will try to engage in the processes of assimilation-accommodation and evaluation in ways that provide high levels of the identity principles. The example given to explain the evaluation process shows how the individual's engagement in the two identity processes might lead to decreased levels of self-esteem. After all, internalised homonegativity is unlikely to facilitate a positive self-conception on the basis of being gay (Williamson, 2000). Although the individual knows that this particular type of evaluation of being gay is aversive for self-esteem, they may actually have limited choice in the matter—dominant and coercive social representations of homosexuality in their social environment (e.g., their valued ethnic group) may compel some to internalise the view that their sexual orientation is a flaw. This view could then initiate a disavowal of that aspect of the self, leading to a lack of psychological integration and equilibrium.

IPT posits that disruption to any of the identity principles due, for instance, to changes in one's social context will result in identity threat which is harmful for psychological wellbeing. The factors that can be seen as potential or actual threats to identity are essentially the stressors that are captured in minority stress theory. IPT would predict that not all stressors will actually result in threats to identity. There are many factors that shape the likelihood of identity threat, such as personality, cognitive abilities, and social context (Jaspal, 2018). This brings us back to the complex content of identity (that is, intersectionality). Identity does not consist of a single characteristic.

In response to identity threat, the individual will engage in varied coping strategies, operating at individual, interpersonal and intergroup levels. For instance, when coming to terms with being gay, some BAME sexual minorities initially deny or re-construe their reality; some may isolate themselves from others in order to avoid stigma; and others may immerse themselves in groups that can provide both social support and access to more positive social representations of their sexual orientation. These examples of coping demonstrate both the variety and complexity of activity in response to identity threat.

Recent developments in IPT have focused upon the concept of identity resilience (Breakwell & Jaspal, 2021). Identity resilience refers to the individual's appraisal of their overall self-esteem, self-efficacy, continuity and positive distinctiveness. This is essentially a trait in that individuals will develop a general sense of their overall level of the four prime identity principles on the basis of many factors, including their past experiences, personality traits, and social context. As a trait, identity resilience is likely to affect the likelihood, extent and severity of identity threat and to influence efficacy of coping strategies. Put simply, a person with high baseline identity resilience may be less susceptible to identity threat when exposed to a hazard to identity (that is, a situation or event that may ordinarily be construed as threatening for identity). They may be more resistant to severe threats and have greater access to varied and effective coping strategies, potentially extinguishing the hazard before it becomes a fully-fledged threat to identity (Jaspal et al., 2022).

It is proposed that IPT provides an integrative framework within which minority stress, intersectionality, threat and coping can be collectively examined.

Stressors and Identity Processes Among BAME Sexual Minorities

Sexual minorities may face a multitude of stressors with the potential to threaten identity and to challenge mental health. It is argued that these stressors may be accentuated in BAME sexual minorities given the additive effect of racism from the White British majority and homonegativity from within their ethnic and/ or religious ingroups. In this section, three potential sources of psychological stress, namely religion, ethnicity/ culture and racism, are described. It is acknowledged that, as group memberships, religion and ethnicity/ culture may also function as protective factors (see Jaspal et al., 2022). However, in this section, we focus on the stigmatising social representations of homosexuality associated with these group memberships which can lead to psychological stress.

Religion

Religion tends to be an important identity component in BAME communities. The social and cultural norms associated with one's religious group may stigmatise homosexuality, making it difficult to assimilate and accommodate it within the identity structure. In their qualitative study of British Pakistani Muslim gay men, Jaspal and Cinnirella (2010) found that individuals struggled to reconcile being gay with their Muslim religious identity because, as a key identity element, their religion served as a 'lens' for evaluating other elements of identity, including their sexuality. This resulted in threats to multiple principles of identity, including psychological coherence, which could be only partially satisfied through the deployment of short-term coping strategies with limited efficacy. For instance, interviewees tended to engage in external attribution in order to assimilate-accommodate and evaluate their sexuality in particular ways. Some reasoned that being gay was determined by Allah (God) and, thus, could and should not be condemned by religious leaders. Conversely, others attributed their sexuality to Shaitan (Satan) and, thus, resisted construing it in terms of an identity and saw it as a mutable behaviour. To support the notion that being gay was akin to a behavioural habit, some interviewees attributed it to 'British culture', which had made them 'become gay'. Incidentally, this line of thinking may be reinforced by the availability of so-called conversion/ reparative therapy practices in some faith groups and organisations, which promote the notion that one's sexual orientation can be successfully changed (Wilkinson & Johnson, 2020). It is easy to see how such practices can accentuate identity conflict and threat as well as a false sense of hope in BAME sexual minorities, potentially decreasing self-efficacy and self-esteem in those who subsequently perceive their conversion/ reparative therapy to have "failed".

In order to resolve threats to psychological coherence, individuals may feel compelled to choose one identity element over the other. In another study, it was found that British Muslim gay men may view being gay as casting doubts on the authenticity of their Muslim identity and that they therefore used a variety of strategies to safeguard the authenticity of their religious identity (Jaspal & Cinnirella, 2014). A key strategy is that of hyper-affiliation, which Jaspal and Cinnirella (2014) define as "accentuated social and psychological identification with a social group in response to threatened group membership" (p. 266). In the context of BAME sexual minorities of religious faith, this strategy may involve attempting to demonstrate—both to oneself and to others— one's commitment to the threatened identity element (i.e., one's religion or ethnicity) and one's 'authenticity' as a member of this group. Some people may adopt norms and values perceived to be associated with it, including the uncritical acceptance of homonegativity. Indeed, some BAME sexual minority individuals are deeply dissatisfied with their sexual orientation and wish to change it, partly to re-establish their relationship with their religion. This amounts to a desire to retain a safe space for their religion within the identity structure.

The experience of identity threat is associated with negative affect. In response to 'hyper-threats' to identity involving multiple principles, BAME sexual minorities of religious faith may experience a variety of negative emotions in relation to their religion and sexuality, including guilt, shame, fear and anger (Jaspal, 2012a; see also Breakwell & Jaspal, 2022). This can be attributed not only to the actual experience of identity threat itself but also to the largely unsustainable, short-term coping strategies that appear to be available to them.

It is noteworthy that, in previous research, sexual minority individuals of Muslim religious faith appear to be particularly susceptible to threats to psychological coherence in that they may construe their religion and sexuality to be incompatible and, on a spiritual level, may experience a sense of conflict (Siraj, 2006). Conversely, those who identify as Sikh or Hindu appear to report fewer challenges in reconciling their religious and sexual identities and may in fact appeal to their religious identities in order to challenge homonegativity that is framed in religious terms (Jaspal, 2012b). More specifically, they may point to the absence of homonegativity in Holy Scripture associated with their religious traditions and interpret this as evidence that there is in fact no religious prohibition of their sexual orientation. Furthermore, some may become more identified with their religion because they perceive it to be more accommodating of their sexuality than their ethnicity, which conversely may be perceived as the true source of homonegativity.

This reflects a strategy for resisting the stressors associated with negative religious representations of one's sexual orientation. Individuals are essentially contesting the validity and veracity of these representations. They are rekindling their relationship with their religious identity in order to challenge stressors (in this case, stigmatising social representations of their sexual orientation), which they instead attribute to their ethnicity and culture.

Ethnicity & Culture

In addition to threats to identity associated with perceived incompatibility between being gay and of religious faith (at an intrapsychic level), BAME sexual minorities may perceive strong cultural pressures to conform to compulsory heterosexuality at a social level. They may believe that the norms, values and social representations associated with their ethnic culture are firmly opposed to their sexuality and, thus, experience threats to identity. In particular, it has been found that cultural honour can be coercively prohibitive of their sexuality, leading BAME sexual minorities to internalise the homonegativity that they face and to conceal their identities from others (e.g., Jaspal, 2020).

McKeown et al. (2010) found that the Black British gay men who participated in their study perceived being Black and gay as incompatible, which itself may be grounded in the belief that being gay is a 'White' phenomenon. In his study of British South Asian gay men, Jaspal (2012b) found that those of Indian descent tended to perceive their family and culture to be unaccommodating of their sexuality which was especially challenging for the continuity principle of identity. Individuals were less concerned about psychological coherence than they were about the continuity of their personal relationships, such as with their parents, siblings and ethnic ingroup members. More specifically, there were concerns about how others would react to their sexuality if they were to come out as gay. This fear of coming out may also lead to difficulties in forming and maintaining interpersonal relationships with significant others, which of course constitute an important source of psychological wellbeing (Bariola et al., 2015). BAME sexual minorities who are not out to the families due to cultural pressures may feel the need to conceal their romantic relationships and to be secretive about them (Jaspal, 2015). This in turn may lead to decreased social support when they experience relationship difficulties and/or dissolution. The threats to identity ordinarily associated with relationship dissolution may be accentuated and access to effective coping strategies curtailed in the absence of social support.

Coercive cultural norms may lead BAME sexual minorities to believe that they must have a heterosexual marriage in order to be fully accepted within their ethnic and cultural ingroups. In some cultures, having an arranged marriage is culturally valued and may result in increased pressure. Jaspal (2014) found that some gay and bisexual men from South Asian communities acquiesced to having an arranged marriage in order to satisfy these cultural norms and also because they believed that this might enable them to change their sexual orientation in the long term. More generally, BAME sexual minorities may feel that their sense of belonging in their ethnic and cultural communities is precarious and in jeopardy and, thus, attempt to safeguard this by complying with the perceived demands of their ingroups.

Although issues of cultural honour are often associated with South Asian cultures, recent research into Latin American communities in London shows the significance of ethnic culture in shaping identity processes. For instance, Jaspal and Williamson (2017) studied the experiences of Colombian gay men living in the UK and found that many had struggled to assimilate and accommodate their sexuality in their identity due to the stigma attached to being gay in Colombian society. Having been exposed to negative, stigmatising social representations of homosexuality since childhood, many had themselves internalised these representations and continued to evaluate their sexuality negatively. For instance, some attempted to locate the 'causes' of their homosexuality and attributed it to adverse childhood experiences, such as sexual abuse from an older male.

Religion and ethnicity are often conflated (see Jaspal, 2012b), but here it is argued that religion and ethnic culture can have differential effects on identity processes among BAME sexual minorities. For some groups and individuals, religion is a more significant identity and source of social representations, but this may not be the case for others. Religion and ethnicity and their respective implications for identity processes need to be examined separately.

Racism

In addition to homonegativity associated with one's religion and/ or ethnic culture, racism represents another significant stressor which can threaten identity among BAME sexual minorities. Several studies show that BAME people report prejudice and discrimination on the basis of their ethnicity and that this can have insidious effects for their mental health (Jaspal et al., 2020), including in BAME sexual minorities specifically (Jaspal et al., 2022).

In addition to racism from the general population, BAME sexual minorities also report racism in LGBT settings. A Stonewall survey of 5375 LGBT people revealed that 45% of BAME respondents reported attending LGBT venues and that 51% of BAME respondents reported experiencing poor treatment or discrimination from others in their local LGBT community – reported rates of discrimination were particularly high in Black individuals (61%) (Bachmann & Gooch, 2018). In a survey of 850 BAME gay men conducted by Gay Men Fighting AIDS (GMFA) (Haggas, 2015), it was found that 80% of Black respondents, 75% of South Asians and 64% of mixed-race respondents indicated that they had personally experienced racism on the gay scene. The survey revealed a broad spectrum of racism, ranging from overt racism to more subtle microaggressions. Bassi (2008) notes that 'on the predominantly white commercial gay scene, gay and bisexual British Asians feel and carry the burden of racialization via the visible marker of their skin colour' (pp. 216–217). It is noteworthy that BAME sexual minorities also report experiences of racism on gay social networking mobile applications, such as Grindr (Jaspal, 2017b).

In his study of British South Asian gay men, Jaspal (2017a) notes that study participants frequented the gay scene because they desired social support from other sexual minorities. They all recounted narratives of stigma and rejection from ethnic and religious ingroup members, which prompted them to seek support from sexual ingroup members. The racism that they encountered on the gay scene constituted a constant threat to identity. Interviewees noted that the gay scene was generally sexualised and that this offered White gay men the pretext of 'sexual preference' to shun or denigrate them. This was clearly harmful for people's self-esteem as some came to internalise the view that their ethnicity constituted a 'flaw' in identity. Although some people challenge the notion that rejecting someone exclusively due to their ethnic appearance is racist, it has in fact been found that this practice is closely associated with general racist attitudes (Callander et al., 2015).

BAME sexual minorities may feel that their ethnic minority identity is more salient than their shared sexual identity (i.e., being gay), which in turn may lead to excessive distinctiveness, rather than a sense of belonging. Indeed, Black British gay men have reported feeling objectified by White gay men on the gay scene, which can make them feel that they are desired exclusively because of their ethnicity (McKeown et al., 2010). People may feel singled out due to their ethnicity and subjected to inappropriate comments, questions and behaviours due to their ethnicity. This is inconsistent with the motive to derive *positive* distinctiveness. BAME sexual minorities may feel unable to challenge or call out others for their racism, which might also challenge feelings of self-efficacy.

Mental Health in BAME Sexual Minorities

Identity threat is of course a habitual experience which all human beings experience. However, it is generally harmful for psychological wellbeing. There are many factors that can influence the relationship between identity threat and mental health outcomes, such as identity resilience, the severity of threat, the availability of coping strategies and the efficacy of the coping strategies deployed. The available evidence suggests that identity threat due to exposure to stressors, such as homonegativity and racism, may result in poor mental health in BAME sexual minorities. This hypothesis is also consistent with minority stress theory.

In their cross-sectional survey study of 289 BAME and White British sexual minorities, Jaspal et al., (2021b) found that BAME respondents reported more discrimination, more ethnicity-related victimisation, and more rejection from significant others (such as parents and siblings) than White British people. Furthermore, BAME respondents reported higher internalised homonegativity and an increased proclivity to conceal their sexual orientation than their White British counterparts. Stressors, such as rejection from significant others and discrimination, were positively associated with psychological distress, depression and suicidal ideation. Crucially, the negative self-schema of internalised homonegativity was positively associated with suicidal ideation. Conversely, outness and help-seeking behaviours were negatively associated with these poor mental health outcomes. There is also evidence that BAME lesbian women are more likely to report engagement in self-harm than gay men (Rehman et al., 2020). This has been attributed to gender-specific marginalisation and adversity, such as gender-based discrimination, intimate partner violence, as well as "invisibility" in LGBT spaces, which further demonstrates the significance of intersectionality. All this research provides preliminary evidence of disproportionate exposure to stressors among BAME sexual minorities which in turn are associated with depressive symptomatology, thereby demonstrating the increased risk of poor mental health in this population.

There is also emerging evidence that a stronger sense of baseline identity resilience is protective against negative affect associated with sexuality-related stressors, such as a negative reaction from significant others (e.g., parents, siblings, friends) to one's coming out (Breakwell & Jaspal, 2022). People who have a higher overall sense of self-esteem, self-efficacy, positive distinctiveness and continuity are less likely to have internalised homonegativity, on the one hand, and less likely to experience negative affect, such as guilt, when recalling a negative coming out experience. In view of the association between negative affect and identity threat, it would appear that having a higher sense of identity resilience enables sexual minorities to resist stressors effectively and to deploy more effective coping strategies before the stressors can cause threats to identity.

Supporting BAME Sexual Minorities

Extant research indicates that BAME sexual minorities may be especially susceptible to stressors associated with their minority identities, which may predispose them to poor mental health outcomes. The key for both practitioners and policymakers is to provide a supportive infrastructure both for reducing the risk of identity threat and for facilitating effective and sustainable coping in those at risk. In this section, the significance of social support and clinical intervention are considered.

Social Support

The most effective strategies for coping with threat focus on the derivation of social support from others and the mobilisation of others who share one's predicament. Social support can enable the threatened individual to disclose aspects of their threatening experience, to exchange confidences and, crucially, to gain exposure to alternative social representations of their sexual orientation. The mobilisation of others in the form of support and pressure groups can perform all of these functions providing immediate relief from threat and, in the long term, by promoting social change. Pressure groups may actively challenge social representations with the potential to threaten identity and to promote alternative cognitive and affective reactions to one's sexual orientation, which enable BAME sexual minorities to evaluate it more favourably and to assimilate and accommodate it within identity.

In recent years, many organisations and communities for BAME sexual minorities have emerged. UK Black Pride was established in 2005 as a gay pride event focusing on LGBT people of African, Asian, Middle Eastern, Latin American and Caribbean heritage. It has broadened its focus to include social networking, advocacy and community outreach.

BlackOut UK is a not-for-profit social enterprise which provides a forum in which Black gay and bisexual men can build a sense of community. The NAZ Project London was founded in the early 1990s to address sexual health inequalities experienced by BAME people, but it has since broadened its focus to include HIV care and support services, counselling and wellbeing services, community programmes and advocacy for BAME people, including those who identify as sexual minorities. There are also smaller regional support groups, such as Dosti in Leicester and Rainbow Noir in the North West. Various groups have emerged that aim to provide support and advocacy for sexual minorities of religious faith, such as Imaan UK (for Muslims), and Sarbat LGBT Sikhs. These organisations play a pivotal role in generating social support and in facilitating a sense of belonging in BAME sexual minorities who, in some cases, report feeling marginalised from their religious, ethnic/ cultural and sexual ingroups.

Clinical Considerations

Later chapters in this book consider different clinical interventions. In this section, we discuss specific points of consideration for those working clinically with BAME sexual minorities. It is important to bear this in mind when reading the later chapters. We describe a fictitious case example that has been created to highlight the complications of focusing exclusively on single axis approaches to oppression when working with BAME sexual minorities at the individual level. The case is explored briefly with reference to minority stress theory, intersectionality and IPT. This case exemplifies how identity conflicts, minority stressors, and intersectional challenges may occur but is not intended to be representative of the BAME sexual minority experience.

'Ahmed'

Ahmed is a 25-year-old South Asian Muslim gay man living in the UK. He lives at home with his parents and is the only son of parents who had emigrated to the UK in the late 1970s. He grew up with two older sisters who

> are now married with children and who live with their husbands, children, and their in-laws. Ahmed left school with excellent A-level grades at 18. He decided against further study and got a part-time job in a warehouse. His salary is low, and therefore he can only contribute a small amount to the bills. For some time, Ahmed knew that he was romantically and sexually attracted to men, though he has felt unable to explore this identity for fear of condemnation by his family and community. His parents have recently been encouraging him to get married and start a family. Ahmed feels confused. He has started to avoid his parents and has been calling in sick at work, spending more and more time alone. Ahmed begins to experience a lot of anxiety and low mood, and he contacts a local counselling centre for assessment.

The case of Ahmed highlights the multiplicity of identity and the associated challenges. There is clearly a risk of identity threat and conflict, where effective coping, and subsequent assimilation and accommodation of Ahmed's different identities into his identity structure, are obstructed. These identity conflicts may then lead to psychological stress due to a lack of psychological coherence (Amiot & Jaspal, 2014). Obstruction to psychological coherence may also lead to a negative appraisal of self-efficacy and self-esteem if Ahmed remains consciously self-defined by both these inter-connected identity elements without access to interpersonal and intergroup support. Coping with this stress alone may entail a variety of different strategies, such as denial, avoidance and suppression of emotion, which in turn may undermine identity integration and psychological wellbeing.

Ahmed is South Asian, gay, and Muslim. His family structure is highly likely to be embedded within a wider community cultural and religious structure with a collectivist orientation. The concepts of kinship ('biraderi'), honour ('izzat'), and shame ('sharam') are important in British South Asian culture (Jaspal & Bayley, 2020) and these important social principles might undermine Ahmed's ability to embrace his sexual identity. It is noteworthy that Ahmed's identities are not only psychologically conflicting but also characterised by intersectional oppression.

Stressors, such as racism, homonegativity, and prejudice and discrimination due to his religious identity, may heighten the risk of identity threat.

The case information notes Ahmed's confusion at the idea of marrying a woman, and that this diverges from his sexual identity. This identity conflict of where he 'belongs' (Vignoles et al., 2002) may lead to an internal impasse where Ahmed does not know how to cope, move forward, or derive meaning and purpose in his life. Ahmed's self-esteem may be impacted due to the internal conflict between fitting into cultural norms, his sexual orientation and identity, and his experience of being in minority groups in the wider social context that may leave him feeling invisible on multiple levels. If Ahmed, aware of both his sexual identity and the concept of familial 'izzat', perceives that he 'should be' finding a wife who may then become part of the family structure, his self-efficacy may be impacted, and he may be confused about his purpose. This in turn may undermine his confidence and perception of control in his life as an in inter-dependent South Asian gay man. As discussed in the previous section, some research has indicated that continuity is more important than having a coherent identity in those of Indian descent (Jaspal, 2012b), and also that cultural pressure has been seen to increase secrecy (Jaspal, 2015). It is also possible that Ahmed will experience the proximal stressor of internalised homonegativity in reaction to his circumstances. In addition, Ahmed may not be able to express his individual distinctiveness and authentic integrated self and, because of all these conflicts, he may subsequently experience both cultural and sexual shame.

Ahmed did excellently at school, but he did not continue his education. The case notes that he 'decided against' further study, though it may be that Ahmed's opportunities for development were limited due to reduced self-esteem, efficacy, and perceived opportunities due to the discrimination against BAME populations (e.g., Jaspal et al., 2021a). Working beneath his competence would limit Ahmed's financial position and may impact upon his sense of achievement, subsequently intensifying negative self-evaluations of efficacy and esteem and minimising the opportunity for psychological distinctiveness and meaning. Ahmed's coping behaviours seem to include social and emotional withdrawal from his family and community, as well as from his job, which may in part culminate in symptoms of anxiety and where repeated no-win cycles lead to learned helplessness and low mood.

When working with patients who experience more than one intersecting identity, it is essential to hold and maintain an awareness of the impact of not just single axis oppressions, but the simultaneous and inter-relating experience of multiple marginalised identities and how this may impact the lived experience and wellbeing of the individuals involved. BAME sexual minorities who belong to more than one oppressed group may end up being categorised into 'one identity or the other' in a single axis binary way which will miss significant intersecting individual experiences. Missing such experiences is likely to add to a patient's identity threat and decreased sense of belonging in the world, thereby imperilling identity integration and psychological wellbeing. It is the co-created nature of the intersection that is so important intra-psychologically, but also interpersonally and socially, including within the dynamics of the patient-practitioner relationship itself.

An effective way of working with groups who have inter-connected, or intersectional identities, is to ask each individual about their unique lived experience of two or more oppressions and to foster an open, non-defensive, and evolving discussion about these experiences, not just in the broader context but also in the context of the one-to-one client-practitioner relationship. Such discussions can then pave the way to identifying possible source of 'support'—that is, what this word means to the patient in their specific context and therefore what 'support' would look like to the patient.

It is especially important to cultivate open discussions about culture, race, sexual identity, gender, and any other aspects of difference in light of the converging or diverging identities of the practitioners themselves. An important practice-based concern here would be to ensure explicitly that all health professionals embark on, and maintain through training and supervision, a committed reflective practice of their own context, perceptions, and experience of difference, of their unconscious biases, position of power as a 'health professional', and appreciation of their own identity processes and how they may intersect interpersonally with those of their patients. Practitioners' personal awareness of their own identities, namely their privileges, oppressions and /or intersectional differences intra- and inter-personally and also socially is important to maintaining a consciousness of equality (e.g., see Turner, 2021). This is a process that can begin in health practitioner training programmes and should raise awareness of the concepts of singular and multiple identities and difference, and explicitly review educational resources that decolonise the relevant curricula. A continuity and commitment of curiosity about our own position in the world at multiple levels and how that position may impact upon others is a hallmark of both good reflective and reflexive practice in any patient-facing discipline.

Conclusion

This chapter focuses on the intersections of ethnicity, religion, and sexuality in the identities of BAME sexual minorities. It draws on elements of minority stress theory, intersectionality and IPT to do so. In line with the concept of intersectionality, it is crucial to note that there are many other categories and identities within this population that impact upon one another. These categories may include age and ageing, sex, gender identity, socio-economic status, health status, occupational status and so on. It is not possible to provide an exhaustive list of all the characteristics that can impinge upon one's identity experience and sense of marginalisation, but it is important to acknowledge that one account will never be truly comprehensive. Individuals' circumstances and life stories are complex and nuanced, and each require specific consideration at the individual, interpersonal, contextual, systemic, and group levels. This is why a serious and sustained multidisciplinary research programme, acknowledging the contribution of distinct academic and practice-orientated research, methods, and clinical practice, is important as we attempt to explore and capture this complexity.

Minority stress theory, intersectionality and IPT are three approaches that can shed light on how scholars and health practitioners understand and work with patients from BAME sexual minorities. Minority stress theory emphasises both distal and proximal stressors that are uniquely experienced, additive, chronic, and socially based, and IPT highlights the underlying psychological processes, motivations, and coping strategies that can exist when conflicting identities begin to converge. The intersectional approach underscores the significance of multiple oppressions and highlights their nuanced and synergistic impact on individuals' lived experience. All these approaches can provide the health practitioner with a broader lens that is both culturally sensitive and affirmative to sexual minorities and that may lead to increased identity resilience and psychological wellbeing in their patients. Furthermore, these approaches may provide the health practitioner, especially those who reside outside the BAME and/or sexual minorities category, with a structure to reflect upon their own positions of privilege, power, and oppression that in turn may enhance their reflective practice. Explicit training and awareness of the complexities that BAME sexual minority individuals might face is crucial, as a lack of this active and continuing awareness would risk significantly increasing the stress, identity threat, and conflict that these groups already experience.

References

Amiot, C. E., & Jaspal, R. (2014). Identity integration, psychological coherence, and identity threat: Linking identity process theory and notions of integration. In R. Jaspal & G. M. Breakwell (Eds.), *Identity process theory: Identity, social action, and social change* (pp. 155–174). Cambridge University Press.

Aspinall, P. (2002). Collective terminology to describe the minority ethnic population: The persistence of confusion and ambiguity in usage. *Sociology, 36*(4), 803–816. https://doi.org/10.1177/0038038502036004 01

Bachmann, C. L., & Gooch, A. (2018). *LGBT in Britain: Hate crime and discrimination.* Stonewall. https://www.stonewall.org.uk/system/files/lgbt_in_britain_hate_crime.pdf

Bariola, E., Lyons, A., & Leonard, W. (2015). The mental health benefits of relationship formalisation among lesbians and gay men in same-sex relationships. *Australian and New Zealand Journal of Public Health, 39*(6), 530–535. https://doi.org/10.1111/1753-6405.12432

Bassi, C. (2008). The precarious and contradictory moments of existence for an emergent British Asian gay culture. In C. Dwyer & C. Bressey (Eds.), *New geographies of race and racism* (pp. 209–222). Ashgate.

Breakwell, G. M. (2015). *Coping with threatened identities*. Psychology Press.

Breakwell, G. M., & Jaspal, R. (2021). Identity change, uncertainty and mistrust in relation to fear and risk of COVID-19. *Journal of Risk Research, 24*(3–4), 335–351. https://doi.org/10.1080/13669877.2020.1864011

Breakwell, G. M., & Jaspal, R. (2022). Coming out, distress and identity threat in gay men in the United Kingdom. *Sexuality Research & Social Policy, 19*(3), 1166-1177. https://doi.org/10.1007/s13178-021-00608-4

Callander, D., Newman, C. E., & Holt, M. (2015). Is sexual racism really racism? Distinguishing attitudes toward sexual racism and generic racism among gay and bisexual men. *Archives of Sexual Behavior, 44*(7), 1991–2000. https://doi.org/10.1007/s10508-015-0487-3

Chryssochoou, X. (2014). Identity processes in culturally diverse societies: How is cultural diversity reflected in the self? In R. Jaspal & G. M. Breakwell (Eds.), *Identity process theory: Identity, social action, and social change* (pp. 135–154). Cambridge University Press.

Collins, P. H. (2015). Intersectionality's definitional dilemmas. *Annual Review of Sociology, 41*, 1–20. https://doi.org/10.1146/annurev-soc-073014-112142

Crenshaw, K. (1991). Mappping the margins: Intersectionality, identity politics and violence against women of color. *Stanford Law Review, 43*(6), 1241–1299. https://doi.org/10.2307/1229039

Haggas, S. (2015). Racism and the gay scene. *FS Magazine, 148*. https://www.gmfa.org.uk/fs148-racism-and-the-gay-scene

Hancock, A. (2007). When multiplication doesn't equal quick addition: Examining intersectionality as a research paradigm. *Perspectives on Politics, 5*(1), 63–79. https://doi.org/10.1017/S1537592707070065

Jaspal, R. (2012a). Coping with religious and cultural homophobia: emotion and narratives of identity threat from British Muslim gay men. In P. Nynäs & A. K. T. Yip (Eds.), *Religion, gender and sexuality in everyday Life* (pp. 71–90). Ashgate. https://doi.org/10.4324/9781315605029-5

Jaspal, R. (2012b). I never faced up to being gay: Sexual, religious and ethnic identities among British South Asian gay men. *Culture, Health and Sexuality: An International Journal for Research, Intervention and Care, 14*(7), 767–780. https://doi.org/10.1080/13691058.2012.693626

Jaspal, R. (2014). Arranged marriage, identity and psychological wellbeing among British Asian gay men. *Journal of GLBT Family Studies, 10*(5), 425–448. https://doi.org/10.1080/1550428X.2013.846105

Jaspal, R. (2015). The experience of relationship dissolution among British Asian gay men: Identity threat and protection. *Sexuality Research & Social Policy, 12*(1), 34–46. https://doi.org/10.1007/s13178-014-0175-4

Jaspal, R. (2017a). Coping with ethnic prejudice on the gay scene: British South Asian gay men. *Journal of LGBT Youth, 14*(2), 172–190. https://doi.org/10.1080/19361653.2016.1264907

Jaspal, R. (2017b). Gay men's construction and management of identity on Grindr. *Sexuality & Culture, 21*(1), 187–204. https://doi.org/10.1007/s12119-016-9389-3

Jaspal, R. (2018). *Enhancing sexual health, self-identity and wellbeing among men who have sex with men: A guide for practitioners.* Jessica Kingsley Publishers.

Jaspal, R. (2019). *The social psychology of gay men.* Palgrave. https://doi.org/10.1007/978-3-030-27057-5

Jaspal, R. (2020). Honour beliefs and identity among British South Asian gay men. In M. M. Idriss (Ed.) *Men, masculinities and honour-based abuse* (pp. 114–127). Routledge. https://doi.org/10.4324/9780429277726-7

Jaspal, R., Assi, M., & Maatouk, I. (2022). Coping styles in heterosexual and non-heterosexual students in Lebanon: A cross-sectional study. *International Journal of Social Psychology, 37*(1), 33–66. https://doi.org/10.1080/02134748.2021.1993117

Jaspal, R., & Bayley, J. (2020). *HIV and gay men: Clinical, social and psychological aspects.* Palgrave Macmillan.

Jaspal, R., & Cinnirella, M. (2010). Coping with potentially incompatible identities: Accounts of religious, ethnic and sexual identities from British Pakistani men who identify as Muslim and gay. *British Journal of Social Psychology, 49*(4), 849–870. https://doi.org/10.1348/014466609X485025

Jaspal, R., & Cinnirella, M. (2014). Hyper-affiliation to the religious ingroup among British Pakistani Muslim gay men. *Journal of Community and Applied Social Psychology, 24*(4), 265–277. https://doi.org/10.1002/casp.2163

Jaspal, R., Lopes, B., & Breakwell, G. M. (2022). Minority stressors, protective factors and mental health outcomes in lesbian, gay and bisexual people in the UK. *Current Psychology.* https://doi.org/10.1007/s12144-022-03631-9

Jaspal, R., Lopes, B., & Breakwell, G. M. (2021a). British national identity and life satisfaction in ethnic minority groups in the United Kingdom. *National Identities, 23*(5), 455–472. https://doi.org/10.1080/14608944.2020.1822793

Jaspal, R., Lopes, B., & Rehman, Z. (2021b). A structural equation model for predicting depressive symptomology in black, Asian, and minority ethnic gay lesbian and bisexual people in the UK. *Psychology and Sexuality, 12*(3), 217–234. https://doi.org/10.1080/19419899.2019.1690560

Jaspal, R., & Williamson, I. (2017). Identity management strategies among HIV-positive Colombian gay men in London. *Culture, Health and Sexuality, 19*(2), 1374–1388. https://doi.org/10.1080/13691058.2017.1314012

McKeown, E., Nelson, S., Anderson, J., Low, N., & Elford, J. (2010). Disclosure, discrimination and desire: Experiences of Black and South Asian gay men in Britain. *Culture, Health & Sexuality, 12*(7), 843–856. https://doi.org/10.1080/13691058.2010.499963

Meyer, I. H. (1995). Minority stress and mental health in gay men. *Journal of Health and Social Behavior, 36*(1), 38–56. https://doi.org/10.2307/2137286

Meyer, I. H. (2003). Prejudice, social stress, and mental health in lesbian, gay, and bisexual populations: Conceptual issues and research evidence. *Psychological Bulletin, 129*(5), 674–697. https://doi.org/10.1037/0033-2909.129.5.674

ONS (2012). 2011 Census: Population estimates for the United Kingdom, March 2011. https://www.ons.gov.uk/peoplepopulationandcommunity/populationandmigration/populationestimates/bulletins/2011censuspopulationestimatesfortheunitedkingdom/2012-12-17#:~:text=The%20population%20of%20the%20UK%20in%202011%20was%2063.2%20million,a%207%20per%20cent%20increase.

ONS (2018). Sexual orientation, UK: 2018. https://www.ons.gov.uk/peoplepopulationandcommunity/culturalidentity/sexuality/bulletins/sexualidentityuk/2018

Ramirez, J. L., & Galupo, M. P. (2019). Multiple minority stress: The role of proximal and distal stress on mental health outcomes among lesbian, gay, and bisexual people of color. *Journal of Gay & Lesbian Mental Health, 23*(2), 145–167. https://doi.org/10.1080/19359705.2019.1568946

Rehman, Z., Lopes, B., & Jaspal, R. (2020). Predicting self-harm in an ethnically diverse sample of lesbian, gay and bisexual people in the United Kingdom. *International Journal of Social Psychiatry, 66*(4), 349–360. https://doi.org/10.1177/0020764020908889

Semlyen, J., King, M., Varney, J., & Hagger-Johnson, G. (2016). Sexual orientation and symptoms of common mental disorder or low wellbeing: Combined meta-analysis of 12 UK population health surveys. *BMC Psychiatry, 16*, 67. https://doi.org/10.1186/s12888-016-0767-z

Siraj, A. (2006). On Being Homosexual and Muslim: Conflicts and Challenges. In L. Ouzgane (Ed.), *Islamic Masculinities* (pp. 202–216). Zed Books.

Turner, D. (2021). *Intersections of priviledge and otherness in counselling and psychotherapy* (1st ed.). Routledge.

Vignoles, V. L., Chryssochoou, X., & Breakwell, G. M. (2002). Evaluating models of identity motivation: Self-esteem is not the whole story. *Self and Identity, 1*(3), 201–218. https://doi.org/10.1080/152988602760124847

Wilkinson, D. J., & Johnson, A. (2020). A systematic review of qualitative studies capturing the subjective experiences of gay and lesbian individuals' of faith or religious affiliation. *Mental Health, Religion & Culture, 23*(1), 80–95. https://doi.org/10.1080/13674676.2020.1724919

Williamson, I. R. (2000). Internalized homophobia and health issues affecting lesbians and gay men. *Health Education Research, 15*(1), 97–107. https://doi.org/10.1093/her/15.1.97

7

Intersecting Identities: Gender and Sexual Diversity

Samantha Martin, Joshua W. Katz,
and Daragh T. McDermott ⓘ

Introduction

Gender and Sexual Minority (GSM) people,[1] in particular trans[2] and non-binary[3] people, are often recognized as an oppressed and marginal-

---

[1] GSM is used throughout this chapter in place of Lesbian, Gay, Bisexual, Transgender, and Queer or Questioning (LGBTQ). This is done in order to acknowledge the multiplicity and diversity of gender and sexual identities. Anyone who does not identify as cisgender and/or heterosexual could consider themselves part of the GSM community.

[2] Trans is used as an abbreviation for transgender in order to denote the diversity of transgender and gender diverse identities (i.e., those whose gender identity or expression is different from their assigned sex at birth; Tebbe et al., 2014).

[3] While individuals who identify as non-binary often fall under the wider 'trans umbrella', the term specifically refers to people who identity with "a fixed gender position other than male or female" (Richards et al., 2017, p. 5). Non-binary people may identify as genderqueer, androgyne, pangender, bigender, genderfluid, agender, neutrois, among many others.

S. Martin
Birmingham City University, Birmingham, UK
e-mail: samantha.martin@bcu.ac.uk

J. W. Katz
University of Saskatchewan, Saskatoon, SK, Canada
e-mail: joshua.katz@usask.ca

© The Author(s), under exclusive license to Springer Nature
Switzerland AG 2023
J. Semlyen and P. Rohleder (eds.), *Sexual Minorities and Mental Health*,
https://doi.org/10.1007/978-3-031-37438-8_7

ized community, vulnerable to poor psychological and physical well-being—this especially being the case for young people (Rimes et al., 2019). Many of these negative outcomes, it would appear, are the result of the stigmatization which GSM experience. Indeed, research suggests that GSM young people experience elevated rates of discrimination and victimization compared to heterosexual and cisgender people on account of their minoritized sexual and/or gender identities (Guasp, 2012; Ellis et al., 2016; METRO Youth Chances, 2016; see also Chapter 3). For example, research conducted with GSM aged 16 to 25 in the United Kingdom found that GSM youth reported having experienced inordinately high levels of verbal (74%), physical (45%), and sexual (18%) abuse (METRO Youth Chances, 2016). Similar findings were reported by DeSmet et al. (2018) who found that non-heterosexual youth aged 12 to 18 were more likely than heterosexual youth to have been the victims of both offline (27.1% vs. 14.0%) and online (11.6% vs. 7.3%) bullying. Further complicating matters for certain GSM, research has demonstrated how transgender and non-binary people are particularly likely to experience acts of discrimination compared to other cisgender[4] members of the GSM community (Grossman et al., 2011; Rimes et al., 2019). For instance, research has shown that while lesbian, gay, and bisexual (LGB) young adults living in the UK do experience elevated rates of hate crimes and victimization (33%), trans young adults are even more susceptible to such occurrences (56%; Bachman & Gooch, 2018). This is emphasized by Grossman et al. (2011) who argue that transgender and non-binary youth experience increased levels of prejudice, discrimination, and hateful language on a daily basis.

As has been discussed in Chapter 3, such experiences often result in negative outcomes for victims, both physical and psychological. These negative outcomes may be exacerbated for gender minorities. For example, substance use has also been found to be significantly more

D. T. McDermott (✉)
Nottingham Trent University, Nottingham, UK
e-mail: daragh.mcdermott@ntu.ac.uk

[4] Cisgender is defined as "people who do not identify as trans or who identify with the sex they were assigned at birth" (McDermott et al., 2018, p. 69).

common among GSMs compared to cisgender sexual minority youth (Reisner et al., 2015). Similarly, Bradlow and colleagues (2017) found that 45% of trans young people had attempted to take their own life compared to 22% of cisgender LGB young persons; worth noting, both of these rates are inordinately high. Such findings are corroborated by other researchers who have demonstrated how trans and non-binary youth may be particularly susceptible to negative mental health outcomes (e.g., Su et al., 2016). Indeed, trans people have also been shown to rate their overall life satisfaction as being lower than that of their cisgender LGB peers (National LGBT Survey, 2018).

While the aforementioned examples of discrimination and their associated health outcomes were by no means meant to serve as an exhaustive list, we wished to provide the reader with a brief snapshot into the often-daily experiences of GSM individuals. Unfortunately, research on gender minorities is sparse compared to that which focuses on cisgender sexual minority individuals.[5] As such, while this chapter will focus on both sexual and gender minorities, where possible, we will highlight gender minorities' discriminatory experiences as well as the associated health implications thereof. Furthermore, this chapter will be broken down into two major sections: first, the various types of discrimination that Gender and Sexual Minority Youth (GSMY) experience will be discussed; and second, we will elucidate upon just a few of the psychological explanations that explain why these forms of discrimination are allowed to perpetuate. In addition, and with respect to both points, critiques of these theories and phenomena will also be provided. Finally, we will conclude this chapter with a note on empowerment.

---

[5] Worth noting, research on sexual minorities is not evenly distributed with much more research focusing on the experiences of gay and lesbian individuals. Bisexuals, in contrast, are often excluded from analyses (Alarie & Gaudet, 2013).

Forms of Discrimination

In Chapter 3, Ellis briefly outlines homophobia, biphobia and hetero-sexism as different forms of social prejudice which impact sexual minority individuals. In addition to these, it is also important to consider those intersecting forms of prejudice and discrimination which GSM individuals face, namely transphobia, cisgenderism and queerphobia.

Transphobia

Hill and Willoughby (2005) define transphobia as an irrational fear of, or emotional disgust towards, individuals who do not conform with society's gender expectations. They further express how trans-phobia includes feelings of revulsion directed towards masculine women, feminine men, crossdressers, and transgender and/or transsexual indi-viduals. Unlike with traditional conceptualizations of homophobia, Hill and Willoughby (2005) also clarify that their use of the term 'phobia' does not imply the presence of a clinical disorder. However, Morrison et al. (2017) argue that "'transphobia' should be conceptualized in a more comprehensive way—that is, stereotypes, prejudice, and discrim-ination directed toward individuals that are or are perceived to be transgender" (p. 395). In 2018, McDermott et al. introduced the concept of transnegativity as an alternative to transphobia that accom-modates the relationship between affective *and* cognitive components of prejudice. Transnegativity in this context is defined as "any prejudi-cial attitudes, discriminatory or victimising behavioural action overtly or covertly directed towards an individual because they are, or are perceived to be, trans" (McDermott et al., 2018, p. 70). While trans persons *do* experience many of the same discriminatory acts as sexual minorities, trans individuals are also at an increased risk to experience trans-specific forms of discrimination as well. Two such examples are deadnaming and misgendering.

Deadnaming refers to the continued use of GSMs (typically trans or non-binary) persons' "names assigned to them in infancy in cases where they have rejected those names" (Turton, 2021, p. 42). Referring to someone using their deadname has been shown to result in feelings of unsafeness, misunderstanding, and/or invalidation (Santos et al., 2021), although the studies conducted on this topic are few. Research indicates that deadnaming is one of the most common forms of bullying that trans and non-binary persons experience. For example, all participants in a study of 169 trans university students attending school in the South-Eastern United States reported having experienced deadnaming (Santos et al., 2021). Further, these students reported that staff used their deadnames in 50% of all interactions. Indeed, even mental health practitioners have been shown to utilize trans persons' deadnames, thus highlighting the widespread prevalence of the practice (Delaney & McCann, 2021). Adding to the issue at hand, many people who use another person's deadname do so unintentionally (Singh, 2020) and repeatedly, even after they have been corrected (sometimes multiple times; Santos et al., 2021). In this way, deadnaming can best be categorized as being microaggressive in nature (Pulice-Farrow et al., 2020). However, deadnaming can also entail expressions of more intentional and/or violent acts of discrimination (Lilienfeld, 2017).

Related to the issue of deadnaming, misgendering serves as another common form of discrimination for trans and non-binary youth. Misgendering in its most common form entails the utilization of inaccurate pronouns that are inconsistent with one's gender identity; however, misgendering also occurs in other situations as well. For instance, misgendering can occur when one is not granted access to a public space (e.g., a bathroom or locker room) on account of their perceived gender identity (McLemore, 2015) or when one is not given the option to use their preferred gender pronoun(s) on legal (or other) documents (James et al., 2016). According to a study conducted by McLemore (2015) with 115 trans individuals living in the United States, most participants reported having experienced some degree of misgendering, which typically resulted in subsequent feelings of stigmatization. While common for many GSM, misgendering appears to be most often directed towards genderqueer individuals (McLemore, 2015). Just as with deadnaming, misgendering often leads to negative psychological consequences for victims. For example, in their study of trans individuals living in and around the United Kingdom, McNeil et al. (2012) found that participants who were frequently misgendered expressed lower levels of self-esteem.

Cisgenderism

Related to the concept of 'transphobia', 'cisgenderism' refers to preju-dicial ideologies that "[deligitimize] people's own designations of their genders and bodies" (Blumer et al., 2013, p. 267). Rather than an indi-vidual attitude, cisgenderism exists as a theoretical perspective that prob-lematizes the categorical distinction between transgender and cisgender, "people who do not identify as trans or who identify with the sex they were assigned at birth" (McDermott et al., 2018, p. 69). Cisgenderism considers trans and non-binary people as 'other' to normative human development and, accordingly, is grounded in notions of transphobia (Ansara & Hegarty, 2012). Today, overt acts of cisgenderism are often challenged in public spaces (McSorley, 2020). However, cisgenderism retains its presence in society as a largely imperceptible process (i.e., as microaggressions), meaning that most cisgender individuals behave in ways that are not always overtly apparent to most cisgender people (Kennedy, 2013). For instance, two of the more common cisgenderist practices include misgendering and pathologizing—a process which only acts to amplify negative attitudes of gender minorities (Riggs et al., 2015). On account of the imperceptibility of and the ease with which cisgenderist acts are enacted, cisgenderism occurs in many domains. For example, family therapy practices often reinforce cisgenderist ideals through the initial consultation process that patients go through (Blumer et al., 2013); more specifically, physicians frequently assume that their patients are cisgender and, accordingly, do not think to inquire about one's gender identity unless prompted to do so. Similarly, a study conducted by Riggs and Bartholomaeus (2018) found that parents of trans youth tended to espouse cisgenderist views as they felt "a falling from [the] certitude" that is afforded the parents of cisgender youth (p. 71).

At this point it is also worth noting how academia is not immune to the various forms of GSM-directed discrimination. For example, academic writing has been criticized as being laden with cisgenderist notions. Indeed, a study conducted by Ansara and Hegarty (2014) sought to identify cisgenderist language in psychology articles and manuals; the authors found evidence to suggest that cisgenderism can take many forms in academic literature including but not limited to the conflation of sex and gender (e.g., treating terms like 'man' and 'male' interchangeably) and a general disregard for people's individual preferences with respect to how they want to be addressed (e.g., the opinions of people who wish to be identified using 'they'/ 'them' pronouns or who would prefer that their names be used in place of pronouns altogether are often ignored). Taken together, all of these cisgenderist acts combine to result in negative psychological consequences for gender minority individuals.

According to the Gender Minority Stress Framework, which serves as an extension of Minority Stress Theory (to be discussed later), trans and gender diverse persons experience risk factors (e.g., distal minority stressors) and protective factors (e.g., access to affirmative healthcare) that influence their mental and physical health both positively and negatively (Tan et al., 2019, 2020).

Queerphobia

"'Queerphobia' describes the discrimination experienced by all LGBTQ + people, including all people who live outside the constraints of cis-heterosexual existences, such as homosexual, homoromantic, lesbian, bisexual, biromantic, trans, pansexual, panromantic, queer, asexual, aromantic, and demisexual people amongst many others" (Marzetti, 2018, p. 702). Marzetti (2018) expands on this definition by expressing how unlike terms like homophobia, biphobia, and transphobia, "queerphobia operates as an umbrella term" (p. 702). Given this, many of the other forms of discrimination discussed in Chapter 3 and here can be said to fall within the category of queerphobia. While little academic literature exists which specifically addresses queerphobic discrimination,[6] that research which does exist suggests that queerphobia is rampant and may be particularly directed at specific GSM subgroups. For instance, in a study of over 1,000 LGBTQ + university students conducted by *The Tab*, trans (41%) and lesbian (39%) individuals reported experiencing higher rates of queerphobic discrimination than either gay (33%) or bisexual (30%) persons (Schifano, 2021). To this extent, and as will be discussed later in terms of intersectionality, these disparities highlight how GSM identities are hierarchically ranked such that certain minoritized individuals are afforded more status and power than are others. While all GSMs may be discriminated against, certain individuals within this community may be *more* susceptible to prejudice and discrimination. With this being said, these exceedingly high percentages for all groups also highlight how queerphobia is a ubiquitous experience for *all* GSMs.

At the Intersection of Gender and Prejudice

Now that we have provided a brief description of the different types of discrimination which trans and gender diverse people experience, we wish to explore the more prominent psychological theories which shed light on experiences of elevated rates of prejudice and discrimination towards gender minorities. In particular, we will examine how concepts related to gender and queer theory are implicated in these prejudicial attitudes and actions. These theories will be framed such that their implications for mental health are prioritized. In addition, critiques of these theories will be levied when and where appropriate.

---

[6] Research instead tends to focus on more specific forms of discrimination with more attention paid to those types of discrimination which affect cisgender, gay, and lesbian individuals, for example homophobia.

Minority Stress Theory

Much of the research which focuses on the wellbeing of GSMs frames discrimination through the lens of Minority Stress Theory. Minority Stress Theory was introduced and defined in Chapter 3, but it is helpful to reconsider it again with specific attention paid to intersecting gender minority identities. Minority stress can result from many different types of events or experiences. For instance, minority stress may be the direct result of overt instances of discrimination, or it may result from internalized negative attitudes in response to expectations of negative interactions (Meyer, 2003). In addition, microaggressions and other seemingly subtle forms of discrimination may lead to added levels of minority stress. To this extent, minority stress can result from either macro or micro forces/processes. Furthermore, individuals who occupy multiple minority positions may be susceptible to added minority stress as these stressors tend to compound stress levels rather than offset them (Austin et al., 2013). Thus, coupled with those stressors which all individuals already experience, members of minority groups often find themselves faced with additional stressors compared to those who do not occupy a minoritized position.

As has been suggested in previous chapters, Minority Stress Theory was originally posited in order to better explain the (often) poorer mental health and physical wellbeing of minoritized persons including members of the GSM community (Holman, 2018). Research tends to support the processes laid out by the theory. For example, sexual minority women have been found to experience significantly higher levels of mental health issues and problematic substance use on account of their minority status (Lehavot & Simoni, 2011). Similarly, Goldberg et al. (2019) found that trans college students experienced numerous minority stressors including but not limited to a lack of family support and an institutional culture that was insensitive towards Gender Minorities (GMs). These stressors, in turn, led participants to experience maladaptive outcomes; indeed, the students in this particular study had dropped out of school (see also Hendricks & Testa, 2012; Hatzenbeuler & Pachankis, 2016, for further discussion of the impact that minority stressors can have on physical and mental health within the GM community). Worth noting, research focusing on trans and gender diverse persons using a Minority Stress Theory framework is relatively novel, although more academics and clinicians are starting to investigate these and other relevant topics (Hendricks & Testa, 2012; Hatzenbeuler & Pachankis, 2016). Taking all of the available evidence into consideration, it is evident that the minority status of GMs has the potential to further cultivate negative outcomes for those who belong to the GM community. And yet, certain scholars have further argued that Minority Stress Theory is insufficient in its attempt(s) to contextualize the negative outcomes experienced by GMs. In particular, it has been argued that the theory may not consider minoritized persons as active participants in their own lives; as well, the very term, minority stress, is actively debated.

While some consider Minority Stress Theory to be a valuable theory in that it directs the conversation away from pathologizing notions of illness and disorder, Wagaman (2015) notes how the theory tends to cast GSM youth as 'victims' who are stripped of their power and agency. Indeed, even Meyer (2003)—who first framed Minority Stress Theory—was conscious of the theory's potential to position minority group members as "passive victims of prejudice" (p. 691). Further complicating matters, Bariola et al. (2017) express how Minority Stress Theory tends to emphasize the negative aspects of GSMYs' mental health rather than highlighting potentially positive aspects thereof. Overall, such trends are not necessarily surprising given the current state of the literature. Indeed, it has been argued that research on GSMs typically approaches persons vis-à-vis a framework of risk, whereby research focuses on GSMs' vulnerabilities as well as their capacity for coping and resiliency rather than on the more positive aspects of individuals' psyches (Wagaman, 2015). In particular, such criticisms are prominent with regard to gender minority youth. Lombardi (2001), for instance, recognizes how access to trans-positive healthcare remains limited despite the many forms of social discrimination that trans people face on a daily basis. Worth noting, healthcare settings are not immune to transphobia and cisgenderism either, as highlighted by research conducted by the likes of Blumer et al. (2013). To this extent, the positive aspects associated with holding a trans or non-binary gender identity are rarely expanded upon or even acknowledged by researchers. Russell et al. (2009) further elucidate upon this point when they state that this focus on risk has overshadowed the many ways in which GSMY are able to develop stable positive identities and enact positive change in their own lives.

Additionally, scholars have also argued that the concept of minority stress does not take into appropriate consideration the effects of ideology and social norms. Riggs and Treharne (2017), for instance, argue that minority stress is not a product of an individual's minority social status; instead, they contend that "'minority stress' refers to how marginalized individuals are stressed by ideologies and social norms which accord them a minority position" (p. 595). More specifically, Riggs and Treharne (2017) contend that ideologies produce stress and that the effects of this stress are different for people with different intersecting identities. To contextualize their thesis in an example, Riggs and Treharne would state that a black lesbian trans woman would experience *different* levels of minority stress than would a cisgender white gay man. This is not to say that the cisgender white gay man does not experience stress on account of his minority status; rather, both individuals experience different levels and types of stress that are unique to their particular circumstances and identities. Given this explanation, layers of stigmatization can be said to 'accentuate' or 'mitigate' levels of minority stress for people with different marginalized identifies. In this way, Riggs and Treharne's version of minority stress can be said to differ from that of multiple minority stress, as highlighted above. Given their position with respect to minority stress, Riggs and Treharne (2017) introduced the concept of 'decompensation', which prioritizes ideologies and social norms, as an alternative explanation for minority stress. Rather than focusing on minoritized persons' abilities to recover from negative events, the purpose of decompensation is to acknowledge the internal and external resources that are available to people with different marginalized identities for coping with oppressive ideologies "that render one's existence unintelligible" (Riggs & Treharne, 2017, p. 15). Concurrently, decompensation attempts to acknowledge the resources that are afforded to other non-GSM marginalized identities on account of layers of privilege such as being white, middle-class, and/or able-bodied. To use an idiom, Riggs and Treharne (2017) describe decompensation as the "straw that broke the camel's back" (p. 15). In this way, decompensation departs from more 'traditional' research on minority stress and the notion that through coping and resilience, one might be able to better protect oneself from minority stressors. In other words, decompensation emphasizes how society not only marginalizes certain populations but also prioritizes how specific identities are privileged over others (Riggs & Treharne, 2017).

Masculinities and Prejudice

While not necessarily a theory, we wish to next discuss the role that masculinities and femininities play with respect to GSM-directed prejudice and discrimination. Much like with Minority Stress Theory, attitudes towards masculinities have come to serve as an explanation for why GSMs are subjected to discriminatory events. Moreover, masculinities have similarly been critiqued as a source of GSM-directed prejudice and discrimination for multiple reasons. In the following sections we will highlight the role that perpetrators' masculinities and femininities play with respect to discrimination and how these interact with the perceived sex and/or gender of the targets of discrimination.

Prejudice towards GSMs has historically been more commonly attributed to cisgender heterosexual men. Research has found that such men tend to exhibit more anti-gay prejudice and behaviours as well as less favourable attitudes towards transgender individuals than their female counterparts (Burn, 2000; Jellison et al., 2004; Nagoshi et al., 2008). For example, McDermott and Blair (2012) conducted a cross-cultural study with heterosexual persons living in Canada, the United States, the United Kingdom, and the Republic of Ireland and found that male participants consistently demonstrated higher levels of homonegativity. Similar findings are also presented by Guasp (2012), who found that gay, lesbian, and bisexual youth tended to be bullied by boys at school, and by Nagoshi et al. (2008) whose study revealed that hypermasculinity was highly correlated with both homophobia and transphobia. Given these findings, it would indeed appear that possessing a more traditional sense of masculinity has the potential to lead individuals to discriminate against their peers. However, there are also facets of GSMs' masculinities which may serve as 'risk factors' for such discrimination.

Indeed, research suggests that violating gender norms is one of the key predictors of prejudice for GSMs, in particular for those whose physical appearance and mannerisms are inconsistent with society's expectations of masculinity and femininity (de Boise, 2015; Herek, 2004). Further problematizing issues, heterosexual men's negative attitudes towards gay men have been linked to their need to maintain traditional gender roles (Jellison et al., 2004; Woodford et al., 2012) as well as to their tendency to view homosexuality as incompatible with and/or a threat to manhood (Falomir-Pichator & Mugny, 2009). To this extent, anti-gay sentiment, it would appear, is engrained within our society; indeed, anti-gay sentiment is regularly cited as being instrumental in the organization and construction of adolescent masculinities (Epstein, 1997). Worth noting, in contrast to gay masculinities, trans men have been found to not be concerned with being perceived as insufficiently masculine, although they do acknowledge the power of hegemonic masculinity and express a desire to be seen as men (Green, 2005). As such, acts of discrimination against GSMs tend to take the form of anti-gay language, which has come to be associated with notions of manhood (Burn et al., 2005; Pascoe, 2005). For instance, Pascoe (2005) found that when boys were called a "fag" by a peer, they interpreted it as a direct attack to their heterosexuality and, by extension, their masculinity. Similarly, a study conducted in the United Kingdom found that the term "gay" is not used by boys to refer to homosexuality but has actually been reappropriated to serve as a signifier that one is not manly (Bridges, 2014).

Given that being gay is often associated with being unmasculine, it should come as no surprise that gay men are often subject to anti-femininity biases (Blair & Hoskin, 2015), sometimes referred to as femmephobia (i.e., "the systematic devaluation of femininity as well as the regulation of patriarchal femininity"; Hoskin, 2019, p. 687) or femiphobia (i.e., "negative feelings toward feminine men"; Miller & Behm-Morawitz, 2016, p. 177; see also Skidmore et al., 2006). As such, in order to avoid being discriminated against on the basis of their sexual orientation, some gay men choose to define themselves as "straight acting"—a less stigmatized group within the gay community (Annes & Redlin, 2012; Bishop et al., 2014; Clarkson, 2006; Sánchez & Vilain, 2012; Taywaditep, 2002). In line with this, gay interview participants in a study conducted by Clarke and Smith (2015) discussed how it is possible to appear "too gay" and, accordingly, spoke to the need to cultivate an authentic appearance that did not 'scream' of being too gay. To this extent, it would appear that some gay men value and, perhaps, feel compelled to outwardly display more traditional forms of masculinity (Sánchez & Vilain, 2012; Sánchez et al., 2010) which can have an adverse impact on a person's identity and sense of mental wellbeing (King et al., 2020).

Such research demonstrates how many cisgender gay men have a vested interest in hegemonic masculinity to the exclusion of 'queerer' forms of manhood such as those associated with being trans, non-binary, and/or feminine. While not necessarily as commonly practiced, these queer forms of masculinity have the potential to be useful in that they offer a chance to "[scrutinize] those processes through which certain bodies, identities, and desires (and not others) become unmarked, normal, and normative" (Milani, 2014, p. 265). In this way, trans and non-binary individuals are given the opportunity to define their own lives and their own masculinities, which can serve as an empowering experience (Halberstam, 2000). Indeed, the introduction of queer theory into the academic lexicon enabled trans people to understand gender as an unfixed entity (Wozolek, 2019). However, queer theory has also been problematic in that it has impeded the lived experiences and realities of some trans persons (Tauchert, 2002). Specifically, understandings of gender as fluid, unfixed, and advocating for the continuous challenge and disruption of gender was in direct contrast to the ways in which many trans individuals chose to live their lives (i.e., as binary transgender men and women who occupied defined gender categories). In this way, queer understandings of gender can also be disempowering for some (Nagoshi et al., 2012). However, such criticisms also led to increased research efforts being placed on trans-specific issues (Nagoshi & Brzuzy, 2010).

Femininities and Prejudice

Discourses of policing gender extend beyond discussions of masculinities. More recently, queer femininities have found themselves as the focal point of a number of vitriolic and divisive debates surrounding sex and gender, and the rights of trans people. These discourses have been mobilised through coordinated groups of women, often described as 'trans-exclusionary radical feminists' (TERFs). Arguments are made in demonstrations, online, and in the press, the aim of which is to reference women's rights, and seemingly promote women's causes whilst platforming explicitly transphobic messages (Lu & Jurgens, 2022; Pearce et al., 2020). These messages aim to convince others that cisgender women are vulnerable to trans women in female spaces (Hines, 2020).

As well as functioning as a regulatory power over queer masculinities, Hoskin (2019) describes how 'femmephobia' acts to police femininity within queer spaces. She states that queer and trans women frequently have to negotiate "dominant cultural ideals of femininity to be validated as women" (Hoskin, 2019, p. 11). One of the key ways in which femininity is policed is through 'biological determinism' whereby bodies assigned female at birth come to reference innate traits and characteristics of femininity. Increasingly, gender essentialist and biological determinist discourses of 'womanhood' have been used to discriminate against queer and trans femininities. Trans-exclusionary feminist groups argue that trans women are not 'real' women due to their not being assigned female at birth. Their beliefs place genitals, reproductive organs, and chromosomal and hormonal make-up as the primary identifiers of authentic gender identity (Hines, 2019; Pearce et al., 2020). These beliefs have been weaponised to exclude trans women from female spaces (Hines, 2020).

This brand of gender essentialism is recognised as a deliberate regression from the queer theorists of the 1980s and 1990s who aimed to disrupt and challenge the sex/gender binary (Hines, 2019). Once again, critics argue that instead of focussing solely on biological markers of male and female sex, we should pay more attention to the meaning(s) that society attributes to the categories of male and female (Hotine, 2021). Trans-exclusionary feminism has been described as one example of 'toxic' or 'rigid femininity' that acts to uphold hegemonic, patriarchal systems of gender (McCann, 2022). McCann (2022) states that the concept of rigid femininities "offers a powerful way to understand how some approaches to gender keep us locked in a toxic gendered system" (p. 22).

One of the primary critiques of trans-exclusionary feminism is that it reproduces the neoliberal, gender normative assumptions of women as vulnerable and helpless to predators, instead of challenging hegemonic perspectives that seek to essentialise bodies based on their reproductive function and potential (Earles, 2018). Furthermore, it intensifies the surveillance on women's bodies, for example through bathroom policing practices (McCann, 2022). Indeed, Hines (2020) notes that such policing practices result in more cisgender women being scrutinised on account of their appearance and in some cases being asked to leave women's toilets because they have been assumed to be trans.

Further critiques of trans-exclusionary feminism talk about the dangerous notion of there being an 'innate' sense of womanhood and how it reproduces racist ideologies. Biological determinism and gender essentialism have historically been weaponised against Black, Indigenous, and women of colour and tend to benefit only those in positions of power (Da Costa, 2021). These strategies of separating bodies and organising them into a hierarchy of authenticity have worked to segregate and subjugate bodies according to race and ethnicity (Hines, 2019). For example, being seen as 'vulnerable' is a position "conditioned by whiteness" (Pearce et al., 2020, p. 681) as Black women are often stereotyped as being dangerously masculine (Patel, 2017). This gender-essentialist logic is now being used to subjugate trans women.

In this way, Da Costa (2021) describes trans-exclusionary feminism as a 'white feminist' discourse. The discourses reproduce white imperialist gender hegemonic, patriarchal power relations that primarily serve "white, cis-straight, wealthy western women" (Da Costa, 2021, p. 317). Such white feminist groups "attempt to organize feminist politics around their particular experiences, and, as a result, exclude and marginalise 'women of difference' from and within feminist spaces." (p. 317). Findings have shown that despite critiques of trans-exclusionary feminism there is evidence of transphobia among some lesbian cis women (Worthen, 2022). However, contrary to the messages espoused by trans-exclusionary women's groups, recent statistics still show that women are more supportive of trans people than are men (Morgan et al., 2020).

A Note on Empowerment

Given the number of young individuals now identifying outside of the traditional categories of heterosexual and homosexual (Diamond, 2008; Savin-Williams, 2006; Thompson & Morgan, 2008; Vrangalova & Savin-Williams, 2010), we wished to conclude this chapter by speaking to the opportunities that queer identities afford those who identify with them. Schwenke (2010) writes how "empowerment starts and is rooted in authenticity and societal acceptance of those of us with 'variant' gender identities—in other words, finding some space to acknowledge our humanity and worth" (p. 188). This can be accomplished in multiple ways. First, GSMs may choose to embrace their minoritized identities. Research with trans participants has shown how possessing a strong sense of pride in oneself and one's trans identity can serve as a protective factor against traumatic life events (Singh & McKleroy, 2011). Second, people outside of the GSM community can choose to actively support and respect GSMs. Findings from a study of sexual minority women and gender diverse persons found that support from allies led to feelings of empowerment and hope for GSMs (Riggle et al., 2018). Taken together, creating spaces of empowerment leads to better physical and mental health outcomes for GSMs. Indeed, studies have demonstrated how empowered GSMs are more likely to receive adequate HIV care (Sevelius et al., 2021) as well as to experience less suicidal ideation (Tucker et al., 2018). In summary, empowering GSMs has been found to provide them with the tools to better deal with various forms of discrimination (Mizock & Mueser, 2014).

Furthermore, most participants found that the strongest sense of support was derived from identifying as part of the feminist community. However, several participants emphasized that this support came specifically from trans-inclusive feminist groups. Worthen (2016) has also argued that transgender and feminist communities share a common rejection of hetero-cis-normativity, or the system of beliefs that places greater value on cisgender and heterosexual identities. Lessons learned from feminist therapy, in particular, may be useful in counselling non-binary individuals. Feminist therapy focuses on oppressive sociocultural forces and power differentials, and may incorporate narrative approaches, thus enabling clients to freely share their lived experiences (Goethals & Schwiebert, 2005; Laird, 1999).

Conclusion

In this chapter, we discussed the various forms of discrimination that GSMs are subject to, with particular emphasis placed on the mental health experiences of GSMY. We then provided brief descriptions of some of the psychological explanations which describe why GSMs are victimized. Finally, we noted the importance of empowerment with respect to GSMs. While much of that research which exists on GSMs adopts a problem-based lens, we wish to conclude by highlighting how GSMs are a resilient community that would benefit from more strengths-based research.

References

Alarie, M., & Gaudet, S. (2013). "I don't know if she is bisexual or if she just wants to get attention": Analyzing the various mechanisms through which emerging adults invisibilize bisexuality. *Journal of Bisexuality, 13*(2), 191–214. https://doi.org/10.1080/15299716.2013.780004

Annes, A., & Redlin, M. (2012). The careful balance of gender and sexuality: Rural gay men, the heterosexual matrix, and "effeminophobia." *Journal of Homosexuality, 59*(2), 256–288. https://doi.org/10.1080/00918369.2012.648881

Ansara, Y. G., & Hegarty, P. (2012). Cisgenderism in psychology: Pathologizing and misgendering children from 1999 to 2008. *Psychology & Sexuality, 3*(2), 137–160. https://doi.org/10.1080/19419899.2011.576696

Ansara, Y. G., & Hegarty, P. (2014). Methodologies of misgendering: Recommendations for reducing cisgenderism in psychological research. *Feminism & Psychology, 24*(2), 259–270. https://doi.org/10.1177/0959353514526217

Austin, S. B., Nelson, L. A., Birkett, M. C., Calzo, J. P., & Everett, B. (2013). Eating disorder symptoms and obesity at the intersections of gender, ethnicity, and sexual orientation in US high school students. *American Journal of Public Health, 103*(2), e16–e22. https://doi.org/10.2105/AJPH.2012.301150

Bachman, C. L., & Gooch, B. (2018). *LGBT in Britain: Trans report*. Stonewall. https://www.stonewall.org.uk/lgbt-britain-trans-report

Bariola, E., Lyons, A., & Lucke, J. (2017). Flourishing among sexual minority individuals : Application of the dual continuum model of mental health in a sample of lesbians and gay men. *Psychology of Sexual Orientation and Gender Diversity, 4*(1), 43–53. https://doi.org/10.1037/sgd0000210

Bishop, C. J., Kiss, M., Morrison, T. G., Rushe, D. M., & Specht, J. (2014). The association between gay men's stereotypic beliefs about drag queens and their endorsement of hypermasculinity. *Journal of Homosexuality, 61*(4), 554–567. https://doi.org/10.1080/00918369.2014.865464

Blair, K. L., & Hoskin, R. A. (2015). Experiences of femme identity: Coming out, invisibility and femmephobia. *Psychology & Sexuality, 6*(3), 229–244. https://doi.org/10.1080/19419899.2014.921860

Blumer, M. L. C., Ansara, Y. G., & Watson, C. M. (2013). Cisgenderism in family therapy: How everyday clinical practices can delegitimize people's gender self-designations. *Journal of Family Psychotherapy, 24*(4), 267–285. https://doi.org/10.1080/08975355.2013.849551

Bradlow, J., Bartram, F., Guasp, A., & Jadva, V. (2017). *School report: The experiences of lesbian, gay, bi and trans young people in Britain's schools in 2017*. Stonewall. https://www.stonewall.org.uk/system/files/the_school_report_2017.pdf

Bridges, T. (2014). A very "gay" straight? Hybrid masculinities, sexual aesthetics, and the changing relationship between masculinity and homophobia. *Gender & Society, 28*(1), 58–82. https://doi.org/10.1177/0891243213503901

Burn, S. M. (2000). Heterosexual use of "fag" and "queer" to deride one another: A contributor to heterosexism and stigma. *Journal of Homosexuality, 40*(2), 1–11. https://doi.org/10.1300/J082v40n02_01

Burn, S. M., Kadlec, K., & Rexer, R. (2005). Effects of subtle heterosexism on gays, lesbians, and bisexuals. *Journal of Homosexuality, 49*(2), 23–38. https://doi.org/10.1300/J082v49n02_02

Clarke, V., & Smith, M. (2015). "Not hiding, not shouting, just me": Gay men negotiate their visual identities. *Journal of Homosexuality, 61*(1), 4–32. https://doi.org/10.1080/00918369.2014.957119

Clarkson, J. (2006). "Everyday Joe" versus "pissy, bitchy, queens": Gay masculinity on StraightActing.com. *The Journal of Men's Studies, 14*(2), 191–207. https://doi.org/10.3149/jms.1402.191

Da Costa, J. C. R. (2021). The "New" white feminism: Trans-exclusionary radical feminism and the problem of biological determinism in western feminist theory. In K. Carter & J. Brunton (Eds.), *TransNarratives: Scholarly and creative works on transgender experience* (pp. 317–334). Women's Press.

de Boise, S. (2015). I'm not homophobic, "I've got gay friends": Evaluating the validity of inclusive masculinity. *Men and Masculinities, 18*(3), 318–339. https://doi.org/10.1177/1097184X14554951

Delaney, N., & McCann, E. (2021). A phenomenological exploration of transgender people's experiences of mental health services in Ireland. *Journal of Nursing Management, 29*(1), 68–74. https://doi.org/jonm.13115.

DeSmet, A., Rodelli, M., Walrave, M., Soenens, B., Cardon, G., & dDe Bourdeaudhuij, I. (2018). Cyberbullying and traditional bullying involvement among heterosexual and non-heterosexual adolescents, and their associations with age and gender. *Computers in Human Behavior, 83*, 254–261. https://doi.org/10.1016/j.chb.2019.02.010

Diamond, L. M. (2008). *Sexual fluidity: Understanding women's love and desire.* Harvard University Press.

Earles, J. (2019). The "penis police": Lesbian and feminist spaces, trans women, and the maintenance of the sex/gender/sexuality system. *Journal of Lesbian Studies, 23*(2), 243–256. https://doi.org/10.1080/10894160.2018.1517574

Ellis, S. J., Bailey, L., & McNeil, J. (2016). Transphobic victimisation and perceptions of future risk: A large-scale study of the experiences of trans people in the UK. *Psychology & Sexuality, 7*(3), 211–224. https://doi.org/10.1080/19419899.2016.1181669

Epstein, D. (1997). Boyz' own stories: Masculinities and sexualities in school. *Gender and Education, 9*(1), 105–116. https://doi.org/10.1080/0954025979721484

Falomir-Pichastor, J. M., & Mugny, G. (2009). "I'm not gay…. I'm a real man!": Heterosexual men's gender self-esteem and sexual prejudice. *Personality and Social Psychology Bulletin, 35*(9), 1233–1243. https://doi.org/10.1177/0146167209338072

Goethals, S. C., & Schwiebert, V. L. (2005). Counseling as a critique of gender: On the ethics of counseling transgendered clients. *International Journal for the Advancement of Counselling, 27*, 457–469. https://doi.org/10.1007/s10447-005-8206-8

Goldberg, A. E., Kuvalanka, K. A., & Black, K. (2019). Trans students who leave college: An exploratory study of their experiences of gender minority stress. *Journal of College Student Development, 60*(4), 381–400. https://doi.org/10.1353/csd.2019.0036

Green, J. (2005). Part of the package: Ideas of masculinity among male-identified transpeople. *Men and Masculinities, 7*(3), 291–299. https://doi.org/10.1177/1097184X04272116

Grossman, A. H., D'Augelli, A. R., & Frank, J. A. (2011). Aspects of psychological resilience among transgender youth. *Journal of LGBT Youth, 8*(2), 103–115. https://doi.org/10.1080/19361653.2011.541347

Guasp, A. (2012). *The school report: The experiences of young gay people in Britain's schools*. Stonewall. https://www.bl.uk/collection-items/school-report-the-experiences-of-young-gay-people-in-britains-schools

Halberstam, J. (2000). Telling tales: Brandon Teena, Billy Tipton, and transgender biography. *a/b: Autho/Biography Studies, 15*(1), 62–81. https://doi.org/10.1080/08989575.2000.10815235

Hatzenbuehler, M. L., & Pachankis, J. E. (2016). Stigma and minority stress as social determinants of health among lesbian, gay, bisexual, and transgender youth: Research evidence and clinical implications. *Pediatric Clinics of North America, 63*(6), 985–997. https://doi.org/j.pcl.2016.07.003

Hendricks, M. L., & Testa, R. J. (2012). A conceptual framework for clinical work with transgender and gender nonconforming clines: An adaptation of the Minority Stress Model. *Professional Psychology: Research and Practice, 43*(5), 460–467. https://doi.org/10.1037/10029597

Herek, G. M. (2004). Beyond "homophobia": Thinking about sexual prejudice and stigma in the twenty-first century. *Sexuality Research & Social Policy, 1*, 6–24. https://doi.org/10.1525/srsp.2004.1.2.6

Hill, D. B., & Willoughby, B. L. B. (2005). The development and validation of the Genderism and Transphobia Scale. *Sex Roles, 53*(7–8), 531–544. https://doi.org/10.1007/s11199-005-7140-x

Hines, S. (2019). The feminist frontier: On trans and feminism. In T. Oren & A. L. Press (Eds.), *The Routledge handbook of contemporary feminism* (pp. 94–109). Routledge.

Hines, S. (2020). Sex wars and (trans) gender panics: Identity and body politics in contemporary UK feminism. *The Sociological Review, 68*(4), 699–717. https://doi.org/10.1177/0038026120934684

Holman, E. G. (2018). Theoretical extensions of Minority Stress Theory for sexual minority individuals in the workplace: A cross-contextual understanding of minority stress processes. *Journal of Family Therapy & Review, 10*(1), 165–180. https://doi.org/10.1111/jftr.12246

Hoskin, R. A. (2019). Femmephobia: The role of anti-femininity and gender policing in LGBTQ+ people's experiences of discrimination. *Sex Roles, 81*(11–12), 686–703. https://doi.org/10.1007/s11199-019-01021-3

Hotine, E. (2021). Biology, Society and Sex: Deconstructing anti-trans rhetoric and trans-exclusionary radical feminism. *Journal of the Nuffield Department of Surgical Sciences, 2*(3).

James, S. E., Herman, J. L., Rankin, S., Keisling, M., Mottet, L., & Anagi, M. (2016). *The report of the 2015 U.S. transgender survey.* National Center for Transgender Equality. https://transequality.org/sites/default/files/docs/usts/USTS-Full-Report-Dec17.pdf

Jellison, W. A., McConell, A. R., & Gabriel, S. (2004). Implicit and explicit measures of sexual orientation attitudes: Ingroup preferences and related behaviors and beliefs among gay and straight men. *Personality and Social Psychology Bulletin, 30*(5), 629–642. https://doi.org/1177/014616720326 2076

Kennedy, N. (2013). Cultural cisgenderism: Consequences of the imperceptible. *Psychology of Women Section Review, 15*(2), 3–11. https://www.aca demia.edu/5112152/Cultural_Cisgenderism_Consequences_of_the_Imperc eptible

King, T. L., Shields, M., Sojo, V., Daraganova, G., Currier, D., O'Neil, A., King, K., & Milner, A. (2020). Expressions of masculinity and associations with suicidal ideation among young males. *BMC Psychiatry, 20*(1), 1–10.

Lehavot, K., & Simoni, J. M. (2011). The impact of minority stress on mental health and substance use among sexual minority women. *Journal of Consulting and Clinical Psychology, 79*(2), 159–170. https://doi.org/10.1037/a0022839

Lilienfeld, S. (2017, June 23). The science of microaggressions: It's complicated. *Scientific American.*

Lombardi, E. (2001). Enhancing transgender health care. *American Journal of Public Health, 91*(6), 869–872. https://doi.org/10.2105/ajph.91.6.869

Lu, C., & Jurgens, D. (2022, July). The subtle language of exclusion: Identifying the toxic speech of trans-exclusionary radical feminists. In *Proceedings of the sixth workshop on online abuse and harms (WOAH)* (pp. 79–91). https://doi.org/ https://doi.org/10.18653/v1/2022.woah-1.8

Marzetti, H. (2018). Proudly proactive: Celebrating and supporting LGBT+ students in Scotland. *Teaching in Higher Education, 23*(6), 701–717. https:// doi.org/10.1080/13562517.2017.1414788

McCann, H. (2022). Is there anything "toxic" about femininity? The rigid femininities that keep us locked in. *Psychology & Sexuality, 13*(1), 9–22. https://doi.org/10.1080/19419899.2020.1785534

McDermott, D. T., & Blair, K. L. (2012). 'What's it like on your side of the pond?': A cross-cultural comparison of modern and old-fashioned homonegativity between North American and European samples. *Psychology & Sexuality, 3*(3), 277–296. https://doi.org/10.1080/19419899.2012.700032

McDermott, D. T., Brooks, A. S., Rohleder, P., Blair, K., Hoskin, R. A., & McDonagh, L. K. (2018). Ameliorating transnegativity: Assessing the immediate and extended efficacy of a pedagogic prejudice reduction intervention. *Psychology & Sexuality, 9*(1), 69–85. https://doi.org//https://doi.org/10.1080/19419899.2018.1429487

McLemore, K. A. (2015). Experiences with misgendering: Identity misclassification of transgender spectrum individuals. *Self and Identity, 14*(1), 51–74. https://doi.org/10.1080/15298868.2014.950691

McNeil, J., Bailey, L., Ellis, S., Morton, J., & Regan, M. (2012). *Trans mental health study 2012.* https://www.scottishtrans.org/wp-content/uploads/2013/03/trans_mh_study.pdf

McSorley, K. (2020). Sexism and cisgenderism in music therapy spaces: An exploration of gender microaggressions experienced by music therapists. *The Arts in Psychotherapy, 71*, Article 101707. https://doi.org/10.1016/j.aip.2020.101707

Merriam-Webster. (n.d.). *Queer Theory.* Merriam Webster. https://www.merriam-webster.com/dictionary/queer%20theory

METRO Youth Chances. (2016). *Youth chances: Integrated report.* Metro. https://metrocharity.org.uk/sites/default/files/2017-04/National%20Youth%20Chances%20Intergrated%20Report%202016.pdf

Meyer, I. H. (2003). Prejudice, social stress, and mental health in lesbian, gay, and bisexual populations: Conceptual issues and research evidence. *Psychological Bulletin, 129*(5), 674–697. https://doi.org/10.1037/0033-2909.129.5.674

Milani, T. M. (2014). Queering masculinities. In S. Ehrlich, M. Meyerhoff, & J. Holmes (Eds.), *The handbook of language, gender, and sexuality* (pp. 260–278). John Wiley & Sons, Inc. https://doi.org/10.1002/9781118584248.ch13

Miller, B., & Behm-Morawitz, E. (2016). "Masculine guys only": The effects of femmephobic mobile dating application profiles on partner selection for men who have sex with men. *Computers in Human Behavior, 62*, 176–185. https://doi.org/10.1016/j.chb.2016.03.088

Mizock, L., & Mueser, K. T. (2014). Employment, mental health, internalized stigma, and coping with transphobia among transgender individuals. *Psychology of Sexual Orientation and Gender Diversity, 1*(2), 146–158. https://doi.org/10.1037/sgd0000029

Morgan, H., Lamprinakou, C., Fuller, E., & Albakri, M. (2020). *Attitudes to Transgender People*. Equality and Human Rights Commission. https://www.equalityhumanrights.com/sites/default/files/attitudes_to_transgender_people.pdf

Morrison, M. A., Bishop, C. J., Gazzola, S. B., McCutcheon, J. M., Parker, K., & Morrison, T. G. (2017). Systematic review of the psychometric properties of transphobia scales. *International Journal of Transgenderism, 18*(4), 395–410. https://doi.org/10.1080/15532739.2017.1332535

Nagoshi, J. L., Adams, K. A., Terrell, H. K., Hill, E. D., Brzuzy, S., & Nagoshi, C. T. (2008). Gender differences in correlates of homophobia and transphobia. *Sex Roles, 59*, 521–531. https://doi.org/10.1007/s11199-008-9458-7

Nagoshi, J. L., & Brzuzy, S. (2010). Transgender theory: Embodying research and practice. *Affilia: Journal of Women and Social Work, 25*(4), 431–443. https://doi.org/10.1177/0886109910384068

Nagoshi, J. L., Brzuzy, S., Terrell, H. K. (2012). Deconstructing the complex perceptions of gender roles, gender identity, and sexual orientation among transgender individuals. (2012). *Feminism & Psychology, 22*(4), 405–422. https://doi.org/10.1177/0959353512461929

National LGBT Survey. (2018). *National LGBT Survey: Research report*. Government Equalities Office. https://assets.publishing.service.gov.uk/government/uploads/system/uploads/attachment_data/file/721704/LGBT-survey-research-report.pdf

Pascoe, C. J. (2005). 'Dude, you're a fag': Adolescent masculinity and the fag discourse. *Sexualities, 8*(3), 329–346. https://doi.org/10.1177/1363460705053337

Patel, N. (2017). Violent cistems: Trans experiences of bathroom space. *Agenda, 31*(1), 51–63. https://doi.org/10.1080/10130950.2017.1369717

Pearce, R., Erikainen, S., & Vincent, B. (2020). TERF wars: An introduction. *The Sociological Review, 68*(4), 677–698. https://doi.org/10.1177/0038026120934713

Pulice-Farrow, L., Gonzalez, K. A., & Lindley, L. (2020). 'None of my providers have the slightest clue what to do with me': Transmasculine individuals' experiences with gynecological healthcare providers. *International Journal of Transgender Health*. https://doi.org/10.1080/26895269.2020.186 1574

Reisner, S. L., Pardo, S. T., Gamarel, K. E., Hughto, J. M. W., Pardee, D. J., & Keo-Meier, C. L. (2015). Substance use to cope with stigma in healthcare among U.S. female-to-male trans masculine adults. *LGBT Health, 2*(4), 324–332. https://doi.org/10.1089/lgbt.2015.0001

Richards, C., Bouman, W. P., & Barker, M.-J. (2017). Introduction. In C. Richards, W. P. Bouman, & M.-J. Barker (Eds.), *Genderqueer and non-binary genders* (pp. 1–8). Palgrave Macmillan.

Riggle, E. D. B., Rostosky, S. S., Drabble, L., Veldhuis, C. B., & Hughes, T. L. (2018). Sexual minority women's and gender-diverse individuals' hope and empowerment responses to the 2016 presidential election. *Journal of GLBT Family Studies, 14*(1–2), 152–173. https://doi.org/10.1080/155 0428X.2017.140853

Riggs, D. W., Ansara, G. Y., & Treharne, G. J. (2015). An evidence-based model for understanding the mental health experiences of transgender Australians. *Australian Psychologist, 50*(1), 32–39. https://doi.org/10.1111/ ap.12088

Riggs, D. W., & Bartholomaeus, C. (2018). Cisgenderism and certitude: Parents of transgender children negotiating educational contexts. *Transgender Studies Quarterly, 5*(1), 67–82. https://doi.org/10.1215/23289252-4291529

Riggs, D. W., & Treharne, G. J. (2017). Decompensation: A novel approach to accounting for stress arising from the effect of ideology and social norms. *Journal of Homosexuality, 64*(5), 592–605. https://doi.org/10.1080/ 00918369.2016.1194116

Rimes, K. A., Goodship, N., Ussher, G., Baker, D., & West, E. (2019). Non-binary and binary transgender youth: Comparison of mental health, self-harm, suicidality, substance use and victimization experiences. *International Journal of Transgenderism, 20*(2–3), 230–240. https://doi.org/10.1080/155 32739.2017.1370627

Russell, S. T., Muraco, A., Subramaniam, A., & Laub, C. (2009). Youth empowerment and high school gay-straight aliances. *Journal of Youth and Adolescence, 38*(7), 891–903. https://doi.org/10.1007/s10964-008-9382-8

Sánchez, F. J., & Vilain, E. (2012). "Straight-acting gays": The relationship between masculine consciousness, anti-effeminacy, and negative gay identity. *Archives of Sexual Behavior, 41*(1), 111–119. https://doi.org/10.1007/s10508-012-9912-z

Sánchez, F. J., Westefeld, J. S., Liu, W. M., & Vilain, E. (2010). Masculine gender role conflict and negative feelings about being gay. *Professional Psychology: Research and Practice, 41*(2), 104–111. https://doi.org/10.1037/a0015805.

Santos, T. C., Mann, E. S., & Pfeffer, C. A. (2021). Are university health services meeting the needs of transgender college students? A qualitative assessment of a public university. *Journal of American College Health, 69*(1), 59–66. https://doi.org/10.1080/07448481.2019.1652181

Savin-Williams, R. C. (2006). Who's gay? Does it matter? *Current Direction in Psychological Science, 15*(1), 40–44. https://doi.org/10.1111/j.0963-7214.2006.00403.x

Schifano, I. (2021, June 25). One in three LGBTQ+ students have experienced discrimination and queerphobia at uni. *The Tab.* https://thetab.com/uk/2021/06/25/one-in-three-lgbtq-students-have-experienced-discrimination-and-queerphobia-at-uni-211509

Schwenke, C. (2010). *Empowerment and Transgender. Development, 53*(2), 187–190. https://doi.org/10.1057/dev.2010.9

Sevelius, J., Chakravarty, D., Neilands, T. B., Keatley, J., Shade, S. B., Johnson, M. O., & Rebchook, G. (2021). Evidence for the model of gender affirmation: The role of gender affirmation and healthcare empowerment in viral suppression among transgender women of color living with *HIV. AIDS and Behavior, 25*(1), 64–71. https://doi.org/10.1007/s10461-019-02544-2

Singh, A. A., & McKleroy, V. S. (2011). "Just getting out of bed is a revolutionary act": The resilience of transgender people of color who have survived traumatic life events. *Traumatology, 17*(2), 34–44. https://doi.org/10.1177/1534765610369261

Singh, K. (2020, December 3). What is deadnaming and why is it harmful? Everything you need to know about deadnaming and why you shouldn't do it. *Fashion Magazine.* https://fashionmagazine.com/flare/what-is-deadnaming-elliot-page/

Skidmore, W. C., Linsenmeier, J. A. W., & Bailey, J. M. (2006). Gender nonconformity and psychological distress in lesbians and gay men. *Archives of Sexual Behavior, 35*(6), 685–697. https://doi.org/10.1007/s/10508-9108-5

Su, D., Irwin, J. A., Fisher, C., Ramos, A., Kelley, M., Mendoza, D. A. R., & Coleman, J. D. (2016). Mental health disparities within the LGBT population: A comparison between transgender and nontransgender individuals. *Transgender Health, 1*(1), 12–20. https://doi.org/10.1089/trgh.2015.0001

Tan, K. K. H., Schmidt, J. M., Ellis, S. J., & Veale, J. F. (2019). Mental health of trans and gender diverse people in Aotearoa/New Zealand: A review of the social determiants of inequalities. *New Zealand Journal of Psychology, 48*(2), 64–72. https://doi.org/10.3390/ijerph17082862

Tan, k. K. H., Treharne, G. J., Ellis, S. J., Schmidt, J. M., & Veale, J. F. (2020). Gender minority stress: A critical review. *Journal of Homosexuality, 67*(10), 1471–1489. https://doi.org/10.1080/00918369.2019.1591789

Tauchert, A. (2002). Fuzzy gender: Between female-embodiment and intersex. *Journal of Gender Studies, 11*(1), 29–38. https://doi.org/10.1080/095892 30120115149

Taywaditep, K. J. (2002). Marginalization among the marginalized: Gay men's anti-effeminacy attitudes. *Journal of Homosexuality, 42*(1), 1–28. https://doi.org/10.1300/J082v42n01_01

Tebbe, E. A., Moradi, B., & Ege, E. (2014). Revised and abbreviated forms of the Genderism and Transphobia Scale: Tools for assessing anti-trans* prejudice. *Journal of Counseling Psychology, 61*(4), 581–592. https://doi.org/10.1037/cou0000043

Thompson, E. M., & Morgan, E. M. (2008). "Mostly straight" young women: Variations in sexual behavior and identity development. *Developmental Psychology, 44*(1), 15–21. https://doi.org/10.1037/0012-1649.44.1.15

Tucker, R. P., Testa, R. J., Simpson, T. L., Shipherd, J. C., Blosnich, J. R., & Lehavot, K. (2018). Hormone therapy, gender affirmation surgery, and their association with recent suicidal ideation and depression symptoms in transgender veterans. *Psychological Medicine, 48*(14), 1–8. https://doi.org/10.1017/S0033291717003853

Turton, S. (2021). Deadnaming as disformative utterance: The redefinition of trans womanhood on *Urban Dictionary*. *Gender and Language, 15*(1), 42–64. https://doi.org/10.1558/genl.18816

Vrangalova, Z., & Savin-Williams, R. C. (2010). Correlates of same-sex sexuality in heterosexually identified young adults. *Journal of Sex Research, 47*(1), 92–102. https://doi.org/10.1080/00224490902954307

Wagaman, M. A. (2015). Changing ourselves, changing the world: Assessing the value of participatory action research as an empowerment based research and service approach with LGBTQ young people. *Child & Youth Services, 36*(2), 124–149. https://doi.org/10.1080/0145935X.2014.1001064

Woodford, M. B., Silverchanz, P., Swank, E., Scerrer, K. S., & Raiz, L. (2012). Predictors of heterosexual college students' attitudes toward LGBT people. *Journal of LGBT Youth, 9*(4), 297–320. https://doi.org/10.1080/19361653.2012.716697

Worthen, M. G. (2016). Hetero-cis–normativity and the gendering of transphobia. *International Journal of Transgenderism, 17*(1), 31–57. https://doi.org/10.1080/15532739.2016.1149538

Worthen, M. G. (2022). This is my TERF! Lesbian Feminists and the Stigmatization of Trans Women. *Sexuality & Culture, 1–22.* https://doi.org/10.1007/s12119-022-09970-w

Wozolek, B. (2019). Implications of queer theory for qualitative research. *In Oxford research encyclopedia of education.* https://doi.org/10.1093/acrefore/9780190264093.013.735

Part II

Interventions

8

Clinical Formulation

Brendan J. Dunlop and James Lea

Introduction

Historically, paradigms for understanding physical or psychological distress were medically based. Psychiatry, working to a medical model of mental distress, understood it as being a result of an underlying biological abnormality or deficit, requiring medical intervention. The assumption therefore is that if a diagnosis is given, then evidence of deficit or abnormality exists. For psychology, counselling and psychotherapy, this is not always as easily translatable, as a plethora of factors can influence psychological wellbeing, at different times and for different reasons.

Medical diagnosis is particularly harmful for sexual minority communities, as it legitimised historical homophobia that permeated society

B. J. Dunlop (✉) · J. Lea
University of Manchester, Manchester, UK
e-mail: brendan.dunlop@manchester.ac.uk

J. Lea
e-mail: James.lea@manchester.ac.uk

© The Author(s), under exclusive license to Springer Nature Switzerland AG 2023
J. Semlyen and P. Rohleder (eds.), *Sexual Minorities and Mental Health*,
https://doi.org/10.1007/978-3-031-37438-8_8

and therefore clinical psychiatry. Up until 1973, homosexuality was classified as a 'mental disorder' (i.e., deficit) within the third edition of the Diagnostic and Statistical Manual of disorders (DSM-III; American Psychiatric Association, 1980). Even though homosexuality had been removed, 'Sexual Orientation Disturbance' was the diagnostic criteria that replaced this, and 'Ego-dystonic Homosexuality' remained as a 'mental disorder' (Spitzer, 1981). Based on the premise upon which medical diagnosis exists, societal and personal understandings of the very *existence* of sexual minority people was that this identity continued to be problematised in that a sexual minority could be distressed about their identity and treated for it. 'Conversion' or 'reparative' therapy was used to 'treat' homosexuality or same-sex attraction, and alarmingly, this abusive practice still goes on today (Bartlett et al., 2001; Government Equalities Office, 2018).

As a result of this historical and current heterosexism and homo/biphobia (see Chapter 3), Frommer (1995) suggested that Lesbian, Gay and Bisexual (LGB) people develop an 'outsider syndrome', whereby they feel "alien within (the) family...and adopt the identity of an outsider even before they can label the nature of this difference" (p. 78). LGB people are not inherently broken, disordered or damaged and do not need to endure ineffective and harmful 'conversion' therapy, therefore understanding psychological distress and mental health challenges from a psychological formulation paradigm, rather than medical diagnosis, is of utmost importance.

In this chapter we shall begin by outlining what formulation is, and why it is important for LGB people (we will use the terms LGB people and sexual minority communities interchangeably throughout). We shall highlight the importance of considering LGB affirmative practice, minority stress, relationships, social, historical, systemic and political factors, and intersectionality, within psychological formulations. After this we shall conside the role played by practitioners within the process of formulation, including the use of sharing lived experience, consideration of any blind spots or unconscious biases, and the need for training. We conclude with a clinical case vignette, to demonstrate how to formulate mental health challenges and experiences for LGB people, incorporating factors that have been discussed.

What Is Formulation?

Clinical psychological formulation is the process of constructing a shared understanding and explanation of how a person's psychological distress and difficulties developed from their life experiences, and how they are maintained in their current life. Psychological theory and research are applied to create this flexible psychological 'story' and guide the development of ways to intervene and help (British Psychological Society; BPS, 2011). For the purposes of this chapter, focus will be given to integrative psychological formulations, that draw upon multiple psychological theories and models (Braham et al., 2015). This is because integrating the fundamental relationships and experiences between the individual person, their original family group and the wider sociocultural context is imperative to understand the psychological distress and needs of LGB people growing and living in a heteronormative and heterosexist world (Downs, 2012). Formulations often provide the basis for hypotheses that can then be tested through intervention (Butler, 1998) and inform the creation of bespoke psychological interventions (Johnstone, 2006). Good practice guidelines for clinical formulation state that they remain person-specific rather than problem-specific, adopt a non-blaming stance, include the person's own strengths and ultimately provide avenues for interventions (BPS, 2011).

Thinking about formulations with LGB people specifically, the BPS (2019) guidelines for working with gender, sexuality and relationship diverse (GSRD) people state that "psychologists are encouraged to recognise that attitudes towards gender, sexuality and relationship diversity are located in a changing sociopolitical context, and to reflect on their own understanding of these concepts" (p. 7). Relevant to the current discussion for formulation with LGB people is that GSRD does not represent a mental disorder, and that mental health practitioners must not offer 'conversion' therapy (BPS, 2019). Above all else, a formulation needs to make sense to the person that it is intended for, and practitioners should therefore be open to the idea that formulations can change over the course of therapy (Johnstone, 2006). Specific unimodal psychotherapy approaches may have different ways of formulating LGB client difficulties (e.g., psychoanalytic, existential or systemic). The primary formulation approach utilised within this chapter is the multi-model approach adopted within clinical and counselling psychology.

Theories and Concepts that Enable Psychological Formulations with LGB People

The next section will explore and explain relevant literature within GSRD psychology and psychotherapy to support psychological formulation work with LGB people. From the outset, it is important to consider the potentially sensitive nature of engaging an LGB person in psychological formulation. A painful experience for LGB people is that their problems are seen as originating purely from 'inside their head', both by themselves and by others Dunlop and Lea (2022a). Psychological formulation can be the medicine to this intrapsychic individual version of distress by including the significant impact of the outside world and society. Many of the stories that the client may need to share will be drenched in shame, marginalisation, othering and oppression coming from the outside in. Pearce and Pearce (1990) in their LUUUTT (Lived, Untold, Unknown, Unheard, Told, Telling) model suggest that mental health practitioners need to be listening out for, and actively asking for the stories that are *Untold, Unknown and Unheard*. Whilst painful, in the authors' experience these are the stories that expand understanding through dialogue and point towards curiosity, connection, containment, understanding, formulation and intervention.

LGB Affirmative Practice in Formulation

A consistent finding in the literature, as discussed in previous chapters, is that simply being LGB in the world is difficult and people experience more psychological distress and mental health difficulties than their heterosexual peers (King et al., 2008; Prell & Traeen, 2018; Ross et al., 2018; Semlyen et al., 2016). It has also been shown that LGB people are more likely to seek out practitioners in mental health services than their heterosexual counterparts (Balsam et al., 2005; Cochran et al., 2003; King et al., 2007), which highlights the importance of conducting assessments and creating psychological formulations in ways that are useful and meaningful to LGB peoples' experience and life. It is important to note that LGB people may encounter institutional heterosexism and homophobia within mental health services (Bartlett et al., 2001; Lea et al., 2010; McFarlane, 1998), and that LGB experience and culture are overlooked in therapy trainings (Butler, 2004; Milton et al., 2002). A playful and necessary jolt in the narrative of this chapter comes from Dominic Davies (1998):

> My mother tongue is "Gay", and I think, feel, and behave more spontaneously and naturally in that language. When I am in the "country" of heterosexuals, then everything I think, say, and do has to go through an interior translator; this can reduce my spontaneity especially with emotions, and result in my being quite guarded and defensive. (p. 117)

Reflecting on this statement feels like a demand for mental health practitioners to educate themselves and develop cultural competence when creating psychological formulations with LGB people. An attitude of LGB affirmative practice is proposed as an alternative to the essentialist heterosexist bias, and attempts to create safe, meaningful and non-pathologising psychological formulations of their difficulties and subsequent intervention for LGB clients (Butler et al., 2008; Coyle & Kitzinger, 2002; Langdridge, 2007; Lea et al., 2010). It is important for practitioners to conceptualise and work with sexuality (Proujansky & Pachankis, 2014) and gender (Gosling et al., 2021, 2022) without unhelpful or stereotyped assumptions, thus aiming to maintain a LGB affirmative stance during formulation work.

A further area relevant to affirmative practice in psychological formulation with LGB people constellates around relationship diversity. It is beyond the scope of this chapter to describe the diverse ways people can be in relation to oneself and to others. However, it is imperative that mental health practitioners do not assume relational styles and/or configurations, for example monogamous couples, and be aware of the cultural norms and privilege afforded to these ways of being in relationship. Whilst others, such as polyamorous relationships, which is when people have open intimate or romantic relationships with more than one person at a time, being seen as less or deviant (Barker, 2019).

LGB Minority Stress in Formulation

The BPS (2019) guidance suggest that practitioners "should strive to understand the ways in which social stigmatisation (e.g., prejudice, discrimination, and violence) pose risks to gender, sexuality and relationship diverse clients" (p. 7). This provides a clear foundation that psychological formulations are built upon this evidence base. The following highlights areas to include in an assessment and creation of a psychological formulation (please refer to Box 8.1 for summary).

As discussed in Chapter 3 and other earlier chapters, the literature suggests that LGB people experience 'minority stress' (Meyer, 1995, 2003, 2010), and it is this that accounts for the increased incidence of psychological distress and mental health difficulties found in this group when compared to heterosexual samples (Timmins et al., 2020). As defined in earlier chapters, minority stress represents unique social and relational stressors not experienced by their socially dominant heterosexual peers, as a result of heterosexism, homo/biphobia, prejudice and stigma (Meyer, 1995, 2003, 2010, 2015). Minority stress is believed to be experienced as distal (external) and proximal (internal) processes, which can be soothed and buffered by resilience factors. We will consider each of these in relation to thinking about formulation. A further development of Meyer's (1995, 2003) Minority Stress Theory (MST), relevant to psychological formulation, is Hatzenbuehler's Psychological mediation framework (2009). This framework posits that direct LGB stigma-related stress may lead to a higher frequency of unhelpful cognitive strategies and difficulties with emotion regulation, which is a clinically relevant predictor of mental health difficulties.

Distal or External minority stressors exist due to any negative treatment, prejudice and stigma from others or organisations that threaten safety or security based on having an LGB identity. Overt examples include discrimination, violence, abuse and victimisation in the world. LGB people are excluded and marginalised in society at individual, relational and institutional levels (Gosling et al., 2021), and often experience being othered from groups and themselves (Dalal, 2006), leading to shame. It could be argued that LGB people inhabit and live the disturbance, distress and disgust given to them by society and those around them (Lea, 2020). Pertinent to this discussion is the external prejudice experienced by LGB people seeking access to mental health services (McNamara & Wilson, 2020). This category also includes microaggressions, which have been described as a "thousand papercuts" (Griffin, 2020; p. 179). Examples include verbal and non-verbal slights, snubs, or insults (whether intentional or unintentional) that communicate hostile, derogatory, or negative messages based solely upon group membership (Nadal et al., 2016; Sue, 2010). An example of this would be a practitioner asking who was the man, and who was the woman in a couple of two men.

Proximal or Internal minority stressors are created as a result of the interaction between the LGB person existing in a society that promotes being heterosexual as the normative or preferred sexuality, i.e., heteronormative. Because the sense of self as 'I' is always born out of the relational 'we' the cognitive, intellectual and emotional architecture of the person is intrinsically influenced by the external heterosexist attitudes (Lea, 2020). The world may be experienced as unsafe and stigmatising, whereby people expect rejection and remain hypervigilant to prejudice and harm to maintain safety and to protect oneself. People may conceal their sexuality as a way to reduce stigma. A further insidious internal process is that LGB people unconsciously internalise the negative social attitudes, shame and disgust from the external world, leading to the experience of internalised oppression: internalised homo/biphobia. These internalised attitudes lead to a pernicious internal distress, whereby the person devalues and feels shame about themselves (Downs, 2012; Meyer, 2003; see also Chapter 13).

These internal processes create significant psychological stress, distress and discomfort for LGB people. *Internalised oppression*, self-stigma and internalised homo/biphobia means that the oppressed person comes to use the methods of the oppressor against themselves. Carroll (2010) found that LGB people with high internalised oppression had lower levels of wellbeing and felt low in mood, experienced significant sexual anxiety, shame and guilt and had lower self-esteem. Internalised homo/biphobia in LGB people means they may feel abnormal, may feel they have to inhabit stereotypes to exist and survive and may also feel disgust towards themselves. This internalised self-stigma may additionally work to actively shame and police other LGB people seen to be contravening heteronormative 'rules', may result in some viewing intimacy as purely sexual, and may leave some LGB people feeling inadequate and desperately lonely.

A further useful construct when formulating the impact of minority stress on LGB people is the idea of *performativity*, proposed by Judith Butler (1990). A persons' sexuality is constructed through reinforced behaviour, language and action, specifically through repeated performances within a specific culture. Performativity can be applied to the process of consciously or unconsciously aligning oneself with the majority group and their power/privilege to survive or achieve. For example, LGB people may perform heterosexuality and heteronormativity to compensate for the shame they feel and minimise threat from the external world. This fuels internalised oppression and feelings of needing to hide ones' identity and being inauthentic. See Box 8.1 for important areas to assess for, and include, within formulation.

Exposure to chronic stress as a result of stigma has been found to undermine LGB peoples' ability to label, understand and regulate their emotions and to utilise helpful cognitive strategies. These difficulties with *emotion regulation* and being trapped in unhelpful *cognitive strategies* influence and seem to increase the experiences of psychological distress and mental health difficulties in LGB people (Hatzenbuehler et al., 2009a; Lewis et al., 2014). LGB people who engaged in cognitive rumination, thinking continuously about their problems, choices and ideas (especially when they are sad or focused on loss) have been shown to predict future low mood and anxiety (Hatzenbuehler et al., 2009b) and psychological distress (Burton et al., 2018; Timmins et al., 2020) in LGB people. Further difficulties with regulating emotions for LGB people could be due to a reduced awareness and acceptance of emotions due to avoidance of feelings, which further compounds the problems as the person only has access to a limited number of coping skills to regulate their emotions: leading to further cyclical emotion dysregulation (Burton et al., 2018). Taken together, this would suggest that stress related stigma and growing up in an invalidating environment (Linehan, 1993, 2015) may reduce the capacity to regulate affect, e.g., flexibly expressing emotions and self-validating emotions. This could leave LGB people vulnerable to psychological distress and mental health difficulties.

Weathering life in a heterosexist world, experiencing minority stress, could make an LGB person believe that their thinking, feeling and identity are wrong, immoral or pathological. This creates fertile grounds for the development of internalised oppression and homo/biphobia, increased vigilance for rejection and victimisation, and defensive attempts to conceal one's minority status and identity; in essence a consuming and internalised experience of distress.

Resilience and protective factors in LGB people can act as a buffer against mental health difficulties, though it remains a struggle for people to grow, develop and live authentically. It is important to remember how difficult it can be for LGB people to live being open about their sexuality, and that this path requires vulnerability and strength in the world—often a difficult balance.

> LGB individuals thrive when they have supportive social networks, accept their emotions and process them with insight, and view the future with hope and optimism. These resilience factors are powerful because they allow LGB individuals to thrive despite societal prejudice. (Kwon, 2013, p. 379)

Because of this, capturing within collaborative formulations the resilience or protective factors that a client has, and how these factors could help to reduce, alleviate, mediate or soothe a particular psychological difficulty, provides a specific avenue for intervention (i.e., the bolstering of this). Important areas of resilience to consider when formulating would be the importance of coping styles (Gosling et al., 2021, 2022); social support and relationship satisfaction, openness about their sexuality, the capacity to flexibly experience and process emotions; hope and optimism for the future (Kwon, 2013); and connection to other

LGB people (Riggle et al., 2008). In that difference, friendship and communion with other LGB people, there is hope and love. There is also a protest in this shared connection: a protest LGB people did not choose, but approach and engage with to live authentically. Organising, connecting and fighting against oppressive systems could be a highly pertinent resilience factor, and one that your client may not have considered themselves.

Box 8.1 Important minority stress areas to assess and discuss during formulation with an LGB person
External:

- Prejudice events from others or organisations
- Discrimination from others or organisations
- Violence from others or organisations
- Abuse and victimisation from others or organisations
- Microaggressions

Internal:

- Expectations of rejection and hypervigilance
- Active concealment of sexuality with whom & where
- Disclosure of sexuality with whom & where
- Internalised oppression, self-stigma, homo/biphobia
- Stigma, emotion dysregulation and cognitive rumination

Further Areas:

- Performativity
- Experience of psychological distress
- Resilience and protective factors

Sociocultural and Systemic Considerations in LGB Formulation

Formulation is so pertinent for sexual minority communities because understanding a multitude of contributing factors for mental health difficulties is essential for developing an awareness of internalised oppression and shame (Downs, 2012), which could allow for the externalising of blame (Macneil et al., 2012). All too often challenges to mental health and wellbeing for LGB people is appraised by others as 'evidence' of deficit and/or psychological instability (Dunlop, 2022), as if the presence of mental health challenges confirms the widely held narratives that LGB people are inherently different to everyone else. Such narratives have historical and political roots and serve to maintain a status quo.

Formulation helps us to understand *what* and *how* a variety of factors and variables lead to mental health difficulties and can provide avenues for LGB-affirmative intervention in therapy (Proujansky & Pachankis, 2014). For sexual minority communities, the social stories that exist in society can have a profound impact on self-concept, identity, mental health and wellbeing. Social stories about sexuality are often created and told by those in powerful and privileged positions, partly to maintain their heteronormative power and privilege through the oppression and marginalisation of non-heterosexual people. It is our opinion that consideration of dominant social stories (Epston & White, 1990) is a crucial facet of integrative formulations for sexual minority communities, as a frame and backdrop from which to understand the development and maintenance of specific mental health challenges Dunlop & Lea (2022a).

Within formulations, client strengths should be captured (Dudley & Kuyken, 2006; Macneil et al., 2012). The reason this is especially important for sexual minority communities is because experiences growing up, and experiences as an adult or older adult, are likely to have been permeated with social stories and narratives of deficit, difference and/or marginalisation. As discussed previously, LGB people can internalise such stories and so can present to practitioners or services with plenty of things that they need help or support with, and perhaps very little attention paid to the strengths, attributes or protective factors that also exist in their lives. Things that may be pertinent for a LGB person's mental health challenges, and should be considered within a formulation, are included in Box 8.2.

Box 8.2 Important psychosocial, systemic, economic and cultural factors to assess and discuss during formulation with an LGB person

- Where and how they grew up (socioeconomic climate, potential for social mobility, access to safe accommodation, reliance on foodbanks/financial benefits) and where they live now
- Who they grew up with (family (non)acceptance of sexuality, friendship groups, early relationships, quality of attachment to caregivers, availability of interpersonal support) and who they live with now
- What social stories they grew up with (appraisal of sexuality diversity, social stories around HIV/AIDS, what it means to be a man/woman) and what stories exist around them now
- Exposure to violence/assault/discrimination (including bullying) and whether this is happening now, or has happened recently
- What the sociopolitical climate is like where they are living (e.g., are LGB people under authority-condoned attack? What rights do LGB people have? What laws exist around freedom of expression?)
- Experience of religion, culture, belief system in relation to being LGB

These types of experiences will undoubtedly impact upon an individual's thoughts, feelings, behaviours and relationships. It is the task of practitioners within formulation to understand how these experiences and consequences may have led to mental health challenges. Importantly, a formulation should help to explain how and why variables and experiences are linked together, so that avenues for intervention can be considered. It is likely that clients will present practitioners with ideas of their own as to why they do the things they do, or their own understandings of how factors and experiences link together for them. Cognitive Analytic Therapy (Ryle, 1995) refers to the formulation process that we engage in therapeutically with our clients therefore as a *reformulation* of their own understanding, and we believe it is important to ensure that you capture your client's understandings during the formulation process.

LGB Intersectionality in Formulation

Kimberlé Crenshaw (1989, 1991), a Black feminist, developed the term 'intersectionality' to describe the experience of inhabiting the junction of multiple marginalised identities, which created a more complex experience of oppression and discrimination. Audre Lorde is an important figure in the world of intersectionality. She self-identified as a Black, Lesbian, mother, warrior and poet. She dedicated her life and creativity to confronting injustices of racism, sexism, classism, heterosexism and homophobia. She believed that "there is no such thing as a single issue struggle, as we do not lead single issue lives" (Lorde, 1984, p. 147). LGB people living with multiple intersecting oppressed characteristics are not living single issue lives, and it is important to psychologically formulate and understand their experience. This is because intersectionality links to minority stress and psychological distress, as all identities are connected to systems of privilege and oppression that give or take away peoples' power. For example, navigating a heteronormative world as a gay man is tricky. When you are a Black gay woman that also happens to be neurodivergent, there are multiple ways in which your experiences of living in a White, heteronormative, patriarchal and ableist world can independently, and as a collective, impact upon health and mental wellbeing. Dunlop and Lea (2022b) provide a set of activities focused upon understanding intersectionality that practitioners may find helpful to consult when formulating with their clients, such as the 'Intersectional Me' worksheet (p. 100).

Understanding *what* intersectional aspects of identity are important to capture in a formulation, as well as *how* these impact upon mental health and wellbeing is a discussion that needs to be had between client and practitioner. Practitioners should not assume which (or how many) marginalised aspects of a client's identity are important for the specific reason they are seeking support. Formulating with, rather than for, is an essential hallmark of formulation (Baird et al., 2017). Collaboration and two-way discussions are crucial for a meaningful shared formulation. Navigating conversations about multiple marginalised identities can be difficult for practitioners. Collaboration in formulation should also apply to formulations of potentially trickier subjects like this, as client involvement in such endeavours can often be lacking for a variety of reasons, including practitioner anxiety (Dunlop, 2019). Chapter 9 further considers a variety of intersecting identities that practitioners may need to consider.

Practitioner Issues in Psychological Formulation with LGB People

Having Appropriate and Affirmative Knowledge and Beliefs

LGB affirmative practice is a belief system or attitude, rather than a therapeutic model, and advocates that practitioners (heterosexual or non-heterosexual) have a substantial knowledge of the issues faced by this diverse group, ensuring culturally competent practice (Crisp & McCave, 2007; Hodges, 2008; Proujansky & Pachankis, 2014—see also Chapter 9). Research suggests that many therapy trainings are heterosexist in nature, leaving LGB issues invisible, and "when there were taught components they were conceptualised as diversity and difference, which again perpetuates heterosexual norms" (Lea et al., 2010, p. 69). It may be helpful for the practitioner to reflect on their possible heterosexual and/or cisgender privilege to support clinical formulation work with GSRD people. Engaging in sufficient specific training and continuing practitioner development to allow meaningful, effective and safe clinical work with LGB people and relationship diversity is paramount (Barker, 2019; BPS, 2019; Lea et al., 2010). It is not the responsibility of clients to educate practitioners, but "to be open to the nuances of their unique lived experience of their relationships" (Barker, 2019, p. 57).

Formulating as an LGB Practitioner

A helping and/or therapeutic relationship is a two-way street. Whilst some may desire or conceptualise the practitioner as being distinct and impartial in the process of formulation and subsequent therapy, this is just not the case. Indeed, the authors of this chapter both identify as gay and/or queer, and attempts to divorce their experiences of being gay from the way in which they have written this chapter, is just not possible. In some ways, it could be argued that being experts by experience, as well as experts by training, was the relational frame of writing this chapter. Reflecting on these factors, it is important to affirm that collaborative formulation itself can be thought of as a process of discovery, moving within professional roles and life experience, as well as an event and outcome to guide intervention (BPS, 2011). Because of this and the potential power of the process, the duty lies with us as practitioners to explore the role of our own histories, beliefs, biases and wishes, so that we can be aware of the impact of our own experiences when we help formulate our client's difficulties. For example, experiences that our clients have endured may resonate with ourselves.

Being a sexual minority practitioner brings with it opportunities and challenges for working with LGB people when considering boundaries and self-disclosure (BPS, 2019; Lea et al., 2010). In the process of formulation, clients may not have the words or labels to conceptualise what has happened to them, may not be able to link thoughts, behaviours, interpersonal patterns or feelings together, and may struggle to be able to articulate how being a sexual minority has impacted upon their difficulties.

An opportunity that comes with being a sexual minority practitioner, is the tool of self-disclosure. Self-disclosure can be thoughts of as "[practitioner] statements that reveal something personal about therapists" (Hill & Knox, 2001, p. 413). Disclosures, or the sharing of lived experiences in an LGB client context, can span a wide spectrum of topics. Crucially, self-disclosure is always a personal choice. It is worth highlighting that research suggests that practitioners who identify as GRSD and disclose their own sexuality (for the benefit of the client in the formulation process) could be incredibly useful, by positively impacting on the therapeutic relationship (Lea et al., 2010; Lovell et al., 2020). The self-disclosure of sexuality in the process of formulation can reduce power differentials, akin to feminist approaches to practitioner self-disclosure (Simi & Mahalik, 1997). It can help the client to understand links in their difficulties, see parts of themselves reflected in their practitioner and find an experience of sameness and connection to another LGB person who can provide a "reasonably positive role model of people who were comfortable and accepting and confident about their own sexuality" (Lea et al., 2010, p. 64). Considering the use of self-disclosure within the process of formulation should be carefully considered, given that this must be in the client's best interests and must be relevant and useful to the formulation process (Dunlop et al., 2021). A framework exists to help practitioners that wish to explore the use of self-disclosure, including disclosure of sexuality, with clients: the *Sharing Lived Experiences Framework* (Dunlop et al., 2021).

How to Create Psychological Formulations with an LGB-Specific Focus

To illustrate some of what has been discussed in this chapter, a fictional clinical vignette ("Robin") now follows. Key aspects of the chapter have been incorporated into this formulation example, to provide an outline of what a good LGB-specific formulation could look like.

Clinical Vignette: Robin

Robin (21 years old) has been referred to mental health services by his GP, who believes Robin should begin medication for his feelings. Robin identifies as White Welsh. The family speak Welsh and have a strong Welsh cultural identity, attending the National Eisteddfod[1] each year. Robin is fluent and proficient in English and has explained that he actually prefers speaking about his difficulties in English, because they feel "a little further away from me and it's easier to talk about them". Robin and his family moved to Manchester when he was 15 years old due to work opportunities for his parents. Robin is a keen football player, can usually

---

[1] Held during the first week of August every year, the National Eisteddfod is a celebration of the culture and language in Wales; for example, music, dance, visual arts and literature.

make friends easily and in school really enjoyed drama classes, though never pursued this.

For the past 12 months, Robin has described feelings of loneliness and sadness, and feeling "like crap because I am a bad person". Prior to this time, Robin had been seeking some support via helplines in relation to his sexuality, though is clear that he does not want to be gay. It seems that Robin feels a lot of shame and guilt for his romantic and sexual feelings, which led him to speak with the family Priest. Unfortunately, this seemed to exacerbate these feelings, as the Priest spoke with his parents and suggested 'conversion' or 'reparative' therapies as a solution. Robin believes that "I will never fit in." Robin works as an IT technician for a major supermarket. He spends lots of time at home on the computer, no longer attends his Church bible study or choir, no longer plays football and often naps during the evening. When asked about this, Robin says that "I want to be on my own, cos I feel disgusting and only upset people". Robin does have some friends from school and college who feel confused that Robin is so worried about possibly being gay. He no longer spends much time with them in person, but when he does he says that "I still have a laugh, but there's this weight in my head and butterflies in my stomach". Robin has told his parents that he has no energy which concerns them as he is intellectually very able.

Robin has spoken about his feelings that he may cut himself, as a way to help himself feel better and get rid of the shame, sadness and worry. He has heard that it can help from other people, and also remembers hearing something about self-flagellation at Church, which he thinks is basically the same thing. Robin is very clear that this is something he has not done yet and does not intend to do anytime soon. When asked if he feels as though he wants to end his life, Robin responds by saying that he has no plans and "I would not do this, as it would be a sin and upset my family".

Robin lives with his parents who are in their late 40's, and his sisters Celin (18 years old), Gwenllian (14 years old) and Elin (10 years old). Robin described where the family live as "a rough (*deprived*) council estate, full of crime and some bad people, though not all of them are bad". The family are all confused and angry about Robin's strange urges and feelings, and concerned about his sadness, saying that "he used to be such a good and polite young man". Robin's mum, Eirlys, works as a support worker in a ward for people with Dementia. Robin's dad, Rhys, works as a construction worker. Parents both work long hours, leaving Robin to cook food and look after his siblings after school until his mum finishes her shift. Robin's family are generally understanding and supportive of him, though not of the possibility that he may be gay. Up until recently, Robin said that he felt close to his family and that they had a good relationship.

Initial Working Psychological Formulation: Robin

It may be useful to begin by making use of the LGB psychological formulation diagram (Fig. 8.1) and to populate the boxes based on the information we know about Robin.

Robin has experienced significant and relentless messages from the external world that heterosexuality is valuable and normal, whilst being gay is sinful and wrong. Robin has become to understand some of the difficulties he is having as being a result of his 'sinful' sexuality. These skewed and destructive stories were further compounded by the fact that his original group, his family, share these prejudiced and discriminatory views about LGB people. It could be speculated that this led Robin to feel shame and doubt his feelings and so he hid an aspect of himself through fear of being shunned. Robin continued to internalise the minority stressors around him and he began to relate to the world and others as unsafe and untrustworthy. Robin holds a strong belief that others will reject him and not accept him for who he is. This fear seems to be somewhat fixed, as it is not eroded by his friendships with people from school and college who accept him for who he is. Behaviourally, Robin seems to withdraw from relational experiences with family, which may be protective to him; though the removal of time with friends seems to further feelings of sadness and isolation. The experience of minority stress and stigma has impacted Robin's ability to trust himself and his feelings, leading to self-doubt and self-invalidation, which has exacerbated feelings of shame, low mood and anxiety in the world. His inability at present to accept himself is projected all around, believing everyone

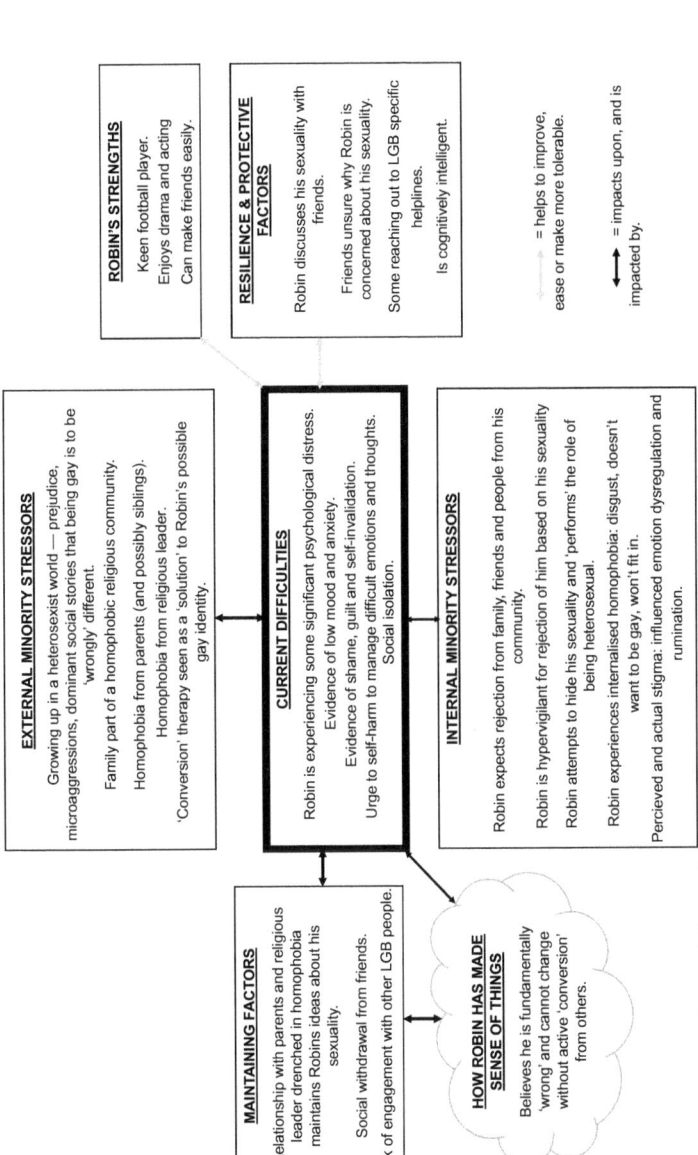

Fig. 8.1 Robin's psychological formulation diagram

ROBIN'S STRENGTHS

Keen football player.
Enjoys drama and acting
Can make friends easily.

RESILIENCE & PROTECTIVE FACTORS

Robin discusses his sexuality with friends.

Friends unsure why Robin is concerned about his sexuality.

Some reaching out to LGB specific helplines.

Is cognitively intelligent.

----▷ = helps to improve, ease or make more tolerable.

◀▬▶ = impacts upon, and is impacted by.

EXTERNAL MINORITY STRESSORS

Growing up in a heterosexist world — prejudice, microaggressions, dominant social stories that being gay is to be 'wrongly' different.

Family part of a homophobic religious community.

Homophobia from parents (and possibly siblings).

Homophobia from religious leader.

'Conversion' therapy seen as a 'solution' to Robin's possible gay identity.

CURRENT DIFFICULTIES

Robin is experiencing some significant psychological distress.
Evidence of low mood and anxiety.
Evidence of shame, guilt and self-invalidation.
Urge to self-harm to manage difficult emotions and thoughts.
Social isolation.

INTERNAL MINORITY STRESSORS

Robin expects rejection from family, friends and people from his community.

Robin is hypervigilant for rejection of him based on his sexuality

Robin attempts to hide his sexuality and 'performs' the role of being heterosexual.

Robin experiences internalised homophobia: disgust, doesn't want to be gay, won't fit in.

Percieved and actual stigma: influenced emotion dysregulation and rumination.

MAINTAINING FACTORS

Relationship with parents and religious leader drenched in homophobia maintains Robins ideas about his sexuality.

Social withdrawal from friends.

Lack of engagement with other LGB people.

HOW ROBIN HAS MADE SENSE OF THINGS

Believes he is fundamentally 'wrong' and cannot change without active 'conversion' from others.

will continue to criticise him and desire him to change his sexuality. Finding it difficult to think about his difference in a way that is not laden with shame creates a situation whereby Robin becomes overwhelmed by his emotions and wants to escape this feeling behaviourally, believeing that self-harm may remove (and therefore solve) his emotional dysregulation. Robin does allow himself to connect with his identity in some small ways, such as discussing his feelings with friends, and also reaching out to LGB helplines. This is positive and protective, as it represents an ember of hope that he is not alone and can consider his life being different, inspite of the pain and oppression he experiences. Robin has several strengths that he may not be able to connect with at the moment, including the fact that he is a good football player and can usually make friends easily.

Conclusion

In this chapter we hope to have provided an overview of the importance of co-constructing meaningful, non-medicalised understandings of psychological distress and mental health difficutlies for LGB people, with important considerations for both the outcome and process of the formulation endeavour. This includes the need to maintain an affirmative approach, to consider minority stressors, to understand a wide range of sociocultural factors relevant to the individual's life and to have a keen eye on the importance of intersectionality. We hope to have also underscored the practitioner issues inherent to the formulation process with LGB communities. Ensuring that practitioners possess the appropriate knowledge and that they engage in appropriate supervision is paramount. Furthermore, reflection upon one's own life stories and experiences as LGB or heterosexual practitioners is needed when considering whether the use of self-disclosure during the formulation process may prove beneficial to a client.

The power of psychological formulation should not be underestimated, and hopefully it is clear in the example of Robin how to incorportate this into clinical practice with LGB people. All too often an LGB client may be well versed in masking, hiding, suppressing and surviving. Having a safe affirmative space to explore and unpack their own story, and to be able to make links between their past, the present and their future, may never have been afforded to them before. This felt sense of connection can be so powerful. We encourage you as the reader, no matter what your therapeutic background or grounding is, to bear this in mind during the formulation process. Often the formulation process can be just as powerful, if not more powerful, than any subsequent intervention.

References

American Psychiatric Association. (1980). *Diagnostic and statistical manual of mental disorders* (3rd ed.). American Psychiatric Association.

Baird, J., Hyslop, A., Macfie, M., Stocks, R., & Van der Kleij, T. (2017). Clinical formulation: Where it came from, what it is and why it matters. *Bjpsych Advances, 23*(2), 95–103. https://doi.org/10.1192/apt.bp.115.014670

Balsam, K. F., Rothblum, E. D., & Beauchaine, T. P. (2005). Victimization over the life span: A comparison of lesbian, gay, bisexual, and heterosexual siblings. *Journal of Consulting and Clinical Psychology, 73*(3), 477–487. https://doi.org/10.1037/0022-006X.73.3.477

Bartlett, A., King, M., & Phillips, P. (2001). Straight talking: An investigation of the attitudes and practice of psychoanalysts and psychopractitioners in relation to gays and lesbians. *The British Journal of Psychiatry: The Journal of Mental Science 179*, 545–549. https://doi.org/10.1192/bjp.179.6.545

Barker, M. (2019). *British Association for Counselling and Psychotherapy (BACP) Good Practice across the Counselling Professions 001 Gender, Sexual, and Relationship Diversity (GSRD).* https://www.bacp.co.uk/media/5877/bacp-gender-sexual-relationship-diversity-gpacp001-april19.pdf

Braham, L., De Boos, D., & Smith, S. (2015). Integrative approaches. In D. L Dawson & N. G. Moghaddam (Eds.), *Formulation in action.* De Gruyter Open.

British Psychological Society. (2011). *Good practice guidelines on the use of psychological formulation.* https://shop.bps.org.uk/good-practice-guidelines-on-the-use-of-psychological-formulation

British Psychological Society. (2019). *Guidelines for psychologists working with gender, sexuality and relationships diversity.* https://www.bps.org.uk/sites/ www.bps.org.uk/files/Policy/Policy%20-%20Files/Guidelines%20for%20p sychologists%20working%20with%20gender%2C%20sexuality%20and% 20relationship%20diversity.pdf

Burton, C. L., Wang, K., & Pachankis, J. E. (2018). Does getting stigma under the skin make it thinner? Emotion regulation as a stress-contingent mediator of stigma and mental health. *Clinical Psychological Science, 6*(4), 590–600.https://doi.org/10.1177/2167702618755321

Butler, J. (1990). *Gender trouble: Feminism and the subversion of identity.* Routledge.

Butler, G. (1998). Clinical formulation. In A. S. Bellack & M. Hersen (Eds.), *Comprehensive clinical psychology.* Pergamon.

Butler, C. (2004). Lesbian and gay trainees: The challenge of personal and practitioner integration. *Lesbian and Gay Psychology Review, 55,* 22–29.

Carroll, L. (2010). *Counselling sexual and gender minorities.* Merrill.

Cochran, S. D., Sullivan, J. G., & Mays, V. M. (2003). Prevalence of mental disorders, psychological distress, and mental health services use among lesbian, gay, bisexual adults in the United States. *Journal of Consulting and Clinical Psychology, 71*(1), 53–61. https://doi.org/10.1037//0022-006x.71. 1.53

Crenshaw, K. (1989). *Demarginalizing the intersection of race and sex: A black feminist critique of antidiscrimination doctrine, feminist theory and antiracist politics.* University of Chicago Legal Forum: Article 8.

Crenshaw, K. (1991). Mapping the margins: Intersectionality, identity politics, and violence against women of color. *Stanford Law Review, 43*(6), 1241–1299. https://doi.org/10.2307/1229039

Crisp, C., & McCave, E. L. (2007). Gay affirmative practice: A model for social work practice with gay, lesbian and bisexual youth. *Child Adolescent Social Work, 24*(4), 403–421. https://doi.org/10.1007/s10560-007-0091-z

Dalal, F. (2006). Racism: Processes of detachment, dehumanization and hatred. *The Psychoanalytic Quarterly, 75*(1), 131–161. https://doi.org/10.1002/j. 2167-4086.2006.tb00035.x

Davies, D. (1998). The six necessary and sufficient conditions applied to working with lesbian, gay and bisexual clients. *The Person-Centred Journal, 5*(2), 111–120.

Downs, A. (2012). *The velvet rage: Overcoming the pain of growing up gay in a straight man's world* (2nd ed.). Da Capo Life Long.

Dudley, R., & Kuyken, W. (2006). Case formulation in cognitive behavioural therapy: A principle-driven approach. In L. Johnstone & R. Dallos (Eds.), *Formulation in psychology and psychotherapy: Making sense of people's problems.* Routledge.

Dunlop, B. J. (2019). A clinical audit of service user and carer involvement in an NHS community mental health team risk assessment tool. *Clinical Audit, 11*, 29–36. https://doi.org/10.2147/CA.S217857

Dunlop, B. J. (2022). *The queer mental health workbook: A creative self-help guide using CBT*. Jessica Kingsley Publishers.

Dunlop, B. J., & Lea, J. (2022a). It's not just in my head: An intersectional, social and systems-based framework in gender and sexuality diversity. *Psychology and Psychotherapy: Theory, Research and Practice, 96*(1), 1–15. https://doi.org/10.1111/papt.12438

Dunlop, B. J., & Lea, J. (2022b). Intersectionality and me. In B. J. Dunlop (Ed.), *The queer mental health workbook: A creative self-help guide using CBT, CFT and DBT*. Jessica Kingsley Publishers.

Dunlop, B. J., Woods, B., Lovell, J., O'Connell, A., Rawcliffe-Foo, S., & Hinsby, K. (2021). Sharing Lived Experiences Framework (SLEF): A framework for mental health practitioners when making disclosure decisions. *Journal of Social Work Practice*. https://doi.org/10.1080/02650533.2021.192 2367

Epston, D., & White, M. (1990). Story, knowledge, power. In D. Epston & M. White (Eds.), *Narrative means to therapeutic ends.* Norton.

Frommer, M. (1995). Countertransference obscurity in the psychoanalytic treatment of homosexual patients. In T. Domencici & R. C. Lesser (Eds.), *Disorienting sexuality* (pp. 65–82). Routledge.

Gosling, H., Pratt, D., & Lea, J. (2022). Understanding self harm urges and behaviour amongst non-binary young adults: A grounded theory study. *Journal of Gay & Lesbian Mental Health*. https://doi.org/10.1080/19359705. 2022.2073310

Gosling, H., Pratt, D., Montgomery, H., & Lea, J. (2021). The relationship between minority stress factors and suicidal ideation and behaviours amongst transgender and gender non-conforming adults: A systematic review. *Journal of Affective Disorders, 303*, 31–51. https://doi.org/10.1016/j.jad.2021.12.091

Government Equalities Office UK. (2018). *National LGBT survey: Summary report*. https://assets.publishing.service.gov.uk/government/uploads/system/uploads/attachment_data/file/722314/GEO-LGBT-Survey-Report.pdf

Griffin, C. L. (2020). *Beyond gender binaries: An intersectional orientation to communication and identities*. University of California Press.

Hatzenbuehler, M. L. (2009). How does sexual minority stigma "get under the skin"? A psychological mediation framework. *Psychological Bulletin, 135*(5), 707–730. https://doi.org/10.1037/a0016441

Hatzenbuehler, M. L., Dovidio, J. F., Nolen-Hoeksema, S., & Phills, C. E. (2009a). An implicit measure of anti-gay attitudes: Prospective associations with emotion regulation strategies and psychological distress. *Journal of Experimental Social Psychology, 45*(6), 1316–1320. https://doi.org/10.1016/j.jesp.2009.08.005

Hatzenbuehler, M. L., Nolen-Hoeksema, S., & Dovidio, J. (2009b). How does stigma "get under the skin"? The mediating role of emotion regulation. *Psychological Science, 20*(10), 1282–1289. https://doi.org/10.1037/a0016441

Hill, C. E., & Knox, S. (2001). Self-disclosure. *Psychotherapy: Theory, Research, Practice, Training, 38*(4), 413–417. https://doi.org/10.1037/0033-3204.38.4.413

Hodges, I. (2008). Queer dilemmas. The problem of power in psychotherapeutic and counselling practice. In L. Moon (Ed.), *Feeling queer or queer feelings? Radical approaches to counselling sex, sexualities and genders* (pp. 7–22). Routledge.

Johnstone, L. (2006). Controversies and debates about formulation. In L. Johnstone & R. Dallos (Eds.), *Formulation in psychology and psychotherapy: Making sense of people's problems*. Routledge.

King, M., Semlyen, J., Killaspy, H., Nazareth, I., & Osborn, D. (2007). *A systematic review of research on counselling and psychotherapy for lesbian, gay, bisexual & transgender people*. British Association for Counselling and Psychotherapy.

King, M., Semlyen, J., Tai, S. S., Killaspy, H., Osborn, D., Popelyuk, D., & Nazareth, I. (2008). A systematic review of mental disorder, suicide, and deliberate self harm in lesbian, gay and bisexual people. *BMC Psychiatry, 8*(1), 70. https://doi.org/10.1186/1471-244X-8-70

Kwon, P. (2013). Resilience in lesbian, gay, and bisexual individuals. *Personality and Social Psychology Review, 17*(4), 371–383. https://doi.org/10.1177/1088868313490248

Langdridge, D. (2007). Gay affirmative therapy: A theoretical framework and defence. *Journal of Gay and Lesbian Psychotherapy, 11*(1/2), 27–43. https://doi.org/10.1300/J236v11n01_03

Lea, J. (2020). A heterosexist matrix: A critical examination of the tripartite matrix and non-heterosexual identities. *Group Analysis North, GANNET, 16*, 14–16. https://www.groupanalysisnorth.com/wpcontent/uploads/2020/09/GANNETJuly2020-1.pdf

Lea, J., Jones, R., & Huws, J. C. (2010). Gay psychologists and gay clients: Exploring practitioner disclosure of sexuality in the therapeutic closet. *Psychology of Sexualities Review, 1*(1), 59–73.

Lewis, R. J., Milletich, R. J., Mason, T. B., & Derlega, V. J. (2014). Pathways connecting sexual minority stressors and psychological distress among lesbian women. *Journal of Gay and Lesbian Social Services, 26*(2), 147–167. https://doi.org/10.1080/10538720.2014.891452

Linehan, M. M. (1993). *Cognitive behavioral treatment of borderline personality disorder*. Guilford Press.

Linehan, M. M. (2015). *DBT skills training manual* (2nd ed.). Guilford Press.

Lorde, A. (1984). *Sister outsider—Essays and speeches*. Crossing Press.

Lovell, J., O'Connell, A., & Webber, M. (2020). Sharing lived experience in mental health services. In L. B. Joubert & M. Webber (Eds.), *The Routledge handbook of social work practice research* (pp. 368–381). Routledge.

Macneil, C. A., Hasty, M. K., Conus, P., & Berk, M. (2012). Is diagnosis enough to guide interventions in mental health? Using case formulation in clinical practice. *BMC Medicine, 10*, 111. https://doi.org/10.1186/1741-7015-10-111

McFarlane, L. (1998). *Diagnosis: Homophobic. The experiences of lesbians, gay men and bisexuals in mental health services*. PACE.

McNamara, G., & Wilson, C. (2020). Lesbian, gay and bisexual individuals experience of mental health services: A systematic review. *The Journal of Mental Health Training, Education and Practice, 15*(2), 59–70. https://doi.org/10.1108/JMHTEP-09-2019-0047

Meyer, I. H. (1995). Minority stress and mental health in gay men. *Journal of Health and Social Behavior, 36*, 38–56.

Meyer, I. H. (2003). Prejudice, social stress, and mental health in lesbian, gay, and bisexual populations: Conceptual issues and research evidence. *Psychological Bulletin, 129*(5), 674–697. https://doi.org/10.1037/0033-2909.129.5.674

Meyer, I. H. (2010). Identity, stress, and resilience in lesbians, gay men, and bisexuals of color. *The Counseling Psychologist, 38*(3), 442–454. https://doi.org/10.1177/0011000009351601

Meyer, I. H. (2015). Resilience in the study of minority stress and health of sexual and gender minorities. *Psychology of Sexual Orientation and Gender Diversity, 2*(3), 209–213. https://doi.org/10.1037/sgd0000132

Milton, M., & Coyle, A., & Legg, C. (2002). Lesbian and gay affirmative psychotherapy: Defining the domain. In A. Coyle & C. Kitzinger (Eds.), *Lesbian and gay psychology: A new perspective.* BPS Blackwell Publishers Ltd.

Nadal, K. L., Whitman, C. N., Davis, L. S., Erazo, T., & Davidof, K. C. (2016). Microaggressions toward lesbian, gay, bisexual, transgender, queer, and genderqueer people: A review of the literature. *Journal of Sex Research, 53*(4–5), 488–508. https://doi.org/10.1080/00224499.2016.1142495

Pearce, W. B., & Pearce, K. A. (1990). Transcendent storytelling: Abilities for systemic practitioners and their clients. *Human Systems, 9*(3–4), 167–185.

Prell, E., & Traeen, B. (2018). Minority stress and mental health among bisexual and lesbian women in Norway. *Journal of Bisexuality, 18*(3), 278–298. https://doi.org/10.1080/15299716.2018.1518180

Proujansky, R. A., & Pachankis, J. E. (2014). Toward formulating evidence-based principles of LGB-affirmative psychotherapy. *Pragmatic Case Studies in Psychotherapy. PCSP, 10*(2), 117–131.

Riggle, E. D. B., Whitman, J. S., Olson, A., Rostosky, S. S., & Strong, S. (2008). The positive aspects of being a lesbian or gay man. *Practitioner Psychology: Research and Practice, 39*(2), 210–217. https://doi.org/10.1037/0735-7028.39.2.210

Ross, L. E., Salway, T., Tarasof, L. A., MacKay, J. M., Hawkins, B. W., & Fehr, C. P. (2018). Prevalence of depression and anxiety among bisexual people compared to gay, lesbian, and heterosexual individuals: A systematic review and meta-analysis. *Journal of Sex Research, 55*(4–5), 435–456. https://doi.org/10.1080/00224499.2017.1387755

Ryle, A. (1995). *Cognitive analytic therapy: Developments in theory and practice.* Wiley.

Semlyen, J., King, M., Varney, J., & Hagger-Johnson, G. (2016). Sexual orientation and symptoms of common mental disorder or low wellbeing: Combined meta-analysis of 12 UK population health surveys. *BMC Psychiatry, 16*(1), 67. https://doi.org/10.1186/s12888-016-0767-z

Simi, N. L., & Mahalik, J. R. (1997). Comparison of feminist versus psychoanalytic/dynamic and other therapists on selfdisclosure. *Psychology of Women Quarterly, 21*(3), 465–483. https://doi.org/10.1111/j.1471-6402.1997.tb00125.x

Spitzer, R. L. (1981). The diagnostic status of homosexuality in DSM-III: A reformulation of the issues. *The American Journal of Psychiatry, 138*(2), 210–215. https://doi.org/10.1176/ajp.138.2.210

Sue, D. W. (2010). *Microaggressions in everyday life: Race, gender and sexual orientation.* Wiley.

Timmins, L., Rimes, K. A., & Rahman, Q. (2020). Minority stressors, rumination and psychological distress in lesbian, gay and bisexual individuals. *Archives of Sexual Behaviour, 49*(2), 661–680. https://doi.org/10.1007/s10508-019-01502-2

9

Sexual, Gender and Relationship Diverse Affirmative Therapy

Catherine Butler⊙, Melissa Brown, Tirtha Kotrial, and Nicola Gunby⊙

Introduction

This chapter focuses on providing culturally competent therapy to clients from Sexual, Gender or Relationship Diverse (SGRD) communities. Sexual diversity might include those who identify as lesbian, gay,

---

C. Butler (✉)
Department of Psychology, University of Exeter, Exeter, UK
e-mail: C.A.Butler@exeter.ac.uk

M. Brown
University of Birmingham, Birmingham, UK
e-mail: mxh1165@student.bham.ac.uk

T. Kotrial
University of the West of England, Bristol, UK
e-mail: tirtha2.kotrial@live.uwe.ac.uk

N. Gunby
University of Bath, Bath, UK
e-mail: Nicola.Gunby@gmmh.nhs.uk

© The Author(s), under exclusive license to Springer Nature Switzerland AG 2023
J. Semlyen and P. Rohleder (eds.), *Sexual Minorities and Mental Health*,
https://doi.org/10.1007/978-3-031-37438-8_9

bisexual, pansexual, queer, kink, etc. Gender diversity might include those who identify as transgender, gender-queer, agender, gender nonbinary, etc. While gender and sexuality are two separate characteristics, they do intersect (see Chapters 7 and 10). Many gender diverse individuals also identify as a minority sexuality identity, the most commonly reported being pansexual or queer (Kuper et al., 2012). Relationship diversity might include those who are polyamorous, non-monogamous, etc. Such individuals might present for therapy specifically about their relationship, gender or sexuality, and wanting a space to talk through these issues from a non-judgemental therapist, or they may present to therapy for a completely different issue, e.g. travel phobia, and so not want their sexual, gender or relationship diversity inappropriately focused on. It is for the therapist to judge when it is, or is not, appropriate to bring issues of sexual, gender or relationship diversity into their questions or formulation. Working collaboratively with the client will create a space where the therapist can ask the client whether this diversity would be useful to bring into the work.

This chapter will focus on why SGRD affirmative therapy is important, what such affirmative therapy might look like and key areas to consider. It should be remembered that there is no blue-print for providing SGRD affirmative therapy, but this chapter suggests some guidelines to work collaboratively with clients to create a space that feels safe for both the client and therapist to explore issues in a non-judgemental way.

SGRD-Affirmative Therapy

Malyon (1982) first used the term 'Gay Affirmative Therapy' to describe a set of organising principles that are trans-theoretical, and so can be adopted when using any therapeutic approach (for examples of this, see Davies & Neal, 1996). However, the term 'Gay Affirmative Therapy' was critiqued for a number of reasons: the use of the term 'Gay' might be taken as excluding anyone who is not a gay man (e.g. lesbians, bisexuals or pansexuals); it is not clear what is being affirmed as (a) all behaviour may not be positive or useful for a client and (b) in terms of whether identity is regarded as fixed or changeable; finally, the term excludes those from gender minorities or with relationship diversity who may also experience mental health issues as a result of discrimination and social exclusion. However, the intention behind the word affirmative was that the therapist is actively promoting and celebrating the client's sexual, gender or relationship choices and identity as equally valid compared to heterosexual, cisgendered, monogamous options that form the majority of British culture. We are therefore using the term 'SGRD-Affirmative' to highlight the need for therapists to be active in their work with clients from sexual, gender and relationship diverse backgrounds, in order to help clients to find a positive and enriching identity and lifestyle, and find the resistance they may need to survive challenges to this from majority culture. A client might belong to all three of these categories or just one, but the same organising principles described in this chapter can be applied regardless of the intersectional presentation of the client.

Why Is SGRD-Affirmative Therapy Needed?

Mental Health and Minority Stress

SGRD individuals' mental health and wellbeing is threatened by discrimination and prejudice (Nel, 2014; Swann et al., 2020—see also Chapter 3); with SGRD populations experiencing higher rates of discrimination (Holman, 2018), assault and harassment (Pepping & Halford, 2014.) These stressors have a major contributing factor to higher rates of depression, anxiety, suicidal ideation, alcohol/substance abuse, smoking, and self-harm (King et al., 2003; Semlyen et al., 2016) for SGRD individuals. This inevitably leads to higher rates of access to therapy than their heterosexual counterparts (Grzanka & Miles, 2016).

As outlined in previous chapters, these stressors have been termed minority stress (Meyer, 2003), representing the clash in values between SGRD group members and dominant society that results in a conflictual social environment of stigma, prejudice (Barnes & Meyer, 2012), oppression and discrimination (Hayes et al., 2011) which, when endured over time, results in mental health problems. For an individual who belongs to more than one minority group, the impact of these stressors can conjugationally be much higher. People who hold multiply marginalised identities, e.g.. SGRDs from ethnic minorities, have been found to report higher levels of distress, depression, and perceived stress when compared to their caucasian SGRD counterparts (Cyrus, 2017; see also Chapter 6). This larger magnitude of psychological distress is experienced as a result of invalidation, insults, exoticization, multiple forms of prejudice and discrimination, including racism in the SGRD communities, and hetero-sexism in their racial/ethnic communities (Bowleg et al., 2003; Balsam et al., 2011; Cyrus, 2017). These intersections are rarely addressed in the literature, with some notable exceptions, and so we therefore consider the intersection of a number of minoritised identities in this chapter.

Legislation

Arguably open-mindedness, compassion and respect should be at the core of any therapeutic or clinical practice. When it comes to considering minority identities however, practitioners also have a legal obligation to provide inclusive and supportive care. The Human Rights Act (1998) was the first UK legislation that protected LGB people from discrimination when using services or at work and paved the way for other legislation changes such as the Adoption and Children's Act change in 2005. Civil Partnership became legal in 2005, allowing LGB people for their first time to legally register their partnerships, and this was followed by the Same-Sex Marriage Act (2014). The Equalities Act (2010) replaced previous single-issue anti-discriminatory laws. Sexual orientation, sex, gender reassignment, and marriage and civil partnerships are all protected characteristics under the Equality Act (2010). This means that under UK law, it is illegal to discriminate against an individual on the basis of any of these characteristics. The Equality Act (2010) moves beyond this however, and states that public sector bodies (e.g., the NHS) also have an Equality Duty to take due regard to the need to promote equality of opportunity, reduce discrimination, and foster relationships between individuals with and without a given protected characteristic. In practice, this means a legal obligation for services to provide SGRD *affirmative* care. Equality duty also extends to fostering an affirmative environment for SGRD staff and colleagues. The NHS in particular are reporting a greater focus on promoting equality and inclusivity within the workforce moving forward, as outlined in the NHS People Plan 2021/2022 (NHS England, 2000). This includes gender, sexual and relationship diversity. Other legislation includes the Protection of Freedoms Act (2012), which allows men who have a previous conviction of consensual gay sex to apply to have this criminal record removed. Therapists are therefore under a legal obligation to provide a non-discriminatory, equal and affirming service to their SGRD clients as to any other clients.

Lack of Training

Therapists should seek to work collaboratively with the client, to create a space to discuss whether their identities and related life choices would be useful to bring into the work. Despite this, evidence suggests that many clinicians do not feel skilled in working with SGRD clients (e.g., Owen-Pugh & Baines, 2014; Salpietro et al., 2019). Studies in the United States have suggested that clinicians are more likely to be less knowledgeable about and have more negative attitudes towards gender diversity compared to sexual diversity (Johnson & Federman, 2014; Logie et al., 2007), with some clinicians holding problematic beliefs about the experiences of gender diverse individuals (Whitman & Han, 2017). Evidence, also from the USA, shows that gender diverse individuals consequently can refrain from seeking help from mental health services (Benson, 2013). A study in Australia analysing data from over 300 clinicians found that knowledge and confidence in working with trans clients is associated with prior experience and training (Riggs & Bartholomaeus, 2016), making training and learning about diversity important for clinicians. Nevertheless, numerous studies highlight a lack of training in this area and indeed in the UK in public sector services, gender, sexual and relationship diversity often falls under general inclusivity and diversity training and is not specifically addressed.

From the therapist perspective, research in the UK has found that trainee counsellors can feel unprepared for working with SGRD clients, including a lack of information on LGBT issues or space to openly explore sex and sexuality within their training (Owen-Pugh & Baines, 2014). Similarly, UK qualified clinical psychologists have reported being unsure when to raise issues of sexuality, lack confidence in discussing these issues and are unsure where to find relevant information and resources (Shaw et al., 2008). Not taking an SGRD-affirmative approach will have a negative impact on the therapeutic relationship (Alessi, 2014), lead to mistrust from clients, possible non-disclosure of SGRD status (Ritter & Terndrup, 2002) in therapy or even prevent clients from accessing therapy altogether (Dardick & Grady, 1980; Hook & Andrews, 2005). Israel et al. (2008) found that experiences of therapy that were perceived as helpful by LGBT clients usually involved work with a therapist that was warm, empathetic, and knowledgeable and helpful in relation to the individual's sexual or gender identity. Unhelpful experiences meanwhile often involved therapists who appeared cold or disinterested, imposed their own values or views upon the client, did not focus on what the client wanted to focus on or, in 21.4% of accounts, responded to the individual's sexual or gender identity in a negative or judgemental way. Unhelpful experiences also included those where individuals were pushed to discuss or disclose topics that they were not ready to. There is evidence that SGRD individuals may find themselves within an 'educator' role in therapy, educating their therapist on either their sexual (Bepko & Johnson, 2000) or gender identity (Motter, 2017; Twist et al., 2017), which is described as unhelpful. This presents practitioners with a need to balance the need for appropriate curiosity and open-mindedness alongside needing to seek out learning and literature on SGRD issues. Without SGRD training forming a part of many therapy training courses, therapists are left seeking their own continued professional development to fill this gap. We hope that this book goes some way in addressing this for the reader, as well as other resources such as guidelines for working with SGRD clients being written by the British Psychological Society (Shaw et al., 2012), American Psychological Association (APA) (2021), and Australian Psychological Society (APS) (2013).

Key Areas to Consider

Coming Out

Coming out and what this means and how it is experienced by the individual has been explored in detail in Chapter 4, where the benefits as well as the potential risks have been outlined. It is important to note that coming out may not always be beneficial or possible to the individual and so careful consideration of these positions should be noted.

A default position to 'come out' can be suggested inadvertently by clinicians, whereby encouragement for the client to navigate and accept a sexual identity can be seen as fully articulated only when disclosed to others (Galarza, 2013). Within these contexts the clinician must be mindful to have cultural awareness and understanding of their clients, in order to ensure they do not risk inviting further psychological or sometimes physical harm as a result of disclosure (Ferguson & Miville, 2017). For example, Chiang et al. (2018) found that in Chinese sexual minorities, although aware of options regarding their sexual identity, many people were not prepared to act on them out of respect for their families' viewpoints and therefore in this context the decision to come out was not appropriate. Clinicians can facilitate this by working with clients to draw upon different attributes of the 'coming out' process, such as assessing the pros and cons, planning the timing, potential consequences, modelling assertive communication, and providing psychoeducation (Duarté-Vélez et al., 2010). These processes often result in the individual becoming more secure with their sexual orientation and through exploration within the therapeutic space they are able to begin the journey of learning to 'pick and choose' when to disclose their sexual orientation (Chiang et al, 2018). By empowering the individual to choose when/if to disclose their sexual identity, they can maximise external support, facilitating growth and personal wellbeing thus reducing any negative impact or discrimination (Chiang et al, 2018). Clinicians must also recognise that the version of the client presented in a therapeutic space may be visible within the safety of the therapeutic context, but it would be inappropriate to extend this into their community for fear of repercussions or further castigation from those who also act as a protective factor for the individual, e.g. in protection from racism (Galarza, 2013).

Not all identities are visible to others and misidentification can occur on multiple levels. Similarly to bisexual or pansexual individuals partnered with opposite sex partners, for partners of trans people, their sexual minority identity can be rendered invisible if their relationship orientation moves from appearing to others as a same-sex relationship to a heterosexual one (e.g., Joslin-Roher & Wheeler, 2009; Moran, 2012). For such couples, there is a conflict between their felt identity and how they may appear to others. Some literature around couples where partners identify as a sexual minority and/or gender diverse shows how such individuals may seek to reaffirm their sexual minority identity through active involvement in the LGBT community and strategic disclosure (Brown, 2009). This might be to counter-balance the loss of recognition as a sexual minority and therefore sometimes LGB community membership (e.g., Pfeffer, 2014), which can happen alongside gaining of heteronormative privilege (and male privilege for the masculine trans individual).

Language

Lev (2004) argues that language can either enable or inhibit the expression of SGRD identities. For some, language and labels might be a means through which people explore their sexual identity (e.g., Pfeffer, 2014). For others however labels may not fully or adequately match one's felt identity or sexuality, rather be a tool by which to express something (i.e., a sexual minority identity) to others (Moran, 2012). There may be no words to describe same-sex love in someone's language of origin (das Nair & Thomas, 2012). Massad (2007) describes the imposition of SGRD labels on some people can feel like colonisation, although regardless of what labels people use to self-identify, they can still experience rejection, discrimination and hate crimes. Language and labels may not always be static throughout a person's life, but an emerging and evolving thing as one's own identity evolves through time and through relationships with others (Moran, 2012).

For some, existing language and categories might not be adequate to express their sexual identities. For example, categories such as lesbian, gay and bisexual are strongly linked to sex and/or gender identity. For gender diverse couples and individuals, sometimes these labels can feel inadequate to express their sexuality (Alegria, 2013; Moran, 2012; Platt & Bolland, 2017). This can result in some adopting new language to express their identities. For example, adopting the term queer rather than lesbian or gay (Brown, 2009), or exploring more creative terms such as *transsensual* (Joslin-Roher & Wheeler, 2009), *heteroflexible* or *situational lesbian* (Alegria, 2013). Some research has highlighted dilemmas around certain terms, for example queer, whereby such terms can be a helpfully inclusive and liberating in that they signify a sexual minority identity without the need to be specific (Chester et al., 2017), but can as a result for some also feel like an empty category (Pfeffer, 2014).

Intersectionality

Whilst Minority Stress theory provides a framework of understanding how various factors can contribute to stress in LGB populations, less is known about the cross-contextual effects of belonging to multiple minority groups and how this can provide unique, culturally specific stressors. Intersectionality considers how multiple oppressions in identity such as race, class, gender and economic status can 'intersect' with one another and overlap (Greene & Flasch, 2019). These compounding characteristics can create obstacles for the individual, which are not often understood or represented within conventional systems of society or articulated within psychological literature. The originals of intersectionality over thirty years ago (Crenshaw, 1991) focused on how experiences of black women were missed by feminism (which ignored race) and anti-racism (which ignored patriarchy). Today, many of the social identities that intersect with sexuality remain ignored or silenced in lived experience and literature (Swank & Fahs, 2013). Purdie-Vaughns and Elbach (2008) refer to this as 'intersectional invisibility': that those who hold multiple subordinate group identities are viewed as atypical by the various groups they belong to. We will briefly address some of the key intersections here, but this is not an exhaustive list and we encourage the reader to further their knowledge through their own research. Previous chapters address some key intersections such as age (Chapter 5), ethnicity (Chapter 6) and gender diversity (Chapter 7) with sexuality.

Visible and Invisible Identities

Ferguson and Miville (2017) refer to 'visibility and invisibility' of different identities. Race is often a visible identity which cannot be concealed, it conveys physical traits, presumed stereotypes and cultural norms, whereas sexual identity can be invisible given heteronormative presumptions that all people are heterosexual. Concealing an identity can result in distress: the individual must consciously and continually adapt to their environment and become hypervigilant to not letting their identity be known. Ferguson and Miville (2017) suggest that those with competing intersections (e.g. race, gender & sexual orientation) may have evolved each identity at different stages of their life, in turn each identity may be developed unevenly. These identities are likely to have been highly influenced by, or dependent on, interactions people have had with friends, family and romantic partners. For those from a racialised ethnic-minority, ethnicity may be the most salient identity, owing to this being a 'visible' identification of who they are and are most likely connected to through family and community; the sexual minority identity may be invisible owing to cultural pressures to conceal.

Race/Racism

The discussion of race and racism is covered in Chapter 6, which outlines the additional marginalisation of sexual minorities from racial/ethnic minority communities as well as the impact of this marginalisation to mental health. Further consideration of this intersection is given here in relation to racial prejudice within the LGBTQ community and some of the unique challenges faced when navigating these communities as an ethnic minority.

Online dating platforms might be considered 'safer' by providing an opportunity to embrace and express one's sexuality with an anonymity that is lacking in person (Hawkins & Watson, 2017). However, such anonymity can extend to unfiltered marginalisation of individuals belonging to racialised ethnic minorities, resulting in explicit sexual rejection or fetishization (Callander et al., 2016). Bhambhani et al. (2020) found that, amongst men seeking men, white men were the most preferred as dating and sexual partners by men of all ethnicities, and black men were least preferred. Similarly, Chiang et al. (2018) identifies prejudices against Asians in online dating, where users would state 'no Asians' on their dating profiles. Those from ethnic minorities have also reported being romantically or sexually rejected either online or in public gay venues because of their skin colour (Bhambhani et al., 2020) and in some instances, made to 'prove' their sexuality by engaging in public displays of affection (das Nair & Thomas, 2012).

Clinicians, if unaware of the existence and effect of these macro-aggressions, may encourage LGB individuals from ethnic minorities to seek partners online or in a real-life setting. Macro-aggressions reinforce the position of oppression and rejection commonly experienced by individuals of a racialised ethnic minority and are further compounded by being rejected within the sexual minority group. The rejection may cause the individual to render their sexual identity invisible and reinforce the belief of unworthiness, resulting in internalised homophobia (David et al., 2019) based on consistent and recurrent rejection from both minority groups. The Rejection Sensitivity Model (Feinstein, 2020) proposes that early experiences of rejection can lead to expectations of future rejection where the individual places high importance on avoiding rejection. For the SGRD ethnic minority, this may result in avoiding specific SGRD spaces.

Some racialised minority groups are stereotypically believed to be overtly homophobic (das Nair & Thomas, 2012). If an individual comes from a supposedly homophobic racialised ethnic group, they are at risk of experiencing the effects of stereotyping and sexual racism from members of SGRD communities who view them as indistinguishable from this ethnic identity. SGRD racialised ethnic minorities can therefore be seen as the aggressors, targets of condemnation, rather than beneficiaries of support usually offered to those who fall victim to acts of homophobia (das Nair & Thomas, 2012). White SGRD individuals may be wary of becoming sources of support to LGB racialised ethnic minorities owing to the negative connotations associated with the wider ethnic group.

Other stereotypes exist when someone from a racial/ethnic minority is visibly gay; for example, East Asian men are assumed to be effeminate (das Nair & Thomas, 2012). Such stereotypical prejudices can create discomfort and a feeling of being unwelcome. Kawale (2003) found that South Asian lesbians/bisexuals enjoyed being in social spaces with South Asian gay/bisexual South Asian men, whereas White lesbian participants preferred women-only spaces. Kawale (2003) reports that this preference was because of a proxy-kinship bond that reinforced feelings of community. This may be caused by the majority of such queer spaces being dominated by white populations, giving them not only hegemony but also a 'natural invisibility' (Kawale, 2003). Thus, this may leave those with racial minority identities, such as the South Asians in Kawale's study, to coalesce in solidarity having a shared experience that may be more visible comparactive to their sexual idenity (Fattoracci et al., 2021).

However, despite many reports of sexual racism, census reports have showed that interracial relationships are more common in sexual minorities compared to heterosexual relationships (Robinson & Frost, 2017). There are a number of ideas proposed as to why this is. The 'minority solidarity assumption' is the belief that members of one minority group are more unprejudiced toward members of other minority groups (Robinson & Frost, 2017), although the research previously mentioned might debunk this idea. Alternatively, it has been proposed that there is a smaller 'dating pool' for people with LGB identities, leading to exploration of dating out of their own racialised ethnic group (Robinson & Frost, 2017). Whether or not either idea is accurate, assumptions cannot be made about mixed-race relationships, but White partners may have their eyes opened to the racism that exists within the LGB community.

Disability

Physically disabled people are often considered asexual (Morris, 1991), while learning disabled people can be considered rampant (Rohleder et al., 2018; Thompson et al., 2001), but in all cases, the assumed norm is heterosexual (O'Toole & Bregante, 1992). When LGB identities are acknowledged within disabled people, these can be viewed as because they have 'failed' to attract on opposite-sex partner (O'Toole, 2000). These general societal views of sexuality are also prevalent in care staff who can be discriminatory, e.g. Clarke and Finnegan (2005) found that 76% of staff would support heterosexual relationships but only 41% would support same-sex relationships. Discrimination can also be found within LGB communities, where there can be an emphasis on social and financial capital and fit, non-disabled bodies (Thompson et al., 2001), and with disability rights groups, where LGB people can be shunned (O'Toole & Bregant, 1992). A lack of support might have started in someone's family of origin, where they may be the only LGB member and/or the only disabled member (Shakespeare, 1996). Shakespeare (1996) found that LGB disabled people were discouraged from exploring sex and relationships compared to their heterosexual siblings. In adult relationships, dating a disabled person may leave a non-disabled person having their choices questioned (Bullard & Knight, 1981), or being seen as a non-sexual carer (O'Toole & Bregante, 1992). Similarly, if two disabled people are dating, it can be assumed that it is because neither has been 'successful' in dating a non-disabled person (Morris, 1991). Where one partner becomes disabled during a relationship, established relationship and sexual patterns may need to adjust and many relationships break down.

Autism

Historically there has been a misconception that autistic individuals are not interested in and cannot have successful and satisfying sexual relationships (Bennett et al., 2018). Thankfully this attitude is changing with greater emphasis being placed on research into autistic sexualities (e.g., Dewinter et al., 2013). Higher numbers of individuals in the autistic population identify as sexual or gender minorities (e.g., Dewinter et al., 2017; Gilmour et al., 2012). One project found that approximately 70% of autistic adults identified as non-heterosexual compared with 30% in the non-autistic sample (George & Stokes, 2018). This includes higher reported rates of asexuality within this population (e.g., Bush et al., 2021). There appear to be some gender differences within this too, which more autistic women reported identifying as a sexual minority than autistic men (Gilmour et al., 2012). As such, autistic individuals may be more likely to require SGRD affirmative information and support. This requires attention and consideration from practitioners working with autistic individuals.

Class

Academic literature into LGB lives often ignores class and assumes the subject is middle-class (das Nair & Hansen, 2012). There are notable exceptions to this (e.g. Keogh et al., 2004; McDermott, 2006; Riggs, 2010; Taylor, 2008, 2010), and these researchers found that class intersected socially and personally for working-class people, often being an organising factor in their lives. An example of this is that butch-femme identities are more common amongst working class lesbian women, but often critiqued and rejected by middle class women (das Nair & Hansen, 2012). Meyer (2010) also found another class difference in how friends and family responded following violent hate crime: middle class survivors were encouraged to report the crime and seek medical/psychological help, working class survivors were encouraged to minimise their violence and consider those who had suffered worse than themselves.

Professionals offering help can be regarded by working class people as not to be trusted and experienced as "bureaucratic, dehumanizing and oppressive" (Strier & Binyamin, 2010, p. 1918). This is particularly so of therapists, who are often themselves middle class and whose professional training is based on the middle-class values of individualism, personal choice and responsibility (Kearney, 2010). This can impact both on the therapeutic relationship and process of therapy, and the content of therapy as the therapist may struggle to understand their clients' lives, for example the constraints people are living under. These constraints might relate to financial stress or life/work balance, or relate specifically to the intersection with sexuality, e.g. in not being able to partake in the consumerism (fashion, gay scene, etc.) that can accompany gay culture (das Nair & Hansen, 2012).

Religion

To be LGB and adhere to a religious faith, can be a polar experience of finding general solace, comfort and protection, but when it comes to one's sexuality, experiencing judgement and condemnation (das Nair & Thomas, 2012). While there are some LGB supportive religious spaces, e.g. churches within Christianity, or in religious texts and temples, e.g. texts, sculptures and paintings in Hinduism, this is not so for other faiths such as Islam. Coming out as LGB may risk expulsion from one's family of origin accompanied by a lack of support financially, emotionally and protectively against issues such as Islamophobia (das Nair & Thomas, 2012). It may therefore not be safe to do so, although this could be accompanied by feelings of isolation. Alternatively, LGB people might be out but feel estranged and unwelcome in communal worship (Cahill, 2011). People may experience a sense of dissonance between their sexual and religious identities (Yip & Khalid, 2010). While it can be hard to find spiritual support within mainstream religious institutions, and LGB support within religious institutions, family and friends, there are third sector organisations that offer support and the opportunity to meet others, e.g. The Jewish LGBT+ Group. However, it may be easier to use such support groups online if someone is fearful of being seen in such a group and thus 'outed'. Alternatively, someone may maintain a sense of spirituality that compliments their sexuality, while rejecting religion (Lease et al., 2005).

Over the past 30 years, there has been an increase in writing from LGB supportive spiritual scholars, which Yip (2010) helpfully synthesises into three main themes: 'defensive apologetics', 'cruising texts' and 'turning theology upside down'. The first theme constitutes where passages that have traditionally been used to condemn homosexuality, are re-contextualised to support it. For example, rather than the story of Sodom and Gomorra in Christianity and Islam being viewed as God's punishment of same-sex sexuality, it is recast as God's punishment of inhospitality. Alternatively, the original religious texts are viewed as specific to the culture and time in which they were written and so inapplicable to modern day life. The flip side of this is 'cruising texts', where writers have sought out examples of same-sex intimacy and eroticism within original religious texts, e.g. in Christianity the intimate relationships between Ruth and Naomi, or between David and Jonathan. The final view is that of an embodied spirituality where sexuality and spirituality are interconnected. Sexuality is linked to not only to sex, but also to relationships, sensuality, commitment, devotion, which reflects the human relationship with God. This latter 'school' has pushed for changes in religious practice such as same-sex marriage. It is therefore possible for some people to be openly LGB and openly religious and proud of both of these identities.

Relationship Diversity

Monogamy is considered the norm in relationships, including many LGB relationships. Relationships that are prized are those of coupledom, love over sex and sexual exclusivity (Moors et al., 2013; Pieper & Bauer, 2005). However, other forms of relationships exist in both heterosexual and LGB communities, and both groups face misunderstandings and prejudice. Even when non-monogamous and polyamorous relationships are recognised, there is often a primary couple dyad assumed (Bairstow, 2017; Barker & Langdridge, 2010). However, there are multiple meanings, definitions and practices across individuals who live diverse relationships and no one-size fits all. Some general categories exist within relationship diversity, but Frank and DeLamater (2010) emphasize that people might be fluid in their identity, relationship arrangements and practice over time. The categories are:

- Polygamy, in some countries one person can marry multiple people;

- Polyamory, an individual has multiple romantic and/or sexual partners but is not married to them (although they might be to one of them);
- Open marriage/relationship, a couples agree to have additional sexual relationships (these might themselves take the form of polyamory or swinging);
- Swinging is similar to an open marriage/relationship but rather than being an agreement between a couple, it extends to an organised behaviour that might be either spontaneously arranged or via an organised club or site;
- Casual relationships refer to where people have an ongoing sexual and/ or romantic connection but they are not exclusive to each other.

This list of possible diverse forms of relationships is not exclusive and therapists should explore a client's unique practices and perspectives on their relationship diversity. Apart from polygamy, which is socially and culturally sanctioned, what all these different relationship forms have in common is that they are misunderstood and have a lack of social acceptance (Balzarini & Muise, 2020). If there is a primary couple within the arrangement, it is important that this couple do not neglect their own relationship and that they work on issues of jealousy when it presents itself.

Key Recommendations for SGRD-Affirmative/ Affirmative Therapy

There are a number of ways that a therapist can be affirmative of SGRD people, considered below.

Considering one's Own Identity

We all have a gender, sexual or relationship identity of some kind. As such, it makes sense that work in this area will bring up different thoughts, feelings and responses for practitioners, regardless of whether they themselves identify with a majority or minority sexuality, gender identity or relationship orientation. Some studies have highlighted discomfort that might arise for therapists from hearing views or experiences of a given identity that might conflict with their own, for example, a gender diverse client expressing ideas of what it means to be a woman that directly conflict with a therapist's sense of what it means to be a woman (Gunby, 2021). In addition, client come with intersecting identities and therapists should also be self-aware of their assumptions and prejudices they hold about all aspects of a client's identities and the additional assumptions that might be held about how these identities intersect.

For practitioners who themselves identify as SRGD, research has highlighted specific issues such as disclosure of their own identity or the issue of a shared space from being members of the same local LGBT community as clients and thus a high likelihood of running into one another socially or knowing people in common (Owen-Pugh & Baines, 2014). Several studies have highlighted issues of the majority culture creating censorship or feeling disinhibited in asking overly-personal questions. For example, in Owen-Pugh and Baines's (2014) study, SGRD practitioners felt their non-SGRD colleagues censored their conversations about sexuality and gender around them. Clinicians can feel a sense trepidation, inhibition, or fear of mis-stepping around discussing sexuality or gender issues both within and outside of the clinical space (e.g. Gunby, 2021). It is clear that work in this area requires practitioners to reflect upon their own experiences and ideas in relation to sexuality, gender and relationships. These reflections might be helped by speaking to a trusted colleague, friend or supervisor and invite challenge and questioning about one's position.

Educating Oneself

Clients can feel the need to educate therapists about sexuality, gender minority and relationship related issues. Through self-reflection and self-knowledge, therapists should be aware of the limits of their knowledge and seek out opportunities to expand this outside of the therapy space. This might be through reading, watching films or documents, training opportunities or joining advocacy or support organisations. To be authentic, this work needs to take place in a therapist's personal life and not just in a work setting. This is an individual journey based on a therapist's own gaps in knowledge, so it is essential that therapists take time to be self-reflexive about what these gaps are so that they can target the learning they need to do now. As a therapist learns more about an area, the types of knowledge and understanding they need will shift and change; it is important to recognise that one never arrives at knowing everything there is to know. The concept of 'cultural humility' (Foronda et al., 2016) is useful here to recognise that this is a lifelong journey.

Considering Language

Therapists should remain aware of the importance and impact of language that is inclusive within services. This includes not assuming that everyone is heterosexual, cisgendered, with just one partner or monogamous, and so not basing conversations and questions from this assumed position. When working with non-binary or gender fluid clients or colleagues, it is important to avoid gender binary language and ask about preferred pronouns. Forms that clients are asked to complete should also be scrutinised to check that they include all identities, or options to self-describe if not practical. Therapists should be aware that terminology may mean different things to different people (e.g., the term 'queer'), as discussed earlier in this chapter. Therapists should attempt to remain curious about individual experiences where appropriate in the therapeutic work, but not to satisfy their personal curiosity (e.g., "I understand the word queer, but I also understand that queer can be used in different ways to mean different things. What does queer mean to you?").

Recommendations When Working with Clients with Multiple Minority Intersecting Identities

Cultural and practical adaptations may need to be made to meet the needs of the SGRD individuals with intersecting minority identities.

Clinicians should remain curious in order to gain an understanding of these needs through the lens of their clients, as well as doing their own research to educate themselves. The therapeutic space may be used for safe exploration where the individual can experiment with different narratives of their visible and invisible identities. It must be noted that making the sexual identity visible outside of the therapeutic space must not be benchmarked as a successful intervention. By empowering the individual to understand their sexuality, this will encourage them to learn how to navigate their world without shame or guilt.

Clinicians should be aware that competence in this area requires continual learning as groups, practices and contexts evolve over time. Clinicians should be cautious of promoting SGRD communities as homogenous supportive groups, and have an understanding of the potential negative consequences that an SGRD client with other minority identities may experience when entering these spaces.

Recommendations for Clinical Practice When Working with Couples and Families

There are likely to be different perspectives and levels of comfort within couples and families in relation to SGRD issues. Experiences of gender and sexuality differ between people and across generations. Experiences of acceptance and rejection are pivotal to an SGRD's well-being and should be explored within a family/couple context as journeys may be shared but they are not the same for the actors involved. However, it should be recognised that a change in one person's identity affects the identity of another (husband to wife, son to daughter). Family members may lose or gain privilege as an SGRD individual 'comes out', and space to explore this is useful.

Therapists should not assume sexual, gender or relationship orientation of either member of a couple. This is especially pertinent due to the sometimes invisible nature of sexual minority identities, and sometimes gender variant identities, and given that it is possible to have mixed-identity relationships (e.g., lesbian ciswoman partnered with a straight trans man). Chapter 14 discusses couple work in more detail.

Conclusion

As this chapter has highlighted, every client is unique and complex and therapists need to approach every client with respect, curiosity and acceptance. The balance between curiosity and acceptance is an interesting one and a recent phenomenon that has emerged from transgender debates is that therapists have been concerned about taking an explorative stance with clients, worried that if they do anything but affirm someone's identity then they will be accused of conversion therapy. This does our clients a disservice as while many clients have spent years working on understanding their identities, some clients are still in the process of doing this and need a therapist who will walk with them on this journey without judgement about where the final end point will be. *Affirming* does not mean *confirming*, and the exploration of a client's unique experiences and meanings of their sexuality, gender and relationships diversity, particularly within their intersecting contexts, is not excluded by taking an affirmative approach. Therapists need to stay open to change and development as our clients are not fixed in time, and neither are the contexts and world in which we coalesce.

References

Alegría, C. A. (2013). Relational and sexual fluidity in females partnered with male-to-female transsexual persons. *Journal of Psychiatric and Mental Health Nursing, 20*(2), 142–149.

Alessi, E. J. (2014). A framework for incorporating minority stress theory into treatment with sexual minority clients. *Journal of Gay & Lesbian Mental Health, 18*(1), 47–66.

American Psychological Association (APA). (2021). *APA guidelines for psychological practice with sexual minority persons.* https://www.apa.org/about/policy/psychological-sexual-minority-persons.pdf

Australian Psychological Society. (2013). *Sexual identity and gender diversity.* https://psychology.org.au/getmedia/e0673849-ff5b-41b0-a16a-14980050c990/information-sheet-sexual-identity-and-gender-diversity.pdf

Balsam, K. F., Molina, Y., Beadnell, B., Simoni, J., & Walters, K. (2011). Measuring multiple minority stress: The LGBT People of Color Microaggressions Scale. *Cultural Diversity and Ethnic Minority Psychology, 17*(2), 163.

Balzarini, R. N., & Muise, A. (2020). Beyond the dyad: A review of the novel insights gained from studying consensual non-monogamy. *Current Sexual Health Reports, 12*, 1–7.

Barker, M., & Langdridge, D. (Eds.). (2010). *Understanding non-monogamies*. Routledge.

Barnes, D. M., & Meyer, I. H. (2012). Religious affiliation, internalized homophobia, and mental health in lesbians, gay men, and bisexuals. *American Journal of Orthopsychiatry, 82*(4), 505–515.

Bairstow, A. (2017). Couples exploring nonmonogamy: Guidelines for therapists. *Journal of Sex & Marital Therapy, 43*(4), 343–353.

Bennett, M., Webster, A. A., Goodall, E., & Rowland, S. (2018). Intimacy and romance across the autism spectrum: Unpacking the "not interested in sex" myth. In M Bennett, A. A. Webster, E. Goodall, & S. Rowland (Eds.), *Life on the autism spectrum*. Springer.

Benson, K. E. (2013). Seeking support: Transgender client experiences with mental health services. *Journal of Feminist Family Therapy, 25*(1), 17–40.

Bepko, C., & Johnson, T. (2000). Gay and lesbian couples in therapy: Perspectives for the contemporary family therapist. *Journal of Marital and Family Therapy, 26*(4), 409–419.

Bhambhani, Y., Flynn, M. K., Kellum, K. K., & Wilson, K. G. (2020). The role of psychological flexibility as a mediator between experienced sexual racism and psychological distress among men of color who have sex with men. *Archives of Sexual Behavior, 49*(2), 711–720.

Bowleg, L., Huang, J., Brooks, K., Black, A., & Burkholder, G. (2003). Triple jeopardy and beyond: Multiple minority stress and resilience among Black lesbians. *Journal of Lesbian Studies, 7*(4), 87–108.

Brown, N. R. (2009). "I'm in transition too": Sexual identity renegotiation in sexual-minority women's relationships with transsexual men. *International Journal of Sexual Health, 21*(1), 61–77.

Bullard, D. G., & Knight, S. E. (1981). *Sexuality and physical disability: Personal perspectives*. Mosby.

Bush, H. H., Williams, L. W., & Mendes, E. (2021). Brief report: Asexuality and young women on the autism spectrum. *Journal of Autism and Developmental Disorders, 51*(2), 725–733.

Cahill, B. (2011). Don't let church leaders drive you away. *National Catholic Reporter, 41*(16), 25.

Callander, D., Holt, M., & Newman, C. E. (2016). 'Not everyone's gonna like me': Accounting for race and racism in sex and dating web services for gay and bisexual men. *Ethnicities, 16*(1), 3–21.

Chester, K., Lyons, A., & Hopner, V. (2017). 'Part of me already knew': The experiences of partners of people going through a gender transition process. *Culture, Health & Sexuality, 19*(12), 1404–1417.

Chiang, S. Y., Fleming, T., Lucassen, M. F. G., Fouche, C., & Fenaughty, J. (2018). From secrecy to discretion: The views of psychological therapists on supporting Chinese sexual and gender minority young people. *Children and Youth Services Review, 93*(1), 307–314.

Clarke, S., & Finnegan, P. (2005). *One law for all? The impact of the Human Rights Act on people with learning difficulties.* Values into Action.

Crenshaw, K. (1991). Intersectionality mapping the margins. *Stanford Law Review, 43*(6), 1241–1260.

Cyrus, K. (2017). Multiple minorities as multiply marginalized: Applying the minority stress theory to LGBTQ people of color. *Journal of Gay & Lesbian Mental Health, 21*(3), 194–202.

Dardick, L., & Grady, K. E. (1980). Openness between gay persons and health professionals. *Annals of Internal Medicine, 93*(1_Part_1), 115–119.

das Nair., R., & Hansen, S. (2012). Social class. In R. das Nair & C. Butler (Eds.), *Intersectionality, sexuality and psychological therapies: working with lesbian, gay and bisexual diversity.* BPS Blackwell

das Nair., R., & Thomas, S. (2012) Race and ethnicity. In R. das Nair & C. Butler (Eds.), *Intersectionality, sexuality and psychological therapies: Working with lesbian, gay and bisexual diversity.* BPS Blackwell.

Davies, D., & Neal, C. (Eds.). (1996). *Pink therapy: A guide for counsellors and therapists working with lesbian, gay and bisexual clients.* Open University Press.

David, E. J. R., Schroeder, T. M., & Fernandez, J. (2019). Internalised Racism: A systematic review of the psychological literature on racisms most insidious consequence. *Journal of Social Issues, 75*(4), 1057–1086.

Dewinter, J., De Graaf, H., & Begeer, S. (2017). Sexual orientation, gender identity, and romantic relationships in adolescents and adults with autism spectrum disorder. *Journal of Autism and Developmental Disorders, 47*(9), 2927–2934.

Dewinter, J., Vermeiren, R., Vanwesenbeeck, I., & van Nieuwenhuizen, C. (2013). Autism and normative sexual development: A narrative review. *Journal of Clinical Nursing, 22*(23–24), 3467–3483.

Duarté-Vélez, Y., Bernal, G., & Bonilla, K. (2010). Culturally adapted cognitive-behavioral therapy: Integrating sexual, spiritual, and family identities in an evidence-based treatment of a depressed Latino adolescent. *Journal of Clinical Psychology, 66*(8), 895–906.

Equality Act 2010, c.15. http://www.legislation.gov.uk/ukpga/2010/15/pdfs/ukpga_20100015_en.pdf

Fattoracci, E. S., Revels-Macalinao, M., & Huynh, Q. L. (2021). Greater than the sum of racism and heterosexism: Intersectional microaggressions toward racial/ethnic and sexual minority group members. *Cultural Diversity and Ethnic Minority Psychology, 27*(2), 176.

Ferguson, A. D., & Miville, M. L. (2017). It's complicated: Navigating multiple identities in small town America. *Journal of Clinical Psychology., 73*(8), 975–984.

Feinstein, B. A. (2020). The rejection sensitivity model as a framework for understanding sexual minority mental health. *Archives of Sexual Behaviour., 49*(7), 2247–2258.

Foronda, C., Baptiste, D.-L., & Reinholdt, M. M. (2016). Cultural humility: A concept analysis. *Journal of Transcultural Nursing, 27*(3), 210–217.

Frank, K., & DeLamater, J. (2010). Deconstructing monogamy. In M. Barker & D. Langdridge (Eds.), *Understanding non-monogamies*. Routledge.

Galarza, J. (2013). Borderland queer: Narrative approaches in clinical work with Latina women who have sex with women (WSW). *Journal of LGBT Issues in Counseling, 7*(3), 274–291.

Gilmour, L., Schalomon, P. M., & Smith, V. (2012). Sexuality in a community based sample of adults with autism spectrum disorder. *Research in Autism Spectrum Disorders, 6*, 313–318.

George, R., & Stokes, M. A. (2018). Sexual orientation in autism spectrum disorder. *Autism Research, 11*, 133–141.

Greene, J. H., & Flasch, P. S. (2019). Integrating Intersectionality into Clinical supervision: A developmental model addressing broader definitions of multicultural competence. *Journal of Counselor Preparation and Supervision., 12*(4), 14.

Grzanka, P. R., & Miles, J. R. (2016). The problem with the phrase "intersecting identities": LGBT affirmative therapy, intersectionality, and neoliberalism. *Sexuality Research and Social Policy, 13*(4), 371–389.

Gunby, N. (2021). *Understanding therapists' experiences of working with Trans clients to inform training and clinical practice within an NHS Secondary Care Psychological Therapies Service* (Unpublished doctoral dissertation). University of Bath Repository.

Hawkins, B., & Watson, R. J. (2017). Viewpoint: LGBT cyberspaces: A need for a holistic investigation. *Children's Geographies, 15*(1), 122.

Hayes, J. A., Chun-Kennedy, C., Edens, A., & Locke, B. D. (2011). Do double minority students face double jeopardy? Testing minority stress theory. *Journal of College Counseling, 14*(2), 117–126.

Holman, E. G. (2018). Theoretical extensions of minority stress theory for sexual minority individuals in the workplace: A Cross-contextual understanding of minority stress processes. *Journal of Family Theory & Review, 10*(1), 165–180.

Hook, A., & Andres, B. (2005). The relationship of non-disclosure in therapy to shame and depression. *British Journal of Clinical Psychology, 44*, 425–438.

Israel, T., Gorcheva, R., Walther, W. A., Sulzner, J. M., & Cohen, J. (2008). Therapists' helpful and unhelpful situations with LGBT clients: An exploratory study. *Professional Psychology: Research and Practice, 39*(3), 361.

Johnson, L., & Federman, E. J. (2014). Training, experience, and attitudes of VA psychologists regarding LGBT issues: Relation to practice and competence. *Psychology of Sexual Orientation and Gender Diversity, 1*, 10–18.

Joslin-Roher, E., & Wheeler, D. P. (2009). Partners in transition: The transition experience of lesbian, bisexual, and queer identified partners of transgender men. *Journal of Gay and Lesbian Social Services, 21*(1), 30–48.

Kawale, R. (2003). A kiss is just a kiss … or is it? South Asian lesbian and bisexual women and the construction of space. In N. Purward & P. Raghuram (Eds.), *South Asian women in the diaspora*. Berg.

Kearney, A. (2010). Class and counselling. In C. Lago & B. Smith (Eds.), *Anti-discriminatory practice in counselling & psychology; Professional skills for counsellors*. Sage.

Keogh, P., Dodds, C., & Henderson, L. (2004). *Working class gay men: Redefining community, restoring identity*. Stigma Research.

King, M., McKeown, E., & Warner, J. (2003). *Mental health and social wellbeing in gay men, lesbians and bisexuals in England and Wales*. Mind.

Kuper, L. E., Nussbaum, R., & Mustanski, B. (2012). Exploring the diversity of gender and sexual orientation identities in an online sample of transgender individuals. *Journal of Sex Research, 49*(2–3), 244–254.

Lease, S., Horne, S., & Noffsinger-Frazier, N. (2005). Affirming faith experiences and psychological health for Caucasian lesbian, gay, and bisexual individuals. *Journal of Counseling Psychology, 52*, 378–388.

Lev, A. I. (2004). *Transgender emergence: Therapeutic guidelines for working with gender-variant people and their families*. Routledge.

Logie, C., Bridge, T. J., & Bridge, P. D. (2007). Evaluating the phobias, attitudes, and cultural competence of master of social work students toward the LGBT populations. *Journal of Homosexuality, 53*, 201–221.

Malyon, A. K. (1982). Psychotherapeutic implications of internalized homophobia in gay men. *Journal of Homosexuality, 7*(2–3), 59–69.

McDermott, E. (2006). Surviving in dangerous places: Lesbian identity performances in the workplace, social class and psychological health. *Feminism and Psychology, 16*(2), 193–211.

Massad, J. A. (2007). *Desiring Arabs*. University of Chicago Press.

Meyer, D. (2010). Evaluating the severity of hate-motivated violence: Intersectional differences among LGBT hate crime victims. *Sociology, 44*(5), 980–995.

Meyer, I. H. (2003). Prejudice, social stress, and mental health in lesbian, gay, and bisexual populations: Conceptual issues and research evidence. *Psychological Bulletin, 129*(5), 674.

Moors, A. C., Matsick, J. L., Ziegler, A., Rubin, J. D., & Conley, T. D. (2013). Stigma toward individuals engaged in consensual nonmonogamy: Robust and worthy of additional research. *Analyses of Social Issues and Public Policy, 13*(1), 52–69.

Moran, C. (2012). '*Whatever it is, it's not lesbian sex!' Transmen and their partners: A conversation about labels, transitioning, sex, and sexuality* (Doctoral dissertation, The Chicago School of Professional Psychology). Retrieved 19 April 2021, from https://search.proquest.com/openview/703509e699f0e28 969f622391d2e5d53/1?pq-origsite=gscholar&cbl=18750&diss=y

Morris, J. (1991). *Pride against prejudice: Transforming attitudes to disability*. The Women's Press.

Motter, B. L. (2017). '*Love is gender blind': The lived experiences of transgender couples who navigate one partner's gender transition* (Doctoral dissertation, University of Northern Colorado). ProQuest Information & Learning.

Nel, J. A. (2014). South African psychology can and should provide leadership in advancing understanding of sexual and gender diversity on the African continent. *South African Journal of Psychology, 44*(2), 124–148.

NHS England. (2000). *Online version of the People Plan for 2020/2021*. https:// www.england.nhs.uk/ournhspeople/online-version/

Owen-Pugh, V., & Baines, L. (2014). Exploring the clinical experiences of novice counsellors working with LGBT clients: Implications for training. *Counselling and Psychotherapy Research, 14*(1), 19–28.

O'Toole, C. J. (2000). The view from below: Developing a knowledge base about an unknown population. *Sexuality and Disability, 18*(3), 207–224.

O'Toole, C. J., & Bregante, J. L. (1992). Lesbians with disabilities. *Sexuality and Disability, 10*(3), 163–172.

Pepping, C. A., & Halford, W. K. (2014). Relationship education and therapy for same-sex couples. *Australian and New Zealand Journal of Family Therapy, 35*(4), 431–444.

Pfeffer, C. A. (2014). "I Don't like passing as a straight woman": Queer negotiations of identity and social group membership. *American Journal of Sociology, 120*(1), 1–44.

Pieper, M., & Bauer, R. (2005). Polyamory and mono-normativity. In L. Méritt, T. Bührmann, & N.B. Schefzig (Eds.), *Mehr als eitte Libe, Polyamouröse Beziehungen.* Orlanda

Platt, L. F., & Bolland, K. S. (2017). Trans* partner relationships: A qualitative exploration. *Journal of GLBT Family Studies, 13*(2), 163–185.

Purdie-Vaughns, V., & Elbach, R. P. (2008). Intersectional invisibility: The Distinctive advantages and disadvantages of multiple subordinate group identities. *Sex Roles, 59*(6), 377–391.

Riggs, D. W. (2010). On accountability: Towards a white middle-class queer 'post identity politics identity politics.' *Ethnicities, 10*(3), 344–357.

Riggs, D. W., & Bartholomaeus, C. (2016). Australian mental health professionals' competencies for working with trans clients: A comparative study. *Psychology & Sexuality, 7*(3), 225–238.

Ritter, K., & Terndrup, A. I. (2002). *Handbook of affirmative psychotherapy with lesbians and gay men.* Guilford Press.

Rohleder, P., Braathen, S. H., & Carew, M. (2018). *Disability and sexual health: A critical exploration of key issues.* Routledge.

Robinson, R. K., & Frost, D. M. (2017). LGBT equality and sexual racism. *Fordham Law Review, 86*(6). https://ir.lawnet.fordham.edu/flr/vol86/iss6/9

Salpietro, L., Ausloos, C., & Clark, M. (2019). Cisgender professional counselors' experiences with trans* clients. *Journal of LGBT Issues in Counseling, 13*(3), 198–215.

Semlyen, J., King, M., Varney, J., & Hagger-Johnson, G. (2016). Sexual orientation and symptoms of common mental disorder or low wellbeing: Combined meta-analysis of 12 UK population health surveys. *BMC Psychiatry, 16*(1), 2–9.

Shakespeare, T. (1996). Disability, identity and difference: In C. Barnes & G. Mercer (Eds.), *Exploring the divide*. The Disability Press.

Shaw, L., Butler, C., & Marriott, C. (2008). Sex and sexuality teaching in UK Clinical Psychology training courses. *Clinical Psychology Forum, 187*, 7–11.

Shaw, E., Butler, C., Langdridge, D., Gibson, S., Barker, M., Lenihan, P., das Nair, R., & Richards, C. (2012). *Guidelines and literature review for psychologists working therapeutically with sexual and gender minority clients*. British Psychological Society.

Strier, R., & Binyamin, S. (2010). Developing anti-oppressive services for the poor: A theoretical and organisational rationale. *British Journal of Social Work, 40*(6), 1908–1926.

Swank, E., & Fahs, B. (2013). An intersectional analysis of gender and race for sexual minorities who engage in gay and lesbian rights activism. *Sex Roles, 68*(11), 660–674.

Swann, G., Stephens, J., Newcomb, M. E., & Whitton, S. W. (2020). Effects of sexual/gender minority and race based enacted stigma on mental health and substance use in female assigned at birth sexual minority youth. *Culture Diversity & Ethnic Minority Psychology., 26*(2), 239–249.

Taylor, Y. (2008). That's not really my theme: Working class lesbians in (and out of) place. *Sexualities, 11*, 523–546.

Taylor, Y. (2010). Complexities and complications: Intersections of class and sexuality. In Y. Taylor, S. Hines, & M. Casey (Eds.), *Theorizing intersectionality and sexuality*. Palgrave Macmillan.

Thompson, S. A., Bryon, M., & Castell, S. (2001). Prospects for identity formation for lesbian, gay or bisexual persons with developmental disabilities. *International Journal of Disability, Development and Education, 48*(1), 53–65.

Twist, J., Barker, M. J., Nel, P. W., & Horley, N. (2017). Transitioning together: A narrative analysis of the support accessed by partners of trans people. *Sexual and Relationship Therapy, 32*(2), 227–243.

Whitman, C. N., & Han, H. (2017). Clinician competencies: Strengths and limitations for work with transgender and gender non-conforming (TGNC) clients. *International Journal of Transgenderism, 18*(2), 154–171.

Yip, A. K. T. (2010). Coming home from the wilderness: An overview of recent scholarship research on LGBTQI religiosity/spirituality in the West. In K. Browne, S. R. Munt, & A. T. K. Yip (Eds.), *Queer spiritual spaces: Sexuality and sacred spaces*. Ashgate.

Yip, A. T. K., & Khalid, A. (2010). Looking for Allah: Spiritual quests of queer Muslims. In K. Browne, S. R. Munt, & A. T. K. Yip (Eds.), *Queer spiritual spaces: Sexuality and sacred spaces*. Ashgate.

10

Queer Trans People and Therapeutic Practice

Shoshana Rosenberg⊙ and Damien W. Riggs⊙

Introduction

When discussing LGBTQ+ people's lives, it is often thought that this initialism refers to a set of separate people: lesbians, gay people, bisexual people, trans people, queer people and so on. However, there are many people who exist at the intersections of several of these identities, most notably trans LGBQ+ people (see Chapter 7). Several studies have shown that trans people have a diverse range of sexualities and choices of sexual partners (Callander et al., 2019; Grant et al., 2010; Riggs & Due, 2013; Strauss et al., 2017). But it does not take a national survey to explicate this point; while some trans peoples may not identify as LGBQ+ (Ansara, 2010), queerness is inextricably linked with transness by the merit of trans and queer peoples' effect on the world. That is to say, queer

S. Rosenberg · D. W. Riggs (✉)
College of Education, Psychology and Social Work, Flinders University, Adelaide, SA, Australia
e-mail: damien.riggs@flinders.edu.au

© The Author(s), under exclusive license to Springer Nature Switzerland AG 2023
J. Semlyen and P. Rohleder (eds.), *Sexual Minorities and Mental Health*, https://doi.org/10.1007/978-3-031-37438-8_10

223

and trans lives, by their mere existence, hold the potential to disrupt western societal binaries and the supposedly rigid lines which demarcate sex, gender, and sexuality as separate fields (Westbrook & Schilt, 2014).

This disruption is not just a matter of theory, but a material fact, something that is exemplified by the reactions that transness, and in particular queer transness, elicits from the broader heterosexual, cisgender public. It is an unfortunate but undeniable fact that one of the most prominent links between transness and queerness is the way these categories continue to be perceived as legitimate threats to straight and cisgender people's safety. You need not look any further than things such as the gay/trans panic defense (Lee & Kwan, 2014) to understand just how deeply homophobia and transphobia are woven into the fabric of many western societies. While queer trans lives are multifaceted and complex, it is difficult not to comprehend these gendered and sexual experiences through the lens of trauma, particularly when it continues to have such dire (and often lethal) consequences (Dinno, 2017; Stotzer, 2017). Queer trans peoples tend to only be remembered and appreciated long after we're gone (Jackson, 2021).

But to reduce the experiences of trans peoples down to our conflicts with a world that privileges cisgender heterosexual people, overlooks some of the nuance of specifically queer trans people. Again, we can understand the existence of these groups by the reactions they receive. While trans people have been subsumed under the collective term LGBTQ+, there are ongoing tensions between trans people (both queer and straight) and lesbian, gay, and bisexual+ cisgender people. These tensions lead to the exclusion of trans people from many aspects of the so-called LGBTQ+ movement, sidelining trans peoples' needs in favour of cisgender LGBQ people's interests (e.g., marriage equality) (Barry et al., 2016; Vidal-Ortiz, 2005). There is also the matter of TERFs (Trans Exclusionary Radical Feminists), many of whom are cisgender lesbians (Hines, 2019), who stand in direct opposition to trans people's rights (Pearce et al., 2020). All of these points of resistance to (particularly queer) transness come from a place of perceived threat; to 'traditional' notions of gayness and womanhood (Weber, 2016), to progress (Feró, 2020), to legibility and societal acceptance (Santana, 2017).

To understand queer trans lived experiences, then, requires us to witness the ways in which the two categories have been systematically wrenched apart, particularly since the rise of the gay rights movement. The fracture points have been many: the appropriation of statedly pro-trans queer activists writings by anti-trans activists (Williams, 2016); the medical de-prioritisation of non-heterosexual trans peoples (which will be discussed in further detail below) (Johnson, 2007); and the perpetuation of stereotypes which essentialise, dichotomise, and obfuscate our understanding of the relationship between trans people's genders and their sexualities (Gazzola & Morrison, 2014), among others.

There is, in a very real sense, a twofold burden for those who are both trans and queer, in that they are doubly perceived as illegible and doubly excluded from communities, categories, and ownership of experiences that are very much theirs to inhabit. This has significant implications not only for how queer trans people are perceived, but what their state of wellbeing looks like: if, for example, (cisgender) lesbians and trans women (regardless of sexuality) experience certain hardships, there is assuredly a multiplication of consequences for a lesbian trans woman. If queer trans people do not fit neatly either in cisgender, heterosexual, or queer groups, the likelihood for social exclusion is high, and with it the tangible impacts on a person's wellbeing (van Bergen et al., 2019; Watson et al., 2016). This double bind queer trans people find themselves in has not only sociological, but psychophysiological impacts.

Medical and Mental Health Needs

Extending the argument of the double bind many queer trans people find themselves in, and the impact this social positioning has on their health, it is particularly important to note the intersections of sexual diversity and transness when considering the history of trans medicalisation. Trans peoples who do not identify as heterosexual have been routinely denied access to gender-affirming healthcare (Johnson, 2007), in large part due to heterosexuality being defined as more "socially desirable" (Auer et al., 2014, p. 10) by medical practitioners and institutions. Trans peoples' validity, in both medical and legal contexts, continues to rely on their relationship to heterosexuality, specifically how successfully they are able to execute it following medical interventions such as surgery (Sharpe, 2006). Failure to become heterosexual as part of a transition process becomes a disruption to receiving gender-affirming care (Bockting et al., 2009), which often carries with it deleterious consequences (Kattari et al., 2020). We see here again the material impact of existing at the intersection of transness and queerness, even within a field of medicine that statedly specialises in providing healthcare to trans peoples.

To discuss the psychophysiological needs of queer trans people therefore requires a kind of reflexivity in healthcare that extends beyond existing best practice guidelines (e.g., Coleman et al., 2012). Current healthcare guidelines continue to distinguish between care provision for (presumed cisgender) lesbians, gay men, and bisexuals and care provision for trans people, whose sexuality is often disregarded in these contexts (Rosenberg, 2017), thereby completely disregarding the significant portion of people who belong to both categories and their unique needs. The iron curtain between how gender and sexuality are handled in healthcare contexts in many ways prevents health practitioners from providing effective practice; current medical understandings of sex, gender, and sexuality carry with them many heterosexist, cisgenderist, bioessentialist, and outdated perspectives which can cause healthcare workers to provide incomplete or even entirely unneeded or unwanted care.

Cisgenderism in particular has myriad consequences across a variety of healthcare fields, including sexual health (Rosenberg et al., 2021), psychology (Ansara & Hegarty, 2012), aged care (Baril & Silverman, 2022), and medicine broadly (Kcomt, 2019). In all cases, the issues rest with a fundamental ignorance or misunderstanding of how trans people engage with and experience their bodies, relationships, and the societies they live within. This trickles down to how healthcare providers navigate working with queer trans people specifically, as the broad social narrative around transness provides few touchstones on how queer trans people lead their lives and the kinds of unique issues they might face. Many of these issues are experienced in the realm of sexual and reproductive health; queer trans peoples may have sexual partners with a variety of genital configurations and genders,[1] which has many implications for how they negotiate safe sex, sexually transmitted infection and blood born virus testing, and pregnancy, to name just a few areas with significant healthcare components. This is especially true if a trans person is in "T4T" sexual or romantic relationships (i.e., two or more trans people in a relationship, see Crowley & Konnelly, 2021), which adds complexity to the issues mentioned above.

But the issues are not merely medical ones; for example, while there are some studies which describe the significantly high rates of intimate partner violence in trans populations (Peitzmeier et al., 2020), little is known about the sexualities of the people involved in those relationships, and how this issue can be addressed in ways that are tailored to variations in sexual dynamics. You do not need to look any further than our ongoing lack of understanding of the intricate dynamics within intimate partner violence in cisgender lesbian, gay, and bisexual relationships to see the implications that a lack of social and clinical knowledge has on health and wellbeing in those populations (Oliffe et al., 2014; Stephenson & Finneran, 2013; Wasarhaley et al., 2017; West, 2002). Even in the authors' own work in the area, the process of educating domestic violence service providers on managing trans peoples who enter their services remains focused on managing transness in general, partly due to the sector lagging behind on even the most basic understandings of trans peoples' needs in the area (Riggs et al., 2016).

We find ourselves at the same cul-de-sac mentioned above in the introduction section: research on, and subsequently clinical practice with, LGBT+ people clusters all trans people as a singular population, largely devoid of sexuality except in the sense that we too experience sexual violence (Brown & Herman, 2015). In flattening any diversity of sexuality by the merit of a person's transness, we deny the nuanced and often complex sexual dynamics of queer trans peoples. This in turn negates our ability to adequately address many of the needs of both trans people who are not heterosexual writ large, as well as those variations between different queer sexualities amongst trans peoples. The issues for a bisexual

---

[1] This is not to say that straight trans people or queer cisgender people may not also have these experiences, but that the likelihood rises significantly in the case of queer trans people.

trans woman may be radically different to those of a gay trans man, or a non-binary lesbian, and their conflation under the singular heading of "trans issues" conceals much of the nuance needed to provide holistic and targeted healthcare.

Nonetheless, we can synthesize some of the pre-existing research on LGBTQ+ medical and mental health issues to produce a picture of queer trans peoples' experiences within these areas. As discussed in Chapter 2, research with (wholly or majority cisgender) queer people suggests that there are high levels of mental health issues (McConnell et al., 2015; Russell & Fish, 2016), especially depression, anxiety, and suicidality. This has been differentiated in some research, with studies that suggest transgender people experience worse mental health outcomes compared to cisgender LGBQ+ people (Su et al., 2016). Other studies have also suggested that queer people experience significant disparities in physical health, such as having lower levels of health-promoting behaviours and higher levels of issues such as substance misuse (Fredriksen-Goldsen et al., 2014b, 2015; Mereish et al., 2014; Wallace & Santacruz, 2017). Many of the studies cited above include trans people, but often fail to note specific needs of trans peoples, and never discuss intersecting populations of queer trans people.

Trans-specific research also provides insight into some of the potential health issues that trans people face, though much of this research lacks the specificity of sexuality and its interplay with the health needs being addressed. Trans people experience significant mental health issues (Carmel & Erickson-Schroth, 2016; Hyde et al., 2013; McCann, 2015; Yarbrough, 2018), with suicidality forming a significant issue, particularly for trans people with little or no social support (Moody & Smith, 2013; Trujillo et al., 2017). Studies have also suggested that trans people are significantly prone to disability and chronic health conditions, as well as having less access to health-promoting behaviours and resources (Downing & Przedworski, 2018; Fredriksen-Goldsen et al., 2014a; Rider et al., 2018). For transgender people who have also undergone gender-affirming surgeries, there are further physical health considerations to be made, namely around pre-operative evaluation, recovery time, loss of function, and the need for revisions for certain surgical interventions (Bernacki & Weimer, 2019; Berry et al., 2012; Callen et al., 2021; Dreher et al., 2018; Küenzlen et al., 2020; Manrique et al., 2018).

In a sense, the disparate nature of much of sexuality-specific and (trans)gender-specific health research is proof in and of itself of the need for addressing the specific needs of queer trans people. There is not only an overlap between the two categories (i.e., queer health needs and trans health needs), but a significant likelihood of a compounding effect for peoples who find themselves belonging to both categories. Queer trans people form a minority within a minority when taking into consideration that the majority of queer people still identify as cisgender (e.g. Hill et al., 2021). People in these positions often find themselves at odds with both broader normative culture and the various subcultures they exist within (Eisenberg et al., 2005). There are pressures at play, as we mentioned above, but also a specific role as people who by their very existence form a resistance to the narratives of the overarching minority group they belong to (Pinto, 2015). The presence of queer trans people therefore adds complexity to a variety of health issues and our approaches to them, which we will expand on in the following section.

Therapeutic Approaches

As we begin exploring some psychological therapeutic approaches to working with queer trans people, it is important to note that trans people's relationship to psychology and psychiatry is complex at best. Therapists often exist as gatekeepers in trans people's lives (Singh & Burnes, 2010), holding a significant amount of power over their clients. There is significant risk of causing psychological harm in therapeutic settings with trans people, particularly when the therapeutic environment is part of an assessment for accessing things such as hormones and gender-affirming surgeries (Ashley, 2019). This is due to the fact that having therapists as gatekeepers for medical interventions upholds two highly problematic perspectives; that trans peoples know less about their gender-affirming medical needs than their psychological professionals, and that cis people (who make up the overwhelming majority of assessing clinicians) have equal or deeper insight into trans peoples' experiences than their transgender clients. With regards to the former, nothing could be further from the truth; in fact, many trans people report having to educate their assessing clinicians on trans medical needs and even bare bones trans knowledge (Baldwin et al., 2018; Bauer et al., 2009; Mizock & Lundquist, 2016). With regards to the latter, the notion of 'experience-as-expertise' (Voronka, 2016) in terms of mental health issues carries through to the expertise of trans peoples (Frost et al., 2019), bringing into question just how much knowledge cisgender clinicians could even have when compared to the deep and rich lived experience of their transgender clients.

With these in mind, arguably the most powerful tool at the disposal of any therapist working with trans people is a sense of humility (Sadusky & Yarhouse, 2020). That is to say, therapeutic relationships must be approached with a mindset that takes into consideration the therapist's potentially significant gaps in knowledge of their clients' experiences. This approach can facilitate a flattening of the power dynamic between therapist and client by maintaining a critical perspective on one's therapeutic approach and addressing clients' individual needs, enacting a therapeutic method that is focused on collaboration as opposed to a top-down clinical perspective (Paine et al., 2015). This approach is even more crucial when working with queer trans people; as discussed so far, there is a significant dearth of research on these intersections of lived experiences, and therefore few established therapeutic frameworks which have been properly evaluated in their efficacy with these peoples. Therapists therefore cannot rely on pre-existing psychological and therapeutic models when working with queer trans people, but instead have to take a self-humbling position wherein their clients' experience-as-expertise holds many of the keys to a therapeutically successful working relationship.

Once again, the necessary tools for working with queer trans people can only be eked out by synthesis, by fusing together research on trans people as a conglomerate and queer people in their various sexual identities and experiences. The usual battery of therapeutic models have been shown to have some positive effects with regards to trans and (presumably cisgender) queer people, such as cognitive behavioural therapy

(CBT) (Austin et al., 2017, 2018; Craig et al., 2013, 2021), dialectical behavioural therapy (DBT) (Sloan & Berke, 2017, 2017), narrative therapy (Chavez-Korell & Johnson, 2010; Nylund & Temple, 2017; Steelman, 2016; Tilsen, 2021), and so on. However, regardless of a clinician's leading therapeutic framework, at the core of all these approaches is the notion that therapy needs to be individualised and focused on a client's unique lifeworld. There is also a need to take into account what a client is hoping to achieve by attending therapy; are they seeking access to gender-affirming medical care or are they looking to explore their gender in the first instance, looking for short-term crisis support (which may or may not be related to their gender and sexuality), or wanting a longer-term holistic therapeutic relationship? These pertinent considerations are crucial in informing one's therapeutic approach, as well as the therapist's requirements regarding self-education (Banks, 2021). More on these issues is covered in Chapter 8 in relation to clinical formulation.

Another essential component to building productive therapeutic relationships with queer trans peoples is confronting the significant knowledge gaps we have discussed so far. The therapist's role then is to consider how their client's experience of transness is augmented by their queerness and vice versa, both in terms of their inner world and their experience of navigating society. None of these matters are adequately addressed in psychological and therapeutic literature, a site of knowledge production that remains dominated by cisgender heterosexuals. But a wealth of insight exists elsewhere, in the autobiographical, fictional, and non-fiction works of queer trans peoples. Trans Bibles such as Julia Serano's *Whipping Girl* (2016), Kate Bornstein's *Gender Outlaw* (1994), and Leslie Feinberg's *Trans Liberation* (1998), to name but a few, lay the groundwork for understanding the evolution of the trans movement and the lived experiences of trans peoples navigating queerness. More contemporary accounts such as Torey Peters' *Detransition, Baby* (2021), the edited collection *Queer and Trans Artists of Colour* (Glennon-Zukoff & Mikalson, 2014), and Laura Jane Grace's *Tranny* (2016) provide more personal and complex accounts of issues such as navigating relationships and understanding gender and sexuality through creativity and self-expression. Resources such as Juno Roche's *Queer Sex* (2018), the incredible contributions contained within *Trans/Love* (Diamond,

2011), the Zoe Belle Gender Collective's *Transfemme* website (2021), and Mira Bellwether's *Fucking Trans Women* (2013) provide hands-on information on the sexual and intimate needs and experiences of trans peoples across the sexual spectrum.

This list is not even remotely exhaustive, but it is illustrative of the fact that knowledge of queer trans experiences cannot be explicated in a single article or study. Rather, it is an assemblage of expertise spanning decades, continents, and genres. Notably, these community resources often trump existing clinical manuscripts in terms of their relevance and availability to queer trans people, by providing information that is developed, written, and disseminated with its audience in mind. Many of these resources are written conversationally, contain information that addresses the specific needs and interests of queer trans peoples, and is often either free or cheap and made widely available. This is in stark contrast to much of academic literature on the subject, which is hidden behind paywalls and often written with cisgender clinicians as the target readers. Trans-led writing and research carries through and amplifies important aspects of trans lives, queer or otherwise, which go unaddressed in the majority of trans academic literature (Rosenberg & Tilley, 2021). This fact needs to be held at the fore of the mind of any clinician seeking to provide appropriate therapeutic services to a queer trans person; they must seek these accounts and immerse themselves in these diverse narratives.

Despite the wide range of available community-led literature and resources on the subject of transness and queerness, these accounts may not cover the experiences of the person sitting before you in your office. As technology evolves, and sociopolitical dynamics shift and change, so too will the lived experiences of queer trans people. This is also true of the ways a person's transition intersects with their sexuality; a trans lesbian with genital dysphoria and no access to gender-affirming surgery will have a vastly different experience of her queer transness compared to a non-binary person with a vulva who relishes penetration. A gay trans man is going to face wildly differing inter- and intrapersonal experiences compared to a straight trans woman, even if the objects of their attraction (and perhaps the sexually-relevant parts of their bodies) are the same. Bodies, histories, identities, and locations coalesce and intersect with gender and sexuality in myriad ways that cannot be accounted for by any one written account, no matter how scientifically rigorous or thorough.

This all may feel like a matter of raising more questions than answering them, and ultimately that is the truth of building therapeutic relationships with people who have these lived experiences. Working with queer trans people is a matter of curiosity and humility, an acknowledgement on behalf of the therapist, even if they are themself a queer trans person, that they do not have all the necessary pieces of information needed to go down a particular therapeutic path. There are no neat boxes, readily-available diagnostic templates, or rigorously tested models. This is true even within our previous work in the area. Namely, the GENDER[2] model, which was developed for working with young trans young people (Riggs, 2019), was formed as a questioning device to assist clinicians in building deeper knowledge of the individuals one might work with, rather than providing a deterministic therapeutic guideline. Applying this device to queer trans people, a therapist might: inquire as to their lived experiences and personal identities; ask about their existing gender and/or sexuality concerns; collaboratively formulate a therapeutic plan; consider what issues may arise as a result of the client's intersections of gender and sexuality (and other people's responses to these intersections), and how to manage them; explore existing support structures, whether it is family and friends or broader gender and sexuality-based communities; and consider how the person's sense of self, both within and beyond gender and sexuality, is supported or disrupted by internal and external factors.

There is also a necessary oscillation at play, between considering a client's gender and sexuality-specific needs, and the broader issues which affect their life as a queer trans person. A person is both affected by, and contains much more than, their gender and sexuality. As mentioned earlier, queer trans peoples may find themselves in a therapist's office for a variety of reasons, and there is as much disservice to avoiding their intersecting experiences of gender and sexuality as there is to hyperfocus on those issues. It is a therapist's duty therefore to understand a person's

---

[2] **G**ender journey and understandings; **E**xpressed concerns; **N**ecessary action; **D**istress management; **E**cologies of support; **R**einforcement and resistance.

whole inner and external ecology, and work towards comprehending how or whether gender and sexuality interplay with their broader lived experience. Ultimately, queer trans people are neither "just like you" (Dugan, 2008), nor are they mythical beings who evade comprehension (Shin, 2014). Our lived experiences can be understood, connected with, and learned from, even if one is a relative outsider.

Conclusion

Queer trans people provide therapists with an opportunity to immerse themselves in several vital aspects of human life: the infinite diversity in infinite combinations that is gender and sexuality, the sense of humility that sits at the core of relating across experiential boundaries, and the empathy and curiosity needed to experience and enact these matters in full. Therapeutic approaches to queer trans people need to focus less on any particular psychological practice model, and turn towards an approach that positions the therapist as knowledge-seeking, permeable, and conscious of the fog surrounding gender and sexuality within psychology as a discipline. In order to parse the haze, there is a need to take a collaborative therapeutic path, with queer trans peoples' experiences leading the way at every turn. For therapists, this means both placing an importance on the perspectives expressed by their queer trans clients, as well as including queer trans literature in their self-education on these issues. Therapists must also strike a balance, understanding gender and sexuality as core, but not sole, factors which affect a person's life. By focusing on how gender and sexuality interplay with a person's historical, personal, relational, and contextual factors, clinicians can form closer and more successful therapeutic relationships with queer trans people.

References

Ansara, Y. G. (2010). Beyond cisgenderism: Counselling people with non-assigned gender identities. In L. Moon (Ed.), *Counselling ideologies* (pp. 123–141). Routledge.

Ansara, Y. G., & Hegarty, P. (2012). Cisgenderism in psychology: Pathologising and misgendering children from 1999 to 2008. *Psychology & Sexuality, 3*(2), 137–160. https://doi.org/10.1080/19419899.2011.576696

Ashley, F. (2019). Gatekeeping hormone replacement therapy for transgender patients is dehumanising. *Journal of Medical Ethics, 45*(7), 480–482. https://doi.org/10.1136/medethics-2018-105293

Auer, M. K., Fuss, J., Höhne, N., Stalla, G. K., & Sievers, C. (2014). Transgender transitioning and change of self-reported sexual orientation. *PLoS ONE, 9*(10), 1–11. https://doi.org/10.1371/journal.pone.0110016

Austin, A., Craig, S. L., & Alessi, E. J. (2017). Affirmative cognitive behavior therapy with transgender and gender nonconforming adults. *Psychiatric Clinics, 40*(1), 141–156. https://doi.org/10.1016/j.psc.2016.10.003

Austin, A., Craig, S. L., & D'Souza, S. A. (2018). An AFFIRMative cognitive behavioral intervention for transgender youth: Preliminary effectiveness. *Professional Psychology: Research and Practice, 49*(1), 1–8. https://doi.org/10.1037/pro0000154

Baldwin, A., Dodge, B., Schick, V. R., Light, B., Schnarrs, P. W., Herbenick, D., & Fortenberry, J. D. (2018). Transgender and genderqueer individuals' experiences with health care providers: What's working, what's not, and where do we go from here? *Journal of Health Care for the Poor and Underserved, 29*(4), 1300–1318. https://doi.org/10.1353/hpu.2018.0097

Banks, J. (2021). *Psychotherapists' approaches to transgender affirmative psychotherapy*. Unpublished Masters thesis, Western University.

Baril, A., & Silverman, M. (2022). Forgotten lives: Trans older adults living with dementia at the intersection of cisgenderism, ableism/cogniticism and ageism. *Sexualities, 25*(1–2), 117–131. https://doi.org/10.1177/1363460719876835

Barry, K. M., Farrell, B., Levi, J. L., & Vanguri, N. (2016). A bare desire to harm: Transgender people and the equal protection clause. *Boston College Law Review, 57*, 507–582. https://lawdigitalcommons.bc.edu/bclr/vol57/iss2/4

Bauer, G. R., Hammond, R., Travers, R., Kaay, M., Hohenadel, K. M., & Boyce, M. (2009). "I don't think this is theoretical; this is our lives": How erasure impacts health care for transgender people. *Journal of the Association of Nurses in AIDS Care, 20*(5), 348–361. https://doi.org/10.1016/j.jana.2009.07.004

Bellwether, M. (2013). *Fucking trans women (issue# 0).* CreateSpace Independent Publishing Platform.

Bernacki, J. M., & Weimer, A. K. (2019). Role of development on youth decision-making and recovery from gender-affirming surgery. *Clinical Practice in Pediatric Psychology, 7*(3), 312–321. https://doi.org/10.1037/cpp0000294

Berry, M. G., Curtis, R., & Davies, D. (2012). Female-to-male transgender chest reconstruction: A large consecutive, single-surgeon experience. *Journal of Plastic, Reconstructive & Aesthetic Surgery, 65*(6), 711–719. https://doi.org/10.1016/j.bjps.2011.11.053

Bockting, W., Benner, A., & Coleman, E. (2009). Gay and bisexual identity development among female-to-male transsexuals in North America: Emergence of a transgender sexuality. *Archives of Sexual Behavior, 38*(5), 688–701. https://doi.org/10.1007/s10508-009-9489-3

Bornstein, K. (1994). *Gender outlaw: On men, women, and the rest of us.* Psychology Press.

Brown, T. N., & Herman, J. (2015). *Intimate partner violence and sexual abuse among LGBT people.* University of California.

Callander, D., Wiggins, J., Rosenberg, S., Cornelisse, V., Duck-Chong, E., Holt, M., & Cook, T. (2019). *The 2018 Australian trans and gender diverse sexual health survey: Report of findings.* The Kirby Institute.

Callen, A. L., Badiee, R. K., Phelps, A., Potigailo, V., Wang, E., Lee, S., Talbott, J., Glastonbury, C., Pomerantz, J. H., & Narvid, J. (2021). Facial feminization surgery: Key CT findings for preoperative planning and postoperative Eealuation. *American Journal of Roentgenology, 217*(3), 709–717. https://doi.org/10.2214/AJR.20.25228

Carmel, T. C., & Erickson-Schroth, L. (2016). Mental health and the transgender population. *Journal of Psychosocial Nursing and Mental Health Services, 54*(12), 44–48. https://doi.org/10.3928/02793695-20161208-09

Chavez-Korell, S., & Johnson, L. T. (2010). Informing counselor training and competent counseling services through transgender narratives and the transgender community. *Journal of LGBT Issues in Counseling, 4*(3–4), 202–213. https://doi.org/10.1080/15538605.2010.524845

Coleman, E., Bockting, W., Botzer, M., Cohen-Kettenis, P., DeCuypere, G., Feldman, J., Fraser, L., Green, J., Knudson, G., & Meyer, W. J. (2012).

Standards of care for the health of transsexual, transgender, and gender-nonconforming people, version 7. *International Journal of Transgenderism, 13*(4), 165–232. https://doi.org/10.1080/15532739.2011.700873

Craig, S. L., Austin, A., & Alessi, E. (2013). Gay affirmative cognitive behavioral therapy for sexual minority youth: A clinical adaptation. *Clinical Social Work Journal, 41*(3), 258–266. https://doi.org/10.1007/s10615-012-0427-9

Craig, S. L., Iacono, G., & Pascoe, R. (2021). The delivery of technology-mediated affirmative Ccgnitive behavioural therapy groups to LGBTQ+ youth during a pandemic: A practice innovation. *Canadian Journal of Community Mental Health, 39*(3), 79–83. https://doi.org/10.7870/cjcmh-2020-020

Crowley, A., & Konnelly, L. (2021, May 21). *The 'transgender couple': Transnormativity, trans separatism, and the discourse of t4t.* Paper presented at the *Lavender languages and linguistic conference.*

Diamond, M. (2011). *Trans/love: Radical sex, love and relationships beyond the gender binary.* Manic D Press.

Dinno, A. (2017). Homicide rates of transgender individuals in the United States: 2010–2014. *American Journal of Public Health, 107*(9), 1441–1447. https://doi.org/10.2105/AJPH.2017.303878

Downing, J. M., & Przedworski, J. M. (2018). Health of transgender adults in the U.S., 2014–2016. *American Journal of Preventive Medicine, 55*(3), 336–344. https://doi.org/10.1016/j.amepre.2018.04.045

Dreher, P. C., Edwards, D., Hager, S., Dennis, M., Belkoff, A., Mora, J., Tarry, S., & Rumer, K. L. (2018). Complications of the neovagina in male-to-female transgender surgery: A systematic review and meta-analysis with discussion of management. *Clinical Anatomy, 31*(2), 191–199. https://doi.org/10.1002/ca.23001

Dugan, K. B. (2008). Just like you: The dimensions of identity presentations in an antigay contested context. In J. Reger, D. J. Myers, & R. L. Einwohner (Eds.), *Identity work in social movements* (pp. 21–46). University of Minnesota Press. https://www.jstor.org/stable/10.5749/j.cttt85v

Eisenberg, A., Spinner-Halev, J., & Eisenberg, A. (Eds.). (2005). Identity and liberal politics: The problem of minorities within minorities. In A. Eisenberg & J. Spinner Halev (Eds.), *Minorities within minorities: Equality, rights and diversity* (pp. 249–270). Cambridge University Press.

Feinberg, L. (1998). *Trans liberation: Beyond pink or blue.* Beacon Press.

Feró, D. (2020). The post-politics of recognition in hegemonic struggles: The road from the new left movements to the crumbling of liberal hegemony. *Intersections, 6*(1). https://doi.org/10.17356/ieejsp.v6i1.563

Fredriksen-Goldsen, K. I., Cook-Daniels, L., Kim, H.-J., Erosheva, E. A., Emlet, C. A., Hoy-Ellis, C. P., Goldsen, J., & Muraco, A. (2014a). Physical and mental health of transgender older adults: An at-risk and underserved population. *The Gerontologist, 54*(3), 488–500. https://doi.org/10.1093/ger ont/gnt021

Fredriksen-Goldsen, K. I., Simoni, J. M., Kim, H.-J., Lehavot, K., Walters, K. L., Yang, J., Hoy-Ellis, C. P., & Muraco, A. (2014b). The health equity promotion model: Reconceptualization of lesbian, gay, bisexual, and transgender (LGBT) health disparities. *American Journal of Orthopsychiatry, 84*(6), 653. https://doi.org/10.1037/ort0000030

Fredriksen-Goldsen, K. I., Kim, H.-J., Shiu, C., Goldsen, J., & Emlet, C. A. (2015). Successful aging among LGBT older adults: Physical and mental health-related quality of Llfe by age group. *The Gerontologist, 55*(1), 154–168. https://doi.org/10.1093/geront/gnu081

Frost, D. M., Fine, M., Torre, M. E., & Cabana, A. (2019). Minority stress, activism, and health in the context of economic precarity: Results from a national participatory action survey of lesbian, gay, bisexual, transgender, queer, and gender non-conforming youth. *American Journal of Community Psychology, 63*(3–4), 511–526. https://doi.org/10.1002/ajcp.12326

Gazzola, S. B., & Morrison, M. A. (2014). Cultural and personally endorsed stereotypes of transgender men and transgender women: Notable correspondence or disjunction? *International Journal of Transgenderism, 15*(2), 76–99. https://doi.org/10.1080/15532739.2014.937041

Glennon-Zukoff, J., & Mikalson, T. (2014). *Queer and trans artists of color: Stories of some of our lives.* CreateSpace Independent Publishing Platform.

Grace, L. J. (2016). *Tranny: Confessions of punk rock's most infamous anarchist sellout.* Hachette.

Grant, J., Mottet, L., Tanis, J., Herman, J. L., Harrison, J., & Keisling, M. (2010). *National transgender discrimination survey report on health and health care.* National Center for Transgender Equality and the Gay and Lesbian Task Force.

Hill, A., Bourne, A., McNair, R., Carman, M., & Lyons, A. (2021). *Private lives 3: The health and wellbeing of LGBTIQ people in Australia.* Latrobe University.

Hines, S. (2019). The feminist frontier: On trans and feminism. *Journal of Gender Studies, 28*(2), 145–157. https://doi.org/10.1080/09589236.2017. 1411791

Hyde, Z., Doherty, M., Tilley, M., McCaul, K., Rooney, R., & Jancey, J. (2013). *The first Australian national trans mental health study: Summary of results*. Curtin University.

Jackson, J. M. (2021). Black feminisms, queer feminisms, trans feminisms: Meditating on Pauli Murray, Shirley Chisholm, and Marsha P. Johnson against the erasure of history. In J. Hobson (Ed.), *The Routledge companion to black women's cultural histories* (pp. 284–294). Routledge.

Johnson, K. (2007). Transsexualism: Diagnostic dilemmas, transgender politics and the future of transgender care. In V. Clarke & E. Peel (Eds.), *Out in psychology: Lesbian, gay, bisexual, trans and queer Perspectives* (pp. 445–464). Wiley.

Kattari, S. K., Bakko, M., Hecht, H. K., & Kinney, M. K. (2020). Intersecting experiences of healthcare denials among transgender and nonbinary patients. *American Journal of Preventive Medicine, 58*(4), 506–513. https://doi.org/10.1016/j.amepre.2019.11.014

Kcomt, L. (2019). Profound health-care discrimination experienced by transgender people: Rapid systematic review. *Social Work in Health Care, 58*(2), 201–219. https://doi.org/10.1080/00981389.2018.1532941

Küenzlen, L., Nasim, S., van Neerven, S., Kühn, S., Burger, A. E., Sohn, M., Rieger, U. M., & Bozkurt, A. (2020). Multimodal evaluation of functional nerve regeneration in transgender individuals after phalloplasty with a free radial forearm flap. *The Journal of Sexual Medicine, 17*(5), 1012–1024. https://doi.org/10.1016/j.jsxm.2020.02.014

Lee, C., & Kwan, P. (2014). The trans panic defense: Masculinity, heteronormativity, and the murder of transgender women. *Hastings Law Journal, 66*, 77–102. https://doi.org/10.2139/ssrn.2430390

Manrique, O. J., Sabbagh, M. D., Ciudad, P., Martinez-Jorge, J., Kiranantawat, K., Sitpahul, N., Nippoldt, T. B., Charafeddine, A., & Chen, H.-C. (2018). Gender-confirmation surgery using the pedicle transverse colon flap for vaginal reconstruction: A clinical outcome and sexual function evaluation study. *Plastic and Reconstructive Surgery, 141*(3), 767–771. https://doi.org/10.1097/PRS.0000000000004122

McCann, E. (2015). People who are transgender: Mental health concerns. *Journal of Psychiatric and Mental Health Nursing, 22*(1), 76–81. https://doi.org/10.1111/jpm.12190

McConnell, E. A., Birkett, M. A., & Mustanski, B. (2015). Typologies of social support and associations with mental health outcomes among LGBT youth. *LGBT Health, 2*(1), 55–61. https://doi.org/10.1089/lgbt.2014.0051

Mereish, E. H., O'Cleirigh, C., & Bradford, J. B. (2014). Interrelationships between LGBT-based victimization, suicide, and substance use problems in a diverse sample of sexual and gender minorities. *Psychology, Health & Medicine, 19*(1), 1–13. https://doi.org/10.1080/13548506.2013.780129

Mizock, L., & Lundquist, C. (2016). Missteps in psychotherapy with transgender clients: Promoting gender sensitivity in counseling and psychological practice. *Psychology of Sexual Orientation and Gender Diversity, 3*(2), 148. https://doi.org/10.1037/sgd0000177

Moody, C., & Smith, N. G. (2013). Suicide protective factors among trans adults. *Archives of Sexual Behavior, 42*(5), 739–752. https://doi.org/10.1007/s10508-013-0099-8

Nylund, D., & Temple, A. (2017). Queer informed narrative therapy: Radical approaches to counseling with transgender persons. In C. Audet & D. Pare (Eds.), *Social justice and counseling* (pp. 151–167). Routledge.

Oliffe, J. L., Han, C., Maria, E. S., Lohan, M., Howard, T., Stewart, D. E., & MacMillan, H. (2014). Gay men and intimate partner violence: A gender analysis. *Sociology of Health & Illness, 36*(4), 564–579. https://doi.org/10.1111/1467-9566.12099

Paine, D. R., Sandage, S. J., Rupert, D., Devor, N. G., & Bronstein, M. (2015). Humility as a psychotherapeutic virtue: Spiritual, philosophical, and psychological foundations. *Journal of Spirituality in Mental Health, 17*(1), 3–25. https://doi.org/10.1080/19349637.2015.957611

Pearce, R., Erikainen, S., & Vincent, B. (2020). TERF wars: An introduction. *The Sociological Review, 68*(4), 677–698. https://doi.org/10.1177/0038026120934713

Peitzmeier, S. M., Malik, M., Kattari, S. K., Marrow, E., Stephenson, R., Agénor, M., & Reisner, S. L. (2020). Intimate partner violence in transgender populations: Systematic review and meta-analysis of prevalence and Correlates. *American Journal of Public Health, 110*(9), e1–e14. https://doi.org/10.2105/AJPH.2020.305774

Peters, T. (2021). *Detransition, baby*. Serpent's Tail.

Pinto, M. (2015). The right to culture, the right to dispute, and the right to exclude. A new perspective on minorities within minorities. *Ratio Juris, 28*, 521–539. https://doi.org/10.1111/raju.12094

Rider, G. N., McMorris, B. J., Gower, A. L., Coleman, E., & Eisenberg, M. E. (2018). Health and care utilization of transgender and gender nonconforming youth: A population-based study. *Pediatrics, 141*(3), e20171683. https://doi.org/10.1542/peds.2017-1683

Riggs, D. W. (2019). *Working with transgender young people and their families: A critical developmental approach.* Springer.

Riggs, D. W., & Due, C. (2013). *Gender identity Australia: The healthcare experiences of people whose gender identity differs from that expected of their natally assigned sex.* Flinders University.

Riggs, D. W., Fraser, H., Taylor, N., Signal, T., & Donovan, C. (2016). Domestic violence service providers' capacity for supporting transgender women: Findings from an Australian workshop. *British Journal of Social Work, 46*(8), 2374–2392. https://doi.org/10.1093/bjsw/bcw110

Roche, J. (2018). *Queer sex: A trans and non-binary guide to intimacy, pleasure and relationships.* Jessica Kingsley Publishers.

Rosenberg, S. (2017). *"I couldn't imagine my life without it": Australian trans women's experiences of sexuality, intimacy, and gender-affirming hormone therapy.* Unpublished Masters thesis, Curtin University.

Rosenberg, S., Callander, D., Holt, M., Duck-Chong, L., Pony, M., Cornelisse, V., Baradaran, A., Duncan, D. T., & Cook, T. (2021). Cisgenderism and transphobia in sexual health care and associations with testing for HIV and other sexually transmitted infections: Findings from the Australian Trans and Gender Diverse Sexual Health Survey. *PLoS ONE, 16*(7), 1–25. https://doi.org/10.1371/journal.pone.0253589

Rosenberg, S., & Tilley, P. J. M. (2021). 'A point of reference': The insider/outsider research staircase and transgender people's experiences of participating in trans-led research. *Qualitative Research, 20*(6), 923–938. https://doi.org/10.1177/1468794120965371

Russell, S. T., & Fish, J. N. (2016). Mental health in lesbian, gay, bisexual, and transgender (LGBT) youth. *Annual Review of Clinical Psychology, 12*, 465–487. https://doi.org/10.1146/annurev-clinpsy-021815-093153

Sadusky, J., & Yarhouse, M. (2020). Cultural humility and gender identity. *Reflections: Narratives of Professional Helping, 26*(2), 107–113.

Santana, A. L. (2017). *Against all odds, I universe you: Academic and personal perspectives on facets of queer identity.* Unpublished PhD thesis, Bard College.

Serano, J. (2016). *Whipping girl: A transsexual woman on sexism and the scapegoating of femininity.* Hachette.

Sharpe, A. (2006). From functionality to aesthetics: The architecture of transgender jurisprudence. In S. Stryker & S. Whittle (Eds.), *The transgender studies reader* (pp. 137–148). Routledge.

Shin, E. (2014). Djuna Barnes, history's elsewhere, and the transgender. *Journal of Modern Literature, 37*(2), 20–38. https://doi.org/10.2979/jmodelite.37.2.20

Singh, A. A., & Burnes, T. R. (2010). Shifting the counselor role from gatekeeping to advocacy: Ten strategies for using the competencies for counseling with transgender clients for individual and social change. *Journal of LGBT Issues in Counseling, 4*(3–4), 241–255. https://doi.org/10.1080/155 38605.2010.525455

Sloan, C. A., & Berke, D. S. (2017). Dialectical behavior therapy as a treatment option for complex cases of gender dysphoria. In M. R. Kauth & J. C. Shipherd (Eds.), *Adult transgender care* (pp. 123–139). Routledge.

Steelman, S. M. (2016). Externalizing identities: An integration of narrative therapy and queer theory. *Journal of Family Psychotherapy, 27*(1), 79–84. https://doi.org/10.1080/08975353.2016.1136549

Stephenson, R., & Finneran, C. (2013). The IPV-GBM scale: A new scale to measure intimate partner violence among gay and bisexual men. *PLoS ONE, 8*(6), 1–17. https://doi.org/10.1371/journal.pone.0062592

Stotzer, R. L. (2017). Data sources hinder our understanding of transgender murders. *American Journal of Public Health, 107*(9), 1362–1363. https:// doi.org/10.2105/AJPH.2017.303973

Strauss, P., Cook, A., Winter, S., Watson, V., Wright-Toussaint, D., & Lin, A. (2017). *Trans-pathways: The mental health experiences and care pathways of trans young people-summary of results*. Telethon Kids.

Su, D., Irwin, J. A., Fisher, C., Ramos, A., Kelley, M., Mendoza, D. A. R., & Coleman, J. D. (2016). Mental health disparities within the LGBT population: A comparison between transgender and nontransgender individuals. *Transgender Health, 1*(1), 12–20. https://doi.org/10.1089/trgh.2015.0001

Tilsen, J. (2021). *Queering your therapy practice: Queer theory, narrative therapy, and imagining new identities*. Routledge.

Trujillo, M. A., Perrin, P. B., Sutter, M., Tabaac, A., & Benotsch, E. G. (2017). The buffering role of social support on the associations among discrimination, mental health, and suicidality in a transgender sample. *International Journal of Transgenderism, 18*(1), 39–52. https://doi.org/10.1080/ 15532739.2016.1247405

van Bergen, A. P., Wolf, J. R., Badou, M., de Wilde-Schutten, K., IJzelenberg, W., Schreurs, H., Carlier, B., Hoff, S. J., & van Hemert, A. M. (2019). The association between social exclusion or inclusion and health in EU and OECD countries: A systematic review. *European Journal of Public Health, 29*(3), 575–582.https://doi.org/10.1093/eurpub/cky143

Vidal-Ortiz, S. (2005). Queering sexuality and doing gender: Transgender men's identification with gender and sexuality. In P. Gagné & R. Tewksbury (Eds.), *Gendered sexualities* (pp. 181–233). Emerald Group Publishing Limited. https://doi.org/10.1016/S1529-2126(02)80008-X

Voronka, J. (2016). The politics of 'people with lived experience' Experiential authority and the risks of strategic essentialism. *Philosophy, Psychiatry, & Psychology, 23*(3), 189–201. https://doi.org/10.1353/ppp.2016.0017

Wallace, B. C., & Santacruz, E. (2017). Health disparities and LGBT populations. In R. Ruth & E. Santacruz (Eds.), *LGBT psychology and mental health: Emerging research and advances* (pp. 177–196). Praeger.

Wasarhaley, N. E., Lynch, K. R., Golding, J. M., & Renzetti, C. M. (2017). The impact of gender stereotypes on legal perceptions of lesbian intimate partner violence. *Journal of Interpersonal Violence, 32*(5), 635–658. https://doi.org/10.1177/0886260515586370

Watson, J., Crawley, J., & Kane, D. (2016). Social exclusion, health and hidden homelessness. *Public Health, 139*, 96–102. https://doi.org/10.1016/j.puhe.2016.05.017

Weber, S. (2016). "Womanhood does not reside in documentation": Queer and feminist student activism for transgender women's inclusion at women's colleges. *Journal of Lesbian Studies, 20*(1), 29–45. https://doi.org/10.1080/10894160.2015.1076238

West, C. M. (2002). Lesbian intimate partner violence: Prevalence and dynamics. *Journal of Lesbian Studies, 6*(1), 121–127. https://doi.org/10.1300/J155v06n01_11

Westbrook, L., & Schilt, K. (2014). Doing gender, determining gender: Transgender people, gender panics, and the maintenance of the sex/gender/sexuality system. *Gender and Society, 28*(1), 32–57. https://doi.org/10.1177/0891243213503203

Williams, C. (2016). Radical inclusion: Recounting the trans inclusive history of radical feminism. *TSQ: Transgender Studies Quarterly, 3*(1–2), 254–258. https://doi.org/10.1215/23289252-3334463

Yarbrough, E. (2018). *Transgender mental health*. American Psychiatric Publishing.

Zoe Belle Gender Collective. (2021). *Transfemme*. https://transfemme.com.au/

11

Cognitive Behaviour Therapy (CBT) for Sexual Minority Adults

Katharine A. Rimes ⓘ

Introduction

Compared to heterosexual people, mental health risk is elevated in those whose sexual orientation is lesbian, gay or bisexual (who may also use other labels such as queer), as detailed in Chapter 2 (see also Semlyen et al., 2016). As discussed throughout this book, Meyer's (2003) minority stress theory proposed social processes contributing to this mental illness excess, including the stressful impact of prejudice, discrimination and victimisation and subsequent effects of rejection expectations, concealment and internalised stigma. Hatzenbuehler's (2009) psychological mediation framework expanded on this to include general psychological processes. He suggested that cognitive, coping/

K. A. Rimes (✉)
Institute of Psychiatry, Psychology and Neuroscience, King's College London, London, UK
e-mail: katharine.rimes@kcl.ac.uk

© The Author(s), under exclusive license to Springer Nature Switzerland AG 2023
J. Semlyen and P. Rohleder (eds.), *Sexual Minorities and Mental Health*,
https://doi.org/10.1007/978-3-031-37438-8_11

emotion regulation and social/interpersonal processes can also be negatively affected by societal stigma and contribute to mental illness. These approaches have informed this chapter.

This chapter provides an overview about cognitive behaviour therapy (CBT), followed by evidence about the hypothesised cognitive and behavioural processes in sexual minority people. Research about treatment outcomes for sexual minorities in routine healthcare is summarised, followed by evidence from studies adapting cognitive behavioural interventions for sexual minority adults. The final section discusses examples of how cognitive behaviour therapy may be adapted to meet the needs of sexual minority adults.

Cognitive Behaviour Therapy

CBT was developed by Aaron T. Beck and other therapists and researchers (e.g. Beck et al., 1979). The underpinning theory suggests that the way that we appraise our ongoing experiences is a key contributory factor in our emotional and behavioural reactions. CBT proposes different levels of cognition. Negative 'core beliefs' or 'unconditional beliefs' or 'schemas' are over-general, negative beliefs about the self, the world or others (e.g. "I am a bad person", "The world is a dangerous place"). 'Unhelpful assumptions' are an intermediate level of conditional beliefs relating to the core belief (e.g. "unless I always put others' needs before my own, then I'm a bad person"). Such beliefs often specify certain behaviours or rules for living that the person should follow, which are aimed at protecting the individual from the distressing activation of their core belief, but which often have unintended negative consequences. Unhelpful beliefs and assumptions are proposed to contribute to cognitive processing biases in attention, memory and interpretation that affect the person's appraisal of ongoing events. This can be evident in the content of their 'negative automatic thoughts', situation-specific thoughts or images such as "none of these people are going to like me". Such thoughts are the most accessible to conscious awareness and are typically the focus at the beginning of therapy. Depending on factors such as the number of sessions available, underlying beliefs may be addressed later too. CBT also addresses responses such as avoidance or rumination, which are often undertaken by the individual with the aim of reducing distress but often maintain or exacerbate the person's difficulties, especially in the longer-term.

Although CBT case formulations will often include contributions from childhood and other earlier life experiences, the key focus is on developing new ways of responding to current problems. CBT is based on a collaborative therapeutic relationship, with the therapist and client working together to address the cognitive and behavioural processes contributing to the presenting problems. Clients are supported to develop skills in evaluating their thoughts and beliefs, re-appraising their experiences, and cultivating new more helpful conditional and unconditional beliefs. Behavioural experiments are used to gather new information and enhance learning, and to test out new more adaptive responses and beliefs. CBT is an evidence-based intervention for many mental health problems and is also used with people with physical health symptoms to help support their coping (Layard & Clark, 2015).

Evidence Regarding Cognitive and Behavioural Contributory Factors in Sexual Minority People

Beliefs

There is some evidence that sexual minority individuals are more likely to have unhelpful beliefs about the self, world or others than heterosexual people. An Iranian study found greater endorsement of seven out of fifteen subscales on the Young Schema Questionnaire, in sexual minority adults relative to matched heterosexual participants: mistrust/abuse; defectiveness/shame, social isolation; emotional inhibition; sacrifice and entitlement (Nematy et al., 2014). Self-esteem and self-acceptance are both lower in sexual minority than heterosexual people (Bridge et al., 2019; Camp et al., 2020). In a UK longitudinal study, Argyriou et al. (2020) found that sexual minority young people had more unhelpful assumptions than heterosexual participants at 17 years and that this mediated higher depressive symptomatology at 18 years. A US longitudinal study with sexual minority women found that daily heterosexism predicted trauma-related cognitions (about the self, world and self-blame) and that these mediated subsequent PTSD symptoms (Dworkin et al., 2018).

Sexual minority individuals may have negative beliefs about their sexual orientation due to internalisation of society's stigmatising attitudes and/or as a result of personal experiences of prejudice and victimisation; this may be heightened in sexual minority individuals who are gender nonconforming (Puckett et al., 2018; Timmins et al., 2020). A meta-analysis found a small to moderate effect size for associations between measures of internalised homophobia and internalising mental health problems (Newcomb & Mustanski, 2010). Similarly, a systematic review found that lower self-acceptance of sexuality was associated with higher levels of minority stressors and poorer mental health (Camp et al., 2020). This review found that general self-acceptance was lower in sexual minority than heterosexual individuals.

Expectations of rejection are higher in sexual minority than heterosexual people (Timmins et al., 2018) and have been shown to prospectively associated with later depressive symptoms (Hatzenbuehler et al., 2008). In relation to beliefs about the future, hopelessness has been found to be higher in sexual minority than heterosexual people (Safren & Heimberg, 1999) and associated with suicide attempts in LGBT youth (Mustanski & Liu, 2013).

Cognitive and Behavioural Processes and Responses

Rumination is higher in sexual minority people compared to heterosexuals (Timmins et al., 2018) and a UK longitudinal study found that this difference can mediate depression disparities (Argyriou et al., 2021). In another UK longitudinal study of LGBTQ + students, unhelpful baseline (Time 1) beliefs about the self, others or the future were associated with more rumination a month later (Time 2), which contributed to later (Time 3) depression and anxiety symptoms (Gnan et al., 2022).

Some avoidant strategies may be the safest option available for sexual minority individuals, especially in the short-term. However, cognitive and behavioural avoidant responses can maintain anxiety and depression in the longer term. In the above-mentioned UK study of LGBTQ + students, avoidance at Time 2 was one of the mediators between unhelpful beliefs at baseline and depression/anxiety symptoms at Time 3 (Gnan et al., 2022).

A specific form of avoidance common in sexual minority individuals is the understandable attempt to conceal sexual orientation to avoid negative evaluations, discrimination or victimisation. Pachankis' (2007) cognitive-affective-behavioural model highlights how concealment can have adverse consequences. It is an effortful process requiring self- and other-monitoring for signs of concealment failures, potentially chronically tiring and impairing of one's performance in tasks or interactions. There is evidence that attempting to conceal one's sexual orientation is associated with greater cognitive depletion (Critcher & Ferguson, 2014). Pachankis (2007) outlines other potential consequences, including impairing interpersonal functioning/relationships, maintaining a threat focus about how others view oneself, preventing potentially positive disconfirmatory feedback about unhelpful beliefs about how others would respond, reducing access to support from other sexual minority people and maintaining shame. A meta-analysis found a small positive association between sexual orientation concealment and internalising mental health problems, but studies conceptualised concealment in very different ways and no conclusions could be drawn about causal directions (Pachankis et al., 2020a). Concealment of minority sexual orientation was more common in bisexual individuals, but showed weaker associations with mental health problems than in gay/lesbian individuals.

Attentional bias towards threat is a key part of cognitive behavioural models as well as minority stress theory (Meyer, 2003). In a US LGBTQ sample, participants reported that hypervigilance was associated with many negative effects including anxiety, exhaustion and social withdrawal (Rostosky et al., 2022).

In summary, there is evidence consistent with the hypothesised cognitive and behavioural processes in sexual minority individuals, which may help explain the disparities in mental health problems compared to heterosexual counterparts.

Treatment Outcomes for Sexual Minorities Compared to Heterosexual Clients in General Mental Healthcare Settings

UK Evidence

As far as the author is aware, there are two UK studies comparing treatment outcomes for sexual minority with heterosexual clients. Rimes et al. (2018) investigated outcomes from four London boroughs in Improving Access to Psychological Therapies (IAPT) services, which provide evidence-based treatments, including CBT, for common mental health problems such as depression and anxiety. IAPT services have since been renamed "NHS Talking Therapies, for anxiety and depression". Rimes et al. (2019) used data from 265,221 clients from all IAPT services in England. Similar results were found, and the latter will be reported here. Compared to heterosexual women, lesbian and bisexual women had poorer treatment outcomes on measures of depression, anxiety, functional impairment, reliable recovery and reliable improvement, after adjusting for baseline scores, sociodemographic variables and treatment characteristics. Bisexual men also had poorer outcomes on these measures compared to heterosexual men, but gay men did not show significant differences to their heterosexual counterparts. Racial minority lesbian/gay or bisexual participants did not show significantly different outcomes to their White lesbian/gay or bisexual counterparts. Treatment disparities were generally largest for the bisexual men, indicating the importance of subgroup analysis by both sexual orientation and sex.

Outcomes Outside of the UK

In a US study, Beard et al. (2017) investigated outcomes for 441 adults with non-psychotic psychiatric disorders receiving in-patient or out-patient treatment based on CBT and dialectical behaviour therapy (DBT). Sexual minority clients did not differ from heterosexual clients on most symptom measures at admission and did not have significantly different treatment response. However, at discharge, bisexual participants had more severe self-injurious and suicidal thoughts, and had lower ratings of quality of care received, after controlling for baseline characteristics and symptoms. No studies were identified that report outcomes for a service providing CBT only.

CBT Adapted for Sexual Minorities

UK Evidence

Little has been published about UK adaptations of CBT for sexual minority individuals. In an Improving Access to Psychological Therapies (IAPT) service in London, two clinical psychologists who are also British Association for Behvioural and Cognitive Psychotherapies (BABCP) accredited therapists developed an eight-session weekly group intervention for sexual minority adults with depression or anxiety (Hambrook et al., 2022). The group was later extended to include gender minority adults. Participants learn about standard CBT methods but with LGBTQ + related examples. The intervention also aims to improve understanding about how stigma experiences may impact mental health via behavioural and cognitive processes. It is facilitated by LGBTQ + therapists and aims to offer a safe space where people can be open about their sexual orientation or gender identity. This is important, given that a survey found that 34% of sexual minority clients referred for IAPT or primary care counselling did not disclose their sexual or gender identity and 44% reported that their sexuality was not discussed in treatment (Foy et al., 2019). An evaluation found the intervention to be acceptable and feasible, and participants showed improvements in measures of depression, anxiety and daily living impairments (Hambrook et al., 2022; Lloyd et al., 2021). However, there was indication of greater dropout for older adults and lower attendance than would be expected for women compared to men, and for ethnic/racial minority compared to

White participants. Furthermore, it has not been compared to a control condition.

A UK pilot study of a six-session individual CBT intervention with 24 sexual minority young adults wanting help for low self-esteem showed promising results (Bridge, 2021 and in press). This used standard CBT techniques and methods from compassion-focused therapy approaches (Gilbert, 2009). The individualised formulation and intervention materials addressed the impact of sexual minority or other stigma/victimisation experiences on beliefs and behaviours relating to low self-esteem. There were some core modules which all participants received (self-criticism and core beliefs) then some others selected collaboratively between therapist and participants based on the formulation (e.g. rumination, avoidance, perfectionism, assertiveness, sexual orientation concealment, building a social support network). The intervention was found to have good acceptability, feasibility and promising improvements in self-esteem, daily functioning, depression and anxiety. Again, a randomised controlled evaluation is needed to compare the intervention to control conditions.

Evidence from Outside of the UK

Pachankis et al.'s (2015) CBT-based intervention for young adult gay/bisexual men aimed to enhance participants' ability to cope with stigma by reducing the minority stress processes of rejective sensitivity, internalised homophobia and concealment. Compared to wait-list, intervention participants showed significant reductions in depressive symptoms, alcohol use problems, sexual compulsivity and condomless sex; results were not significant for anxiety (Pachankis et al., 2015). Pachankis et al. (2020b) adapted the intervention for young adult sexual minority women. Group comparisons indicated greater reductions in depression and anxiety in the treatment than the waitlist group but no significant differences for alcohol use or suicidality.

Neither study found significant group differences for either universal processes (rumination, emotional regulation, perceived social support, assertiveness) or minority stress processes (rejection sensitivity, conceal-ment, internalised stigma and gay-related stress, except for unexpectedly higher perceived social support in the women's waitlist group. In the men's study, pre-post intervention comparisons in the intervention group showed reductions in the expected directions for the universal processes except for emotion regulation, and for minority stress processes except for concealment; effect sizes were generally large and a future study should have a larger sample size to investigate these processes. In contrast, in the women's study, pre-post comparisons indicated significant reduc-tions only for emotion dysregulation ($d = 0.66$) and rumination ($d = 0.70$). Overall, the effect sizes for minority stress processes in the women's study were small (mean $d = 0.25$) and for universal processes were small-to-medium ($d = 0.48$).

Pachankis et al. (2022) reported that their intervention was not statis-tically superior to either LGBQ-affirmative counselling or HIV testing/counselling for HIV transmission risk behaviour, depression, anxiety, substance use, suicidality or various mental health diagnoses.

Third-Wave CBT Approaches

A systematic review of Acceptance and Commitment Therapy (ACT) approaches for LGBTQI + individuals identified five uncontrolled studies (Fowler et al., 2022). There were some promising findings, but all studies were rated as methodologically weak. An uncontrolled US pilot study found an online mindfulness-based stress reduction intervention to be acceptable, feasible and associated with preliminary indications of some reduction in perceived stress (Jabson Tree & Patterson, 2019). For DBT, see Chapter 12.

Conclusions About CBT Protocols Adapted for Sexual Minority Adults

A summary of key research findings is presented in Box 11.1. The limited current research does not provide strong evidence to support the use of CBT protocols specifically adapted for sexual minority adults over standard CBT. No research has compared adapted versus standard CBT in relation to acceptability, retention or outcomes. The highest quality studies of adapted protocols found reductions for some of the psychological symptoms assessed but the evidence of reductions in minority stress processes targeted was less strong, especially for sexual minority women. This is particularly concerning given the evidence already described that in the UK National Health Service Talking Therapies for anxiety and depression programme, sexual minority women have poorer outcomes in standard interventions than their heterosexual counterparts (Rimes et al., 2019). Further research is required into how to improve CBT for sexual minority women in particular. It is possible that adapted CBT for sexual minority women needs to address the psychological impact of the increased child and adulthood abuse, violence and victimisation experienced by sexual minority women compared to heterosexual women (McGeough & Sterzing, 2018; Roberts et al., 2010; Schneeberger et al., 2014) or other forms of stigma and social disadvantage that co-occur with their sexual minority status, such as sexism (Dworkin et al., 2018). Research could also investigate whether sexual minority women may benefit from more intense or longer duration CBT.

Box 11.1: Summary of Key Research Findings

- Cognitive and behavioural processes suggested to contribute to mental health problems are found at elevated rates in sexual minority adults. This may be at least partly due to minority stress experiences. However, current evidence is drawn from cross-sectional studies and stronger research designs are needed to investigate causal directions.
- A study using national data from England from services which provide evidence-based treatments including CBT, found that compared to their heterosexual counterparts, poorer treatment outcomes were evident for lesbian women, bisexual women and bisexual men. Gay men did not show significantly different treatment outcomes than heterosexual men.
- Promising results were found in UK studies of two interventions specially adapted for sexual minority adults, but these were uncontrolled studies.

- Two US randomised studies of transdiagnostic CBT, adapted to address minority stressors, for sexual minority young men and women, found larger reductions in depression and anxiety in the intervention group compared to the waitlist control group but no significant group differences for the minority stress or universal cognitive behavioural processes targeted. A third study of the same intervention compared to counselling or HIV testing found no significant group differences for HIV risk behaviours or mental health.

Providing CBT for Sexual Minority Adults

Therapist Knowledge and Beliefs

UK adults who had received CBT or another evidence-based treatment reported that they felt their therapists often lacked knowledge about sexual minority experiences, demonstrated heteronormative assumptions, neglected discussions about how their experiences as a sexual minority individual had impacted on their mental health and sometimes pathologised their sexual orientation (Morris et al., 2022). This is consistent with findings from an earlier systematic review of psychotherapy experiences (King et al., 2007). It is important for therapists to be aware of their own beliefs and experiences relating to sexual orientation and how these could impact on their interpretation of the client's difficulties, the therapeutic relationship and other therapy processes. This is not only the case for therapists with negative views or who have knowledge of the harm of homophobia/biphobia. Some therapists may have an unrealistically positive or optimistic approach to minority sexual orientation, which could be perceived as invalidating or even put clients at risk if they encourage behavioural experiments in unsafe contexts. The therapist should consider how the client's ongoing minority stressors may impact on their ability to benefit from therapy. Extra training may be required. Clinical supervision should also be used for therapist reflection and further learning. Optimising one's clinical practice with sexual minority clients is an ongoing process, as the therapist learns from their work with people with widely different experiences and in a changing social context.

Assessment and Formulation

In Chapter 8, issues of minority stress factors and social-cultural consideration to be made in clinical formulation were discussed. In this chapter, we focus on CBT formulation specific to sexual minority clients. The formulation involves the application of cognitive behavioural theory and research to develop a collaborate understanding of the client's presenting problems, which guides the treatment plan. UK research indicates that many therapists do not ask about whether the client's sexual orientation could play any role in their presenting difficulties (Morris et al., 2022). This could be due to a fear of seeming prejudiced or pathologising minority sexual orientation, or displaying a lack of understanding about the experiences of sexual minority people and how these may impact on mental health and therapy processes. It means that important information may be missed about the role of sexuality-related processes in the development or maintenance of the problem. It also risks making the client feel that the therapist is not interested in their sexual orientation, has negative views about it or considers it irrelevant. This may make it more difficult for the client to trust the therapist, feel understood or consider it safe to talk about their sexual orientation or minority stress processes.

The impact of one's sexual orientation should be discussed for possible inclusion in the longitudinal formulation. For example, there is longitudinal research evidence that compared to heterosexual people, sexual minority adults were more likely to be gender nonconforming in childhood, showing play or appearance preferences considered atypical for children of their sex (e.g. Li et al., 2017). Childhood gender nonconformity is associated with increased risk of child abuse and peer and emotional problems abuse (e.g. Warren et al., 2019, 2022), perhaps through acting as a visible marker of difference, and may contribute to core beliefs about being unacceptable, flawed or different to others.

Society-wide ideals regarding beauty or sexual attractiveness can be experienced in both similar and different ways by sexual minority adults (e.g. Bridge et al., 2022b) with potential impact on core beliefs relating to being ugly, unattractive, undesirable and so on.

Sexual minority individuals who are finding it difficult to accept their orientation are particularly likely to have negative attitudes towards same-sex attractions or the meaning of those in the eyes of others. People who are questioning their sexual orientation may also be facing these beliefs and attitudes for the first time and may require support too. Even those who accept their sexual orientation or see it positively may at the same time have negative beliefs about the consequences of about open about one's sexual orientation, trying to find a same-sex partner, or parenting or growing older as a sexual minority person. These areas may well be more challenging for a sexual minority person than a heterosexual person, but beliefs may be excessively negative or place limitations on the person progressing in valued life domains.

Regarding *maintaining factors*, one example is the chronic impact of stress relating to one's sexual orientation, for example as a result of fear or experienced victimisation or prejudice and monitoring the environment for safety. This may not be fully realised by sexual minority individuals, as it is a part of their daily lives and they may not have known anything different. For this and other reasons such as shame or fearing lack of understanding, clients may not spontaneously mention such effects.

It may be more difficult for sexual minority adults to utilise or cultivate positive coping responses such as assertiveness, socialising with like-minded peers or seeking social support in the context of societal stigma, prejudice, discrimination and victimisation. In such contexts, general unhelpful behaviours such as avoidance, rumination and excessive substance use may be more likely to develop (see Hatzenbuehler, 2009).

Sexual orientation concealment may protect the individual from some stigma experiences but can have a wide range of negative effects (see Pachankis et al., (2020a)) which may be important to include in the formulation. Sexual-orientation contexts and peers should also be considered. For example, using drugs or alcohol as a coping mechanism may be more likely and harder to address if the main venues for meeting other sexual minority people involve these substances. The increased substance use within some sexual minority contexts may also normalise behaviours, so that people do not acknowledge a problem or seek try to help until problematic use has got more severe.

Unhelpful underlying beliefs and rules are often associated with unhelpful coping or compensatory strategies, but the relationship is not always immediately apparent and may require guided discovery. For example, a belief such as "My sexual orientation makes me inferior to others and vulnerable to rejection" may be associated with an unhelpful assumption such as "Unless I perform to a very high standards at work and in my personal life, others will reject me because I'm already viewed as being inferior due to be gay", which is accompanied by unhelpful perfectionist behaviours.

As with the development of unhelpful beliefs, supporting the client to reflect on how the sexual orientation experiences have impacted on the development of helpful and unhelpful behavioural responses may help them develop greater understanding and a more self-compassionate approach to their current difficulties. These should be considered in the context of experiences of other types of prejudice and discrimination for example in relation to sex, race, religion and so on. Everyone's developmental, family, community and sociocultural context is different and consideration is required regarding the impact of experiences of homophobia/biphobia for the client's own systems. It is also important to acknowledge that stigma-related stressors continue through the life course (see Chapter 5).

Psychoeducation

Psychoeducation materials can be checked for heterosexism and adapted using examples and additional information relevant to sexual minority individuals.

Working with Negative Automatic Thoughts

The therapist should be alert for negative thoughts relating to, or impacted by, sexuality-related factors. If the level of distress does not seem to be in proportion to the thought expressed, the therapist could explore if there could be other negative thoughts, which the person may find difficult to identify or disclose. Internalised stigma may result in thoughts such as "Having these sexual feelings is disgusting/immoral/a sin" or "This sexual attraction means I'm letting down my family and community". People can also report self-critical thoughts about their coping ability e.g. "I should be able to accept my sexuality" or "Other people cope much better than I do" (Bridge et al., 2022b). It may also be difficult to acknowledge to the self or the therapist that they have negative thoughts about other sexual minority individuals, for example as an effect of internalising society's negative attitudes towards same-sex behaviour or gender nonconformity. The therapist could encourage disclosure by talking about how societal attitudes can have strong effects on us and that we all have prejudices, which can include internalised stigma.

Addressing Conditional Beliefs and Rules

As when working with any type of unhelpful assumption, attitude or rule, the therapist can support the client to reflect on the understandable contexts in which the belief developed, and the advantages and disadvantages of the belief and associated behaviours. For example, striving to meet consistently high standards in a valued life area (e.g. "If I'm not consistently highly successful in XYZ, then others will consider me a total failure because of my sexuality") may have helped them to achieve higher standards and feel less of a failure. A belief that "If I conceal my same-sex attractions, I won't be rejected or victimised" may have been the safest belief in a homophobic/biphobic school and family context. However, when such conditional beliefs specify outcomes that are unattainable, held in a rigid, inflexible manner that does not allow for changing contexts, and associated with unhelpful compensatory behaviours, they can have a range of negative consequences which outweigh potential benefits; this could include highly negative automatic thoughts and associated distress when the conditions are not met. Once a collaborative, compassionate understanding of the beliefs and behaviours has been developed, which may incorporate the impact of stigma or victimisation experiences relating to sexual orientation, the therapist and client can work together on the development of a new more adaptive belief. Potential new beliefs can be evaluated against previous experience as well as learning through specifically targeted behavioural experiments to gain new information.

Addressing Maintaining Behaviours/Processes

Standard CBT methods such as exposure and behavioural experiments can be applied for helping the client to reduce unhelpful responses and cultivate more helpful ones. Beliefs relating to unhelpful maintaining factors should be identified to inform behavioural experiments. Examples of beliefs relating to avoidant behaviours could be "If I try going to LGBTQ + events, I'll be judged as unattractive and be left out" or "If I try to get support from Mum about relationship difficulties with my partner, she will just blame it on being a lesbian and won't be any help".

When planning behavioural experiments or exposure, as usual in CBT, the client should be supported to consider possible outcomes. In the case of sexual minorities practising being more open about their sexual orientation, there can be safety issues to consider regarding possibility of verbal, physical and sexual victimisation. Sexual minority young people are also at increased risk of being made homeless (Corliss et al., 2011). Many sexual minority individuals find that others can detect their sexual orientation even if they try to conceal it. Some have become avoidant of situations to an extent that impairs their life (e.g. never using public transport) or they utilise other safety-seeking behaviours that bring negative consequences. This may require careful discussion about the pros, cons and risks of different behaviours and whether their strategies could be modified while maintaining safety.

For some sexual minority individuals, avoiding discussing their sexual orientation may be associated with a more generalised avoidance of discussing personal information or their feelings. Behavioural experiments testing out specific unhelpful beliefs about the consequences of being more open can be undertaken. People often find it preferable to do this in a graded manner, for example starting with individuals either most trusted or for whom the potential negative consequences are perceived to be less severe, and with less personal or distressing content.

If the client is ruminating excessively about the causes of their sexual orientation, the therapist could help identify the associated beliefs, such as whether they belief this could lead to some way of changing their sexual orientation. There may be a need for self-acceptance work within a compassionate framing that there is no evidence that adult same-sex attractions are amenable to intervention attempts (Fish & Russell, 2020). Rumination can also be addressed using cognitive behavioural methods for perseverative processing (Watkins et al., 2011).

Cultivating Effective Coping Responses

Sexual minority individuals often have previous or ongoing experiences that may make it more challenging to develop or employ effective coping responses. CBT can aim to improve the effectiveness and utilisation of existing strategies and expand the range of coping methods. Two examples are provided here.

For some sexual minority individuals, it has been more challenging to develop assertiveness skills due to underlying beliefs about being unworthy, bad or socially unacceptable. It is important to identify beliefs about using assertive behaviours. For example, the individual may believe "If I try to stand up to my mother's excessive demands, she will use my sexual orientation to shame or pressurise me" or "If I don't do everything that my family want, they will reject me because of my sexual orientation" or "If I stand up for myself with X, they will 'out' me". Such beliefs may or may not be currently correct, which can be evaluated by guided discovery and behavioural experiments. The client may need support in learning adaptive ways of coping if their feared consequence is correct.

Social support skills and networks can also be more challenging for sexual minority individuals to develop and maintain, especially those who conceal their sexual orientation or live outside of larger cities. Although more support is now available due to online resources, the limitations of purely online support should be acknowledged. The client may benefit from further developing their social support skills using standard CBT methods, or social support access through multiple means including LGBTQ + groups or organisations, LGBTQ + individuals or allies within their existing family/friend/work networks. Behavioural experiments may indicate that even people who were initially not supportive may become so over time, especially if the client feels able to share their experiences and feelings to help others understand. Some find volunteering and social justice work has a positive impact on their social support and positive sexuality identity; again an experimental approach can be encouraged so that possible negative effects are also addressed, such as greater exposure to stigma processes.

Working with Core Beliefs

Depending on factors such as the presenting problem and number of sessions available, addressing core beliefs may or may not be necessary or feasible. When negative core/unconditional beliefs are addressed, the therapist can collaboratively support the client to reflect whether their experiences as a sexual minority individual have contributed to their development or maintenance. Messages from family, peers or their socio-cultural group, either explicit or implicit, that having same sex attractions is bad, wrong, disgusting, immoral and so on, may have had a strong impact. Experiences of stigma, discrimination or victimisation would also be expected to contribute to negative over-general beliefs about other people (e.g. "Other people will reject me", "Others would be better off if I didn't exist", the world (e.g. "The world is dangerous place") or the future (e.g. "The future is hopeless"). Discussing the challenges of developing positive core beliefs in stigmatising contexts may help the client to become more open to the possibility that their beliefs are not necessarily true, and help them to develop greater self-compassion. Identifying sexual minority role models may be helpful in the cultivation of positive and accepting self-beliefs, and improving access to social support from accepting others may also be important (Bridge et al., 2022a). The challenges of maintaining positive self-beliefs in the context of ongoing stigma and realities of being different from the majority, should be acknowledged.

Conclusion

Research suggests that many unhelpful cognitive and behavioural processes are elevated in sexual minority individuals compared to heterosexual peers, and that minority stress experiences and child abuse may contribute to these differences. Therefore, there is a good rationale for CBT. Research into CBT outcomes for sexual minorities compared to heterosexuals using standard CBT, and adaptations to CBT for sexual minority adults is limited but increasing. Research so far indicates that sexual minority women benefit less than sexual minority men from routine or adapted CBT. CBT therapists and their clients may benefit from greater understanding and attention to the impact of experiences relating to minority sexual orientation on mental health problems, the therapeutic relationship and therapy processes.

References

Argyriou, A., Goldsmith, K. A., & Rimes, K. A. (2021). Mediators of the disparities in depression between sexual minority and heterosexual individuals: A systematic review. *Archives of Sexual Behavior, 50*(3), 925–959. https://doi.org/10.1007/s10508-020-01862-0

Argyriou, A., Goldsmith, K. A., Tsokos, A., & Rimes, K. A. (2020). Psychosocial mediators of the relations between sexual orientation and depressive symptoms in a longitudinal sample of young people. *Psychology of Sexual Orientation and Gender Diversity, 7*, 142–153. https://doi.org/10.1037/sgd0000369

Beard, C., Kirakosian, N., Silverman, A. L., Winer, J. P., Wadsworth, L. P., & Björgvinsson, T. (2017). Comparing treatment response between LGBQ and heterosexual individuals attending a CBT- and DBT-skills-based partial hospital. *Journal of Consulting and Clinical Psychology, 85*(12), 1171–1181. https://doi.org/10.1037/ccp0000251

Beck, A. T., Rush, A. J., Shaw, B. F., & Emery, G. (1979). *Cognitive therapy of depression.* Guilford Press.

Bridge, L. (2021). *Self-esteem in sexual minority young adults: An investigation of factors affecting self-esteem and development of a new psychological intervention to improve low self-esteem.* Unpublished PhD dissertation, King's College London.

Bridge, L., Langford, K., McMullen, K., Rai, L., Smith, P., Rimes, K. A. (in press). *Acceptability, feasibility, and preliminary efficacy of a compassion-based cognitive behavioural intervention for low self-esteem in sexual minority young adults.* Clinical Psychology & Psychotherapy.

Bridge, L., Smith, P. A., & Rimes, K. A. (2019). Sexual orientation differences in the self-esteem of men and women: A systematic review and meta-analysis. *Psychology of Sexual Orientation and Gender Diversity, 6*(4), 433–446. https://doi.org/10.1037/sgd0000342

Bridge, L., Smith, P., & Rimes, K. A. (2022a). Self-esteem in sexual minority young adults: A qualitative interview study exploring protective factors and helpful coping responses. *International Review of Psychiatry, 34*(3–4), 257–265. https://doi.org/10.1080/09540261.2022.2051446

Bridge, L. P., Smith, P., & Rimes, K. A. (2022b). Sexual minority young adults' perspectives on how minority stress and other factors negatively affect self-esteem: A qualitative interview study. *International Review of Psychiatry, 34*(3–4), 383–391. https://doi.org/10.1080/09540261.2022.2051444

Camp, J., Vitoratou, S., & Rimes, K. A. (2020). LGBQ+ self-acceptance and its relationship with minority stressors and mental health: A systematic literature review. *Archives of Sexual Behavior, 49*, 2353–2373. https://doi.org/10.1007/s10508-020-01755-2

Corliss, H. L., Goodenow, C. S., Nichols, L., & Austin, S. B. (2011). High burden of homelessness among sexual-minority adolescents: Findings from a representative Massachusetts high school sample. *American Journal of Public Health, 101*(9), 1683–1689. https://doi.org/10.2105/AJPH.2011.300155

Critcher, C. R., & Ferguson, M. J. (2014). The cost of keeping it hidden: Decomposing concealment reveals what makes it depleting. *Journal of Experimental Psychology: General, 143*(2), 721–735. https://doi.org/10.1037/a0033468

Dworkin, E. R., Gilmore, A. K., Bedard-Gilligan, M., Lehavot, K., Guttman-nova, K., & Kaysen, D. (2018). Predicting PTSD severity from experiences of trauma and heterosexism in lesbian and bisexual women: A longitudinal study of cognitive mediators. *Journal of Counseling Psychology, 65*(3), 324–333. https://doi.org/10.1037/cou0000287

Fish, J. N., & Russell, S. T. (2020). Sexual orientation and gender identity change efforts are unethical and harmful. *American Journal of Public Health, 110*(8), 1113.

Fowler, J. A., Viskovich, S., Buckley, L., Dean, J. A., & J.A. (2022). A call for action: A systematic review of empirical evidence for the use of Acceptance and Commitment Therapy (ACT) with LGBTQI+ individuals. *Journal of Contextual Behavioral Science, 25*, 78–89. https://doi.org/10.1016/j.jcbs.2022.06.007

Foy, A., Morris, D., Fernandes, V., & Rimes, K. A. (2019). LGBQ+ adults' experiences of improving access to psychological therapies and primary care counselling services: Informing clinical practice and service delivery. *The Cognitive Behaviour Therapist, 12*, e42. https://doi.org/10.1017/S1754470X19000291

Gilbert, P. (2009). Introducing compassion-focused therapy. *Advances in Psychiatric Treatment, 15*(3), 199.

Gnan, G., Rahman, Q., & Rimes, K. (2022). Cognitive and behavioral factors contributing to distress in LGBTQ+ students: A prospective mediation study. *International Review of Psychiatry, 34*(3–4), 274–281. https://doi.org/10.1080/09540261.2022.2058871

Hambrook, D., Benjamin, L., Aries, D., & Rimes, K. (2022). Group intervention for sexual minority adults with common mental Health problems: Preliminary evaluation. *Behavioural and Cognitive Psychotherapy, 50*(6), 575–589. https://doi.org/10.1017/S1352465822000297

Hatzenbuehler, M. L. (2009). How does sexual minority stigma "get under the skin"? A psychological mediation framework. *Psychological Bulletin, 135*(5), 707–730. https://doi.org/10.1037/a0016441

Hatzenbuehler, M. L., Nolen-Hoeksema, S., & Erickson, S. J. (2008). Minority stress predictors of HIV risk behavior, substance use, and depressive symptoms: Results from a prospective study of bereaved gay men. Health psychology: official journal of the Division of Health Psychology. *American Psychological Association, 27*(4), 455–462. https://doi.org/10.1037/0278-6133.27.4.455

Jabson Tree, J. M., & Patterson, J. G. (2019). A Test of feasibility and acceptability of online mindfulness-based stress reduction for lesbian, gay, and bisexual women and men at risk for high stress: Pilot study. *JMIR Mental Health, 6*(8), e15048. https://doi.org/10.2196/15048

King, M., Semlyen, J., Killaspy, H., Nazareth, I., & Osborn, D. (2007). *A systematic review of research on counselling and psychotherapy for lesbian, gay, bisexual & transgender people.* British Association for Counselling and Psychotherapy.

Layard, R., & Clark, D. M. (2015). What works for whom? Chapter 10 in *Thrive: How better mental health care transforms lives and saves money* (pp.153–179). Princeton University Press. https://doi.org/10.2307/j.ctv c77595

Li, G., Kung, K. T. F., & Hines, M. (2017). Childhood gender-typed behavior and adolescent sexual orientation: A longitudinal population-based study. *Developmental Psychology, 53*(4), 764–777. https://doi.org/10.1037/dev000 0281

Lloyd, C. E., Rimes, K. A., & Hambrook, D. G. (2021). LGBQ adults' experiences of a CBT wellbeing group for anxiety and depression in an improving access to psychological therapies service: A qualitative service evaluation. *The Cognitive Behaviour Therapist, 13,*. https://doi.org/10.1017/S1754470X200 00598

McGeogh, B. L., & Sterzing, P. R. (2018). A systematic review of family victimization experiences among sexual minority youth. *Journal of Primary Prevention, 39,* 491–528.

Morris, D., Fernandes, V., & Rimes, K. (2022). Sexual minority service user perspectives on mental health treatment barriers to care and service improvements. *International Review of Psychiatry, 34*(3–4), 230–239. https://doi.org/10.1080/09540261.2022.2051445

Meyer, I. H. (2003). Prejudice, social stress, and mental health in lesbian, gay, and bisexual populations: Conceptual issues and research evidence. *Psychological Bulletin, 129*(5), 674–697. https://doi.org/10.1037/0033-2909.129.5.674

Mustanski, B., & Liu, R. T. (2013). A longitudinal study of predictors of suicide attempts among lesbian, gay, bisexual, and transgender youth. *Archives of Sexual Behavior, 42*(3), 437–448. https://doi.org/10.1007/s10 508-012-0013-9

Nematy, A., Fattahi, K., Khosravi, Z., & Khodabakhsh, R. (2014). A Comparison of early maladaptive schemata among homosexual, bisexual and heterosexual people in Iran. *Journal of Gay & Lesbian Mental Health, 18*(4), 361–374. https://doi.org/10.1080/19359705.2014.908334

Newcomb, M. E., & Mustanski, B. (2010). Internalized homophobia and internalizing mental health problems: A meta-analytic review. *Clinical Psychology Review, 30*, 1019–1029. https://doi.org/10.1016/j.cpr.2010. 07.003

Pachankis, J. E. (2007). The psychological implications of concealing a stigma: A cognitive-affective-behavioral model. *Psychological Bulletin, 133*(2).

Pachankis, J. E., Harkness, A., Maciejewski, K. R., Behari, K., Clark, K. A., McConocha, E., Winston, R., Adeyinka, O., Reynolds, J., Bränström, R., Esserman, D. A., Hatzenbuehler, M. L., & Safren, S. A. (2022). LGBQ-affirmative cognitive-behavioral therapy for young gay and bisexual men's mental and sexual health: A three-arm randomized controlled trial. *Journal of Consulting and Clinical Psychology, 90*(6), 459–477. https://doi.org/10. 1037/ccp0000724

Pachankis, J. E., Hatzenbuehler, M. L., Rendina, H. J., Safren, S. A., & Parsons, J. T. (2015). LGB-affirmative cognitive-behavioral therapy for young adult gay and bisexual men: A randomized controlled trial of a transdiagnostic minority stress approach. *Journal of Consulting and Clinical Psychology, 83*(5), 875–889.

Pachankis, J. E., Mahon, C. P., Jackson, S. D., Fetzner, B. K., & Bränström, R. (2020a). Sexual orientation concealment and mental health: A conceptual and meta-analytic review. *Psychological Bulletin, 146*(10), 831.

Pachankis, J. E., McConocha, E. M., Clark, K. A., Wang, K., Behari, K., Fetzner, B. K., Brisbin, C. D., Scheer, J. R., & Lehavot, K. (2020b). A transdiagnostic minority stress intervention for gender diverse sexual minority women's depression, anxiety, and unhealthy alcohol use: A randomized controlled trial. *Journal of Consulting and Clinical Psychology, 88*(7), 613.

Puckett, J. A., Feinstein, B. A., Newcomb, M. E., & Mustanski, B. (2018). Trajectories of internalized heterosexism among young men who have sex with men. *Journal of Youth and Adolescence, 47*, 872–889. https://doi.org/ 10.1007/s10964-017-0670-z

Rimes, K. A., Broadbent, M. T. M., Holden, R., Rahman, Q., Hambrook, D., Hatch, S. L., & Wingrove, J. (2018). Comparison of treatment outcomes between lesbian, gay, bisexual and heterosexual individuals receiving a primary care psychological intervention. *Behavioural and Cognitive Psychotherapy, 46*, 332–349. https://doi.org/10.1017/S13524658170 00583

Rimes, K. A., Ion, D., Wingrove, J., & Carter, B. (2019). Sexual orientation differences in psychological treatment outcomes for depression and anxiety:

National cohort study. *Journal of Consulting and Clinical Psychology, 877*, 577–589. https://doi.org/10.1037/ccp0000416

Roberts, A. L., Austin, S. B., Corliss, H. L., Vandermorris, A. K., & Koenen, K. C. (2010). Pervasive trauma exposure among US sexual orientation minority adults and risk of posttraumatic stress disorder. *American Journal of Public Health, 100*(12), 2433–2441. https://doi.org/10.2105/AJPH.2009.168971

Rostosky, S. S., Richardson, M. T., McCurry, S. K., & Riggle, E. D. B. (2022). LGBTQ individuals' lived experiences of hypervigilance. *Psychology of Sexual Orientation and Gender Diversity, 9*(3), 358–369. https://doi.org/10.1037/sgd0000474

Safren, S. A., & Heimberg, R. G. (1999). Depression, hopelessness, suicidality, and related factors in sexual minority and heterosexual adolescents. *Journal of Consulting and Clinical Psychology, 67*(6), 859–866. https://doi.org/10.1037/0022-006X.67.6.859

Schneeberger, A. R., Dietl, M. F., Muenzenmaier, K. H., Huber, C. G., & Lang, U. E. (2014). Stressful childhood experiences and health outcomes in sexual minority populations: A systematic review. *Social Psychiatry and Psychiatric Epidemiology, 49*(9), 1427–1445. https://doi.org/10.1007/s00127-014-0854-8

Semlyen, J., King, M., Varney, J., & Hagger-Johnson, G. (2016). Sexual orientation and symptoms of common mental disorder or low wellbeing: Combined meta-analysis of 12 UK population health surveys. *BMC Psychiatry, 16*, 67. https://doi.org/10.1186/s12888-016-0767-z

Timmins, L., Rimes, K. A., & Rahman, Q. (2018). Minority stressors, rumination, and psychological distress in monozygotic twins discordant for sexual minority status. *Psychological Medicine, 48*, 1705–1712. https://doi.org/10.1017/S003329171700321X

Timmins, L., Rimes, K. A., & Rahman, Q. (2020). Minority stressors, rumination and psychological distress in lesbian, gay and bisexual individuals. *Archives of Sexual Behavior, 49*, 661–680. https://doi.org/10.1007/s10508-019-01502-2

Warren, A.-S., Goldsmith, K. A., & Rimes, K. (2019). Childhood gender-typed behavior and emotional or peer problems: A prospective birth-cohort study. *Journal of Child Psychology and Psychiatry, 60*(8), 888–896. https://doi.org/10.1111/jcpp.13051

Warren, A. S., Goldsmith, K. A., & Rimes, K. A. (2022). Childhood gender-typed behaviour, sexual orientation, childhood abuse and post-traumatic stress disorder: A prospective birth-cohort study. *International Review of*

Psychiatry, 34(3–4), 360–375. https://doi.org/10.1080/09540261.2022.206 4211

Watkins, E., Mullan, E., Wingrove, J., Rimes, K., Steiner, H., Bathurst, N., Eastman, R., & Scott, J. (2011). Rumination-focused cognitive–behavioural therapy for residual depression: Phase II randomised controlled trial. *British Journal of Psychiatry, 199*(4), 317–322. https://doi.org/10.1192/bjp.bp.110. 090282

12

Dialectical Behaviour Therapy for Sexual Minority Populations

Jake Camp

Introduction

As outlined in Chapter 2, individuals identifying as sexual minorities and sexuality diverse (that is, LGBQ+) have been shown to have a significantly higher risk of mental ill-health and are more likely to engage in self-harming and suicidal behaviours compared to their heterosexual peers (King et al., 2008; Meyer, 2003; Semlyen et al., 2016). Sexual minorities also present with increased difficulties with emotion dysregulation from a young age (Hatzenbuehler et al., 2008; Kapatais et al., 2022). As discussed in earlier chapters, LGBQ+ groups are suggested to experience varying stressors related to their minority status and living

J. Camp (✉)
Institute of Psychiatry, Psychology, & Neuroscience, King's College London, London, UK
e-mail: Jake.Camp@slam.nhs.uk; Jake.camp@kcl.ac.uk

National & Specialist CAMHS, DBT Service, South London and Maudsley NHS Foundation Trust, London, UK

J. Semlyen and P. Rohleder (eds.), *Sexual Minorities and Mental Health*, https://doi.org/10.1007/978-3-031-37438-8_12

in environments that privilege heterosexual-majority ideologies, on top of typical stressors experienced by majority groups. In addition, sexual-minority individuals are thought to experience gender-based stressors due to the increased likelihood of gender diversity outside of typified dominant binary gender norms (Gordon & Meyer, 2007; Skerven et al., 2019). The burden of such additive minority-based stress likely contributes to the higher vulnerability of LGBQ+ individuals to mental health difficulties and self-harming behaviours (King et al., 2008; Meyer, 2003). Therefore, sexual-minority individuals living in heterosexist environments and experiencing minority stress may be more likely to experience difficulties that Dialectical Behaviour Therapy (DBT) addresses (such as self-harm and emotion dysregulation). Thus, DBT may be well positioned to effectively target difficulties that burden the LGBQ+ population.

This chapter will outline the ways in which DBT may be a potentially viable option for supporting sexuality-diverse or -minority individuals experiencing psychological distress. Details will be provided regarding how the underlying transactional biosocial model may compliment minority stress models (for example, Meyer, 2003) in understanding how distress develops within this population and how to use this model to support clients to understand themselves and feel validated. Additionally, the application of DBT skills and principles to LGBQ-associated difficulties, how the structure of delivery is useful and can be optimised, and specific suggestions for therapists supporting sexual minority groups will be discussed. The chapter will conclude with a summary of the current research investigating the application of non-adapted DBT and LGBQ-affirmative adaptations for sexuality-diverse individuals.

Dialectical Behaviour Therapy

DBT was initially developed by Marsha Linehan (1993) for highly suicidal individuals who experienced difficulties regulating intense emotional pain. DBT is a principle-based intervention structured around behaviourism, validation, Zen, and dialectical philosophies. Comprehensive DBT is comprised of four modes of treatment: weekly individual therapy sessions, weekly group skills training, between-session telephone support and skills coaching, and therapist team consultation groups (Linehan, 1993). DBT aims to support individuals to work towards to their version of 'a life that is worth living', usually inclusive of value-congruent occupation, supportive relationships, and good-enough environments to inhabit (that is: something to do, somewhere to live, and people to love). It is underpinned by a transactional biosocial model (see Fig. 12.1), which suggests that difficulties regulating emotions is the key contributor to dysregulation in other areas, such as in behaviour, relationships, cognitions, and sense of self. The biosocial model posits that individuals at risk of emotion dysregulation may have a biological or temperamental sensitivity to emotions, where they experience increased sensitivity and are more reactive to emotion cues, and have a slower return to baseline compared to the average population (Linehan, 1993). It has also been suggested that trait anxiety and impulsivity have similar pathways to the development of symptoms associated with emotion dysregulation (Grove & Crowell, 2019). An emotion sensitivity, over time, shapes how the person interacts with their environment. The environment often does not fit well with the needs of someone with any such 'sensitivity' or difference. Thus, this often increases the likelihood of the 'sensitive' person experiencing their environment—the developmentally-important people around them—as invalidating.

An invalidating environment, the 'social' part of the model, is an environment that regularly rejects or ignores primary adaptive emotions and internal experiences, and overly attends to extreme or 'dysfunctional' displays of emotion, thus teaching a child from an early age that their internal experiences are unacceptable and invalid, and that they need to escalate their response to get their needs met (Linehan, 1993). Another aspect of the invalidating environment is the oversimplification of problem-solving complex human experiences and emotions (Linehan, 1993). Invalidating environments tend to reinforce the need for more extreme emotion-driven behaviours to get needs met and punishes normative 'adaptive' emotion-based expressions. The transactional aspect of the model suggests that the external expression of emotion by the individual and the invalidation from the environment interact continuously and reciprocally, over time amplifying the intensity and nature of emotional experience and expression, and thus the intensity and nature of invalidation. This chronic transaction between a 'sensitivity' and an invalidating environment can prevent the development and cause the breakdown of adaptive skills to regulate emotional pain, including the capacity to label and modulate emotions (Grove & Crowell, 2019; Linehan, 1993). It also increases difficulties with accurately and effectively expressing emotions, thus further increasing the likelihood that others will not understand the internal experiences of the person, leading to an increased likelihood that they will invalidate them (Fruzzetti et al., 2005).

Chronic exposure to an invalidating environment ultimately results in the internalisation of invalidation, producing self-invalidation. Self-invalidation further compounds the mistrust of internal experiences and prevents the development of effective skills to regulate painful emotions and experiences (Linehan, 1993). Impairment in the ability to regulate intense and painful emotions then increases the likelihood of dysregulation in other areas of the person's life. This model is further expanded below in relation to how it is applied to sexual-minority populations (Fig. 12.1).

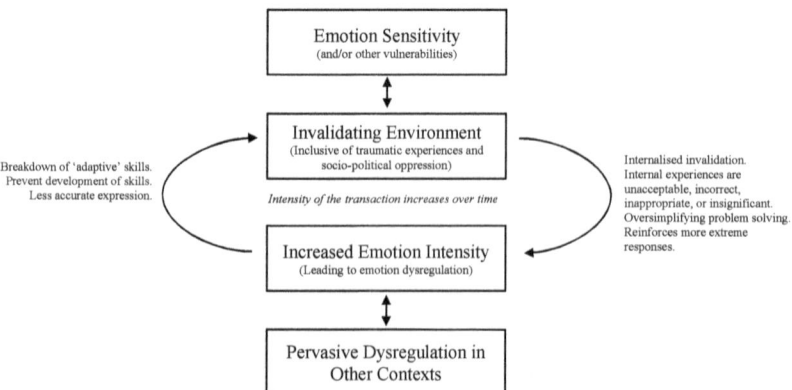

Fig. 12.1 The biosocial transactional model (*Source* Adapted from the model as described by: Fruzzetti et al., 2005; Grove & Crowell, 2019; Linehan, 1993)

DBT attempts to reduce emotion dysregulation, as a key treatment target, by supporting the person to develop adaptive skills to modulate emotions and experiences where possible, balanced with tolerating and accepting aspects which cannot be changed in the moment. All principles and skills in DBT are guided by the core dialectic: acceptance and change. On the change end of the dialectic exist skills to help regulate emotions and get needs met from others while maintaining relationships and self-respect. On the acceptance end exist skills around validation (self- and other-directed), mindful awareness of experience and acceptance of reality. Dialectics is the philosophy which underpins the DBT model and represents the notion that there are many truths, that potentially opposite truths can exist simultaneously, and that everything is inter-related and caused.

DBT has a relatively strong evidence-base for a number of outcomes. The most researched outcome is self-harm and suicidal behaviours in adult populations, within which DBT has demonstrated efficacy (see Chen et al., 2021; DeCou et al., 2019for reviews). In addition, DBT is also evidenced to be effective in reducing symptoms associated with a diagnosis of borderline personality disorder (BPD) (Some issues related to this diagnosis and LGBQ+ individuals are discussed further below), emotion dysregulation, depression, anxiety, eating disorders and substance use disorders (Ben-Porath et al., 2020; Chen et al., 2021; Haktanir & Callender, 2020; Neacsiu et al., 2014). DBT has also been adapted for adolescent populations and demonstrated efficacy in reducing self-harming behaviours, suicidal ideation, BPD symptoms, emotion dysregulation and depression symptoms (see Bahji et al., 2021; Johnstone et al., 2022; MacPherson et al., 2013 for reviews). DBT is recommended by the UK National Institute of Health and Care Excellence (NICE, 2009) for the management of self-harm and for adults with a diagnosis of BPD where self-harm is present, and for adolescents engaging in self-harming behaviours and experiencing emotion dysregulation (NICE, 2022).

Both DBT for adults and adolescents is accessible via the UK National Health Service (NHS). Comprehensive DBT (including all four treatment modes) is often a secondary or tertiary specialist intervention, reflecting the higher intensity of the intervention for more severe mental health difficulties. DBT-informed interventions, including group-only or individual-only formats, are also often delivered at lower-tiered services where there is less need for intensive interventions, however it is noteworthy that while group-only DBT interventions have emerging evidence supporting its effectiveness, particularly in lower-severity population (for example, Linehan et al., 2015), it is the comprehensive model which is most robustly evidenced.

The Application of DBT for Sexual Minorities

While DBT was originally developed for highly suicidal clients and later identified as a helpful treatment for BPD, its principle-based approach (as opposed to manualised) and generalisability of these principles means that is it widely considered a transdiagnostic intervention that, among other things, targets emotion dysregulation and other common maintenance factors in psychopathology, which has the flexibility to incorporate minority-associated needs (for example, Cohen et al., 2021). Therefore, DBT may be applicable for a number of difficulties that sexual minorities are at risk of beyond self-harm and suicidal behaviours, such as difficulties with substance use, impulsive behaviours, and specifically managing minority stress (King et al., 2008; Oginni et al., 2020; Pachankis et al., 2015; Rodriguez-Seijas et al., 2019). The principle-based nature of DBT also makes it an ideal candidate for adaptation to sexual-minority groups experiencing distress. DBT principles guide how the intervention is delivered and allow for personalisation depending on what the client needs, meaning it could be adapted for both minority-specific difficulties and general difficulties for sexual minorities. The core principles include the transactional biosocial model to explain how psychological distress may develop, validation and acceptance principles to reduce the effects of the invalidating environment, behavioural change principles (skills training, exposure, cognitive modification, contingency management) to help reduce maladaptive and increase skilful behaviours, problem solving, and a dialectical philosophy to help increase flexibility of thinking and approach (Linehan, 1993). Below is further detail of the application of DBT principles and modes to LGBQ+ clients.

The Transaction Biosocial Model

The Transactional Biosocial Model is thought to fit well with minority stress theory in the understanding of how sexual-minority groups may be at increased risk of mental ill-health (see Fig. 12.2 for adapted model for sexual minorities with potential generalisation to other minoritised groups). While the biosocial theory suggests the presence of a biological vulnerability to emotion sensitivity (alongside other possible predisposing temperamental factors like trait impulsivity), it is suggested that in the face of chronic oppression and invalidation, such as that experienced by minoritised groups, it could be that minority stress may be sufficient alone to cause a skill breakdown and the development of emotion dysregulation (Cohen et al., 2021; Skerven et al., 2021). Therefore, belonging to one or more minoritised group may be sufficient alone to transact with an invalidating and oppressive environment to result in difficulties with emotion dysregulation, and that this transaction may be amplified as the number of minoritised intersectional characteristics increases. Congruently, Marsha Linehan (1993), in her original version of the biosocial model, suggested that both traumatic experiences/invalidation and socio-political oppression (for example, sexism) constitute extreme versions of an invalidating environment. This has since been expanded to LGBQ+ groups, where the invalidating environment for these individuals will, to some degree, be defined by societal stigma and oppression towards their minoritised identities (Cohen et al., 2021; Pantalone et al., 2019; Skerven et al., 2019, 2021; Tilley et al., 2022). Experiences of stigma enacted by others and structural stigma from the wider societal structures communicates to LGBQ+ individuals that aspects of their identity and experience are unacceptable and invalid, and that at worse will lead to social rejection and persecution. Such experiences of invalidation and oppression are hence often internalised. Receiving and internalising ideology that your identity is invalid and unacceptable, and likely to lead to punishing consequences, can result in increased shame and distress, as well as core beliefs about the self as unworthy and unlovable, and others as dangerous and unaccepting (Meyer, 2003; Pantalone et al., 2019). The chronic stress and heightened emotional arousal from experiences of invalidation and oppression is likely to prevent the development of adaptive emotion regulation abilities and cause a deterioration of any effective skills that do develop (Linehan, 1993; Skerven et al., 2021). In addition, abuse, victimisation and violence are extreme forms of invalidation, which are significantly more likely to occur towards sexual-minority individuals compared to heterosexual groups (Balsam & Hughs, 2013). Therefore, the biosocial model may be a useful formulaic framework for understanding how sexual minority individuals are likely at increased risk of developing emotion dysregulation, and thus dysregulation in other areas of life, due to a high likelihood of experiencing the full spectrum of invalidation from their environment, regardless of whether an emotion sensitivity or temperamental disposition is present.

Within this model, the development of emotion dysregulation via the transactions between the invalidating/oppressive environment and oppressed/minoritised characteristics (such as sexuality diversity) is suggested to contribute, in a reciprocal and dynamic way, to dysregulation in other areas, including in the behaviour (for example, impulsive and self-harming), interpersonal (for example, relationship instability and fear of abandonment), self (for example, confused sense of self),

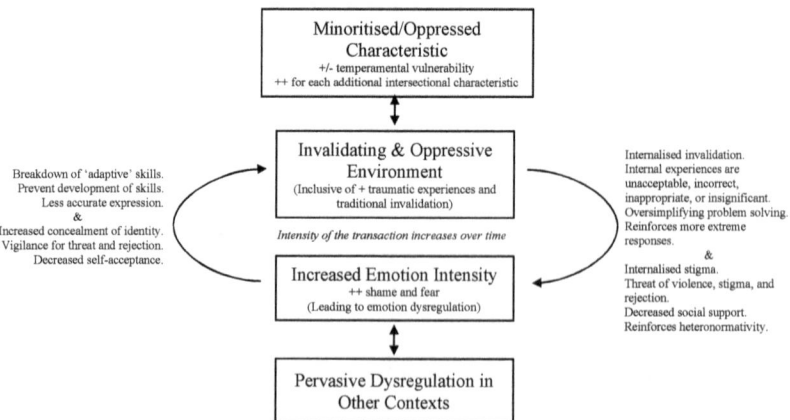

Fig. 12.2 The biosocial transactional model applied to sexual minorities (*Source* Adapted from the model as described by: Fruzzetti et al., 2005; Grove & Crowell, 2019; Linehan, 1993, Inclusive of Minority Stressors from Minority Stress Theory [Meyer, 2003])

and cognitive (for example, maladaptive thinking patterns and dissociation; Linehan, 1993) domains. Indeed, sexual minorities are shown to be at increased risk of commonly targeted difficulties within this model mapped onto the aforementioned areas of dysregulation, including: self-harming and potentially impulsive *behaviours* (King et al., 2008; Oginni et al., 2020; Pachankis et al., 2015; Rodriguez-Seijas et al., 2019), fear of rejection and difficulties maintaining *relationships* (Doyle & Molix, 2015; Meyer, 2003), difficulties with *self*-acceptance and *identity* confusion (Camp et al., 2020; Morgan, 2013), and *cognitive* self-criticism and 'hypervigilance' for threat (Hatzenbuehler, 2009), further supporting the potential application of the biosocial model and the impact of the increased prevalence of emotion dysregulation in LGBQ+ groups (Hatzenbuehler, 2009).

These areas of dysregulation were originally developed to explain the symptoms and difficulties that, together, were described diagnostically as BPD or emotionally unstable personality disorder (EUPD; Bohus et al., 2021; Linehan, 1993). It is important to note that while there is evidence suggesting inflated rates of BPD/EUPD in LGBQ+ populations, that this is considered to be partly due to diagnostic bias, given the overlap between minority-stress-associated presentations of distress and the pathologisation of normative experiences for sexual-minority individuals (Eubanks-Carter & Goldfried, 2006; Rodriguez-Seijas et al., 2021). Therefore, this chapter does not seek to suggest that BPD will need to be present, nor that this is the core focus of applying DBT to LGBQ+ individuals, however that the areas of 'dysregulation' within this model may be applicable to common difficulties experienced by sexual minorities and at the same time may be helpfully targeted by DBT. Additionally, the model may fit well for those with co-occurring difficulties associated with BPD/EUPD and minority stress. Other difficulties which do not fall clearly into these broad categories of dysregulation could be added, depending on what made most sense to the client, and thought would need to be given by therapists regarding the application of effective, complimentary, intervention(s) for said targets.

Nonetheless, the aforementioned areas of difficulty, mapped onto the areas of dysregulation described by Linehan's (1993) biosocial model, are those often described by minority stress (Meyer, 2003) and psychological mediation (Hatzenbeuhler, 2009) theories. As discussed in previous chapters, minority stress theory suggests that distal (external) stressors such as discrimination and stigma (the invalidating environment) alongside proximal (internal) stressors (for example, the internalisation of the invalidating environment, identity concealment, and expectations of rejection), develop as a result of an oppressive stigmatising environment, and this causes significant stress for sexual-minority individuals (Meyer, 2003). The internalisation of heterosexist and anti-LGBQ+ societal messages, akin to internalised invalidation in DBT, further exacerbate this stress even in the absence of external invalidation and results in self-stigma and self-invalidation (Cohen et al., 2021; Meyer, 2003; Skerven et al., 2021). These stressors then increase the likelihood of painful emotions, which may tip into clinical levels of distress or mental health disorders via common psychological processes implicated in the development of mental health difficulties (psychological mediation framework; Hatzenbeuhler, 2009)—namely *emotion dysregulation* in this model. Emotion dysregulation, according to the transactional biosocial model, then reciprocally initiates and maintains dysregulation in other processes commonly implicated in mental health difficulties such as high self-criticism or maladaptive behavioural attempts to cope with such distress (for example, using mood-altering substances), thus increasing the likelihood of distress and limiting the development of adaptive coping strategies. All areas of dysregulation are thought to transact with one another in a continuous and reciprocal way, increasing the intensity of the transaction and thus distress over time—further contributing to the breakdown of skills (Linehan, 1993).

The transactional processes in the biosocial model may also add to the existing minority stress models, which are considered interactional rather than transactional (Sloan et al., 2017). The transactional model suggests that aspects of the individual and the environment influence one another continuously, reciprocally, and with changing intensity and nature over time. The interactional minority stress model, however, suggests that a variable at one level gets triggered by another variable, and that this relationship is relatively stable in nature and intensity over time (Sloan et al., 2017; see Fig. 12.3). For example, it may be inferred from minority stress models that one experience of homophobic slurs by a passer-by will have a particular emotional impact on the person and interact with other existing vulnerabilities (for example, internalised homophobia and expectations of rejection), in a way that is relatively stable over time. Each similar stigma-related event thereafter would have an additive effect alongside other stressors and predisposing factors, which if they reached a certain threshold may result in clinical levels of psychological distress. Whereas, a transactional model suggests that the same incident would have a constantly different and likely inflated impact on the person depending on the accumulation of similar experiences and internalisation of these experiences over time, and the effect would reciprocally impact the next occurrence of the event (for example, via internalising and expecting invalidation, thus making it more likely that such events will enter awareness and by cognitive processes which highlight memories of past similar events). This is not to say that the 'responses' by minoritised individuals cause increased stigma, but that the response may have an impact on the nature or perception of future experiences. Such transactions would still have an additive effect on stress, as is the case with interactional models. However, the nature of the relationship would change over time in a complex fashion, which may increase the impact of the original cue (that is, a homophobic slur in this example). This alludes to how distress may become much higher than would 'fit the facts' of a particular present situation alone, and that the person may become more 'sensitive' to the cue(s), or even so in the absence of the original cue(s), over time. Therefore, the transactional aspect of the DBT biosocial model may help to expand the understanding of how minority stress from an invalidating and oppressive environment may influence the experience of LGBQ+ individuals, and that this experience will further continuously and reciprocally influence their social environment, and that the intensity and nature of the relationship between each will change over time. It also helps consider the transactional dynamic of intersecting issues, such as cultural and social norms (see Chapter 6).

The biosocial model is explicitly taught to clients and used throughout DBT in order to help clients build an understanding of, and validate how, their difficulties may have developed over time. When using this model with LGBQ+ individuals, it is important to validate how

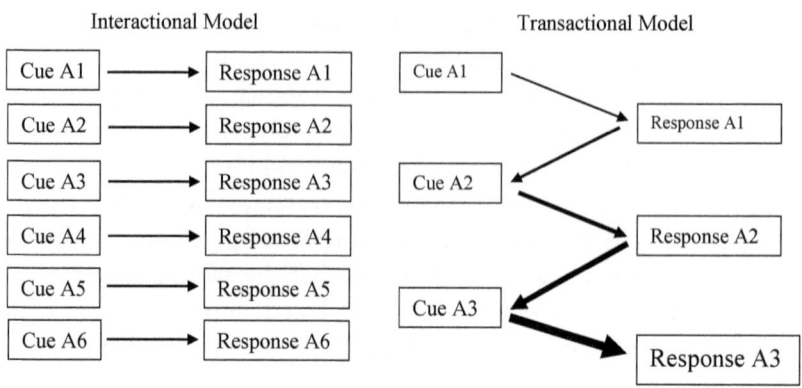

Fig. 12.3 Shows how the relationship between each occurrence of a cue (demarked by numbers) and the responses is stable for the interactional model and relatively one-directional, whereas it is reciprocal and continually changing in the interactional model

aspects of 'dysregulation', such as rejection sensitivity and concealment of identity, may at times be valid and appropriate, albeit not ideal, responses within a heterosexist and unsafe environment (Feinstei et al., 2020; Rodriguez-Seijas et al., 2021). The acknowledgement of the invalidating environment for sexual minority clients, inclusive of minority stressors and understandable responses to these stressors, may help cultivate awareness of how their self-stigma and self-invalidation developed. Thus, supporting them to detach from self-blame and self-invalidation towards being aware of the impact of minority stress and the invalidating environment—increasing self-validation and compassion (Cohen et al., 2021). It may also support with empowering minoritised individuals to understand the impact of their wider socio-political environment and consider avenues for activism and interventions for affirmative and anti-oppressive social change. Indeed, the integration of minority stress information has been piloted in early studies (Cohen et al., 2021; Skerven et al., 2021) and has been cited in qualitative research with young LGBQ+ individuals in DBT as relevant for their treatment with a desire for more focus on these topics (Camp, Morris, Wilde, Smith, & Rimes, accepted). Self-validation and self-compassion are likely to be helpful precursors to regulating emotional pain and connecting with experiences of acceptance, community connection and joy, to improve quality of life and take further steps towards a life worth living (Camp et al., 2020; Ceatha et al., 2021; Helminen et al., 2022; Jaspal et al., 2022).

DBT Skills

DBT assumes a skill deficit in managing emotional pain and the consequential dysregulation in other areas. Therefore, one key principle of DBT is skills training to empower individuals to accept and change aspects of their experience and social environment. These skills are highly adaptable to LGBQ-specific experiences and suggestions around how to adapt the skills to stigma-related experiences are detailed in the literature (Camp, Morris et al., accepted; Cohen et al., 2021; Pantalone et al., 2019; Skerven et al., 2019; Skerven et al., 2021).

The skills which lie at the acceptance end of the dialectic include mindfulness and distress tolerance. DBT mindfulness skills aim for the person to build non-judgmental awareness of the present moment and strengthen attentional control, with a focus on targeting dysregulation in the self and cognitive domains (Linehan, 2015). A potential use of mindfulness skills for sexual minority individuals is to help them develop a non-judgmental awareness of their internal experiences and identity, diffuse from maladaptive thinking patterns derived from internalised stigma, develop self-compassion despite the invalidating environment, and get the most out of affirmative experiences by being mentally present and unmindful of worries/expectations of rejection. Mindfulness skills also encourage the connection with the 'wise mind', a useful reference for tapping into a person's inherent wisdom and supporting with the integration of 'reasonable' (that is, fact and logic) and 'emotional' (that is, emotion and felt senses) parts of our minds and experiences. These skills may be particularly helpful for sexual minorities to help them balance their emotions and reason/logic in the face of stigma-related situations, and use 'wise mind' to make difficult decisions.

Distress tolerance skills primarily aim to reduce behavioural dysregulation by replacing impulsive and self-harming behaviours and urges with more adaptive coping to help individuals tolerate distress and accept reality (Linehan, 2015). These skills may be useful for sexual minorities to help them tolerate understandable distress when they experience stigma or self-stigma and to help them not act on urges that may make things worse in the medium- to long-term (for example, self-harm and suicide attempts). This is with the caveat that DBT assumes that while it may not be the fault of the person that they feel distressed, which is important for stigma- and oppression-related experiences, they will need to find a way to tolerate distress in order to not do anything that would make their situation worse and so they can access what they need to navigate life, which is sadly likely to include heterosexism. Additionally, this skillset equips individuals with skills to help them accept reality as it is in the moment, especially when it cannot be changed, to prevent valid emotional pain from turning into unnecessary suffering (Linehan, 2015). It is likely adaptive, to some degree, to be able to accept or at least tolerate the consequences of living in a heterosexist world, as this is the reality at the current time (Cohen et al., 2021). Furthermore, reality acceptance is suggested to be a necessary precursor to change (Linehan, 1993). Therefore, increasing reality acceptance, where appropriate, may help increase the capacity for advocating for change in the socio-political environment for LGBQ+ individuals. Reality acceptance alongside mindful non-judgmental awareness skills may also support in the development of self-acceptance for LGBQ+ individuals and challenge internalised heterosexism. While reality acceptance sits within the distress tolerance skillset, which is primarily targeted at behavioural dysregulation and associated urges, it is thought that these skills have a much wider applicability and usefulness to navigating life problems and dilemmas (Linehan, 2015). Mindfulness and distress tolerance skills may, therefore, be effective for LGBQ+ individuals experiencing difficulties in self-, cognitive- and behaviour-based dysregulation, alongside generally supporting the development of acceptance.

It is important that acceptance-based skills are balanced with change-based skills, as the consequence of a polarised focus on acceptance skills can create hopelessness and a lack of change where it is needed. At the same time, a polarised focus on change-based skills can re-create the invalidating environment and increase blame towards the oppressed individual. The change-based skills include those in the emotion regulation and interpersonal effectiveness skillsets. Emotion regulation aims to help people reduce vulnerability to painful emotions and directly modulate emotions where needed (Linehan, 2015). These skills may help LGBQ+ individuals reduce vulnerability to difficult emotions as a result of minority stress by maintaining aspects of wellbeing such as balanced eating and sufficient sleep, as well as increasing the frequency of pleasant and mastery-based activities which are congruent with their values, affirming, and provide connection to similar others (Linehan, 2015). Case management principles of balancing consultation to the client and environmental interventions may further aid sexual minorities in accessing affirmative environments and spaces by supporting them to make the necessary steps towards these goals while balancing this with stepping in as professionals or supportive others when the environment feels too powerful. The addition of the 'cope ahead' skill may also help sexual minorities cope ahead of time with difficult situations such as disclosing their sexual orientation to others, managing stigma-related situations and anxiety in anticipation of entering LGBQ+ spaces. Skills to help modulate emotions may also be helpful in supporting LGBQ+ individuals to 'check the facts' when experiencing fear of rejection or other situations that may cue emotions, and working out whether the intensity and duration of their emotion-based response is justified. If not, the use of 'opposite action' provides LGBQ+ individual with an effective skill, utilising behaviour- and body-based bottom-up processes to modulate unjustified or ineffective emotional arousal, which may be particularly useful for unjustified and toxic shame caused by the internalisation of anti-LGBQ+ stigma, and ineffective anxiety when trying to access affirmative spaces. This of course needs to be balanced with considerations around when it is safe to act opposite to shame and/or anxiety where this means disclosing identity in environments that may include threats of harm, which is important to support the LGBQ+ person to weigh up when using these skills. Moreover, problem solving skills may be helpful for navigating multiple complex problems that arise for LGBQ+ individuals living in heterosexist environments, including how to manage and advocate against stigma, coming out to others, navigating challenges such as surrogacy, and accessing affirming spaces and building connection with similar others.

These skills are complimented by the interpersonal effectiveness skills, which aim to support the person to get their needs met while maintaining their relationships and self-respect, increasing self-validation, and ending destructive relationships where needed (Linehan, 2015). This skillset intends to emphasise the importance of the relational aspects of wellbeing in how we use social support and co-regulation, alongside the potential negative impact others can have, especially on minoritised individuals. This is an important skillset for sexual minorities, as their experiences and consequential fear of rejection or, worse, persecution for advocating for their needs in a heterosexual world may make it difficult for them to feel safe enough to ask for what they need and to say no. This could make them more vulnerable to fall towards the more extreme options of interpersonal intensity. On one end, some may be more likely to engage in more passive communication around their needs, resulting in a sacrifice of self-respect and said needs. On the other end, LGBQ+ individuals may be at risk of engaging in more aggressive communication, sacrificing relationships and self-respect. Neither polarity is thought to be effective if used often, if at all. Therefore, balancing relationship objectives and practicing the effective intensity of communication on the passive-aggressive continuum may support with more assertive communication when advocating for their needs and for LGBQ-affirmative changes in society, as well as recruiting allies to support this endeavour. In addition, the skill of self-validation may be key for reducing some of the effect of the invalidating environment and for reducing internalised stigma and self-blame, especially if they are able to connect with the understandable distress born from the invalidating environment. This skill is also thought to directly modulate emotional arousal (Fruzzetti & Shenk, 2008).

These skills, carefully balanced between acceptance and change, may help LGBQ+ individuals manage minority-specific stress alongside general stress in both a treatment and a prevention context. An assumption in DBT is that, while the emotional pain experienced by the individual may not be their fault, it is incumbent on them to do something differently to change it, as the external world and wider society is not as easily in our control as our internal world and more immediate actions (Linehan, 1993). This can be a helpful mantra for LGBQ+ individuals receiving DBT, alongside heavy validation for the burden of minority stress, to help them build the motivation to learn skills to manage, even though their exposure to the invalidating environment is not their fault, in order to get them to a place where they feel capable of changing the external world in whatever way they can. This may be complimented by other assumptions in DBT, including that the person's life as it is currently is unbearable, that they are trying their best to solve their problems and at the same time need to try harder to achieve what they want (with support of course), and that they cannot fail in DBT (the treatment can fail but not the client; Linehan, 1993).

A Dialectical and Validating Philosophy

Dialectics is a philosophical underpinning of DBT and encompasses the idea that multiple potentially-conflicting truths (most simply put: the thesis and antithesis) can exist simultaneously and that being 'dialectical' is to consider these truths, particularly what is being left out, use them to reach a middle path (better described as a 'synthesis'); and that everything is inter-related (cause and effect; Linehan, 1993). The way in which this philosophy may be applied to distress in gender-minority groups is detailed elsewhere and has applicability to sexual minority individuals, especially if there is intersectional gender diversity (Sloan et al., 2017). As discussed above, the skills and principles in DBT are grouped around the core dialectic in DBT: acceptance and change. Individuals who have experienced an invalidating environment, especially those who have experienced this in relation to their identity and core aspects of themselves, may find purely change-based approaches difficult as they risk further invalidating internal experiences, oversimplifying problem solving in the face of complex stressors and societal oppression, and communicating that it is the oppressed individual who needs to change rather than the environment (Cohen et al., 2021). Therefore, it is likely that DBT suits the needs of chronically-invalidated individuals, such as sexual minorities, as it encourages and utilises a balance of acceptance of how things are in the moment (for example, that the world is largely heterosexist) and change where it is possible (for example, advocating for social justice and equity anyway). Acceptance and validation may be particularly powerful for helping validate and acknowledge the realities of emotional pain and help accept the self in a world that privileges heterosexuality and subjugates queerness. In addition, the use of dialectics (considering multiple truths, finding a middle path) may help LGBQ+ individuals to increase cognitive flexibility, which may have a positive impact on wellbeing and support with accepting the complex and changing nature of sexuality diversity. Another important dialectical dilemma for supporting minoritized clients in oppressive and heterosexist socio-political environments, particularly important for psychological therapies aiming to support individuals to reduce their own distress, is balancing empowering the client to reduce their own difficulties while not underplaying the role of the wider environment in contributing to their distress. Thus, emphasising the need for change outside of the individual, with congruent relevant interventions and support from the therapist. The core dialectical dilemmas in DBT (for example, active passivity and apparent competence; Linehan, 1993) can also be used to help understand particular patterns of clients and help them to find an effective synthesis. Finally, a dialectical position by therapists can help them accept seemingly opposing behaviours and motives by the client, as both being true at once, which can be particularly helpful for working with 'maladaptive' behaviours such as self-harm (for example, accepting that this is both their best attempt to cope and at the same time they want things to be different). Therapists may also benefit from taking a dialectical approach to the dynamic nature of their clients' identity, particularly sexual identity, where this may change over time.

DBT Structure, Treatment Hierarchy, & Consultation Agreements

As discussed above, DBT has four modes of treatment, all with different aims. It is thought that the skills group aspect of the model, which aims to support the development of adaptive skills, may be well suited to LGBQ+ individuals (Cohen et al., 2021). This is because safe and affirming group spaces may support with social connection with accepting others, which may be helpful for developing relationships and curative for internalised stigma, as supported by the experiences of LGBQ+ young people in DBT (Camp, Morris et al., accepted). However, if group interventions also include people from majority groups, it is important that facilitators take care to make the space safe and affirming, with appropriate safety signals and structures in place (Skerven et al., 2019). It is considered that teaching in DBT skills groups needs to be adapted for the participants. In particular for LGBQ+ individuals, thought may need to be given to how to tailor examples and materials to varied aspects of diversity, while also providing safety signals within the group such as clear indications of supporting LGBQ+ rights (Camp, Morris et al., accepted).

The individual therapy mode of DBT aims to increase motivation, support problem solving and facilitate the application of adaptive skills to the person's life. This mode may be helpful for ensuring the personalisation of skills for LGBQ+ individuals' needs, especially those skills groups that are not able to personalise content to sexual-minority experiences. A lack of specific application of skills to LGBQ-associated dilemmas has been cited as a potential barrier to the generalisability of skills in this way, and thus conscious and explicit application may be necessary when relevant (Camp, Morris et al., accepted). This may include practicing skills and solutions for difficulties associated with LGBQ + experience and also checking in with LGBQ + clients if particular skills fit with their context, both as a sexuality diverse individual and considering any other relevant intersectional characteristics. In addition, individual sessions are structured around a hierarchy of treatment targets, which prioritises the targeting of life-threatening and therapy-interfering behaviours, respectively. Only when they are not present, is it recommended to dedicate session time to other lower-order targets. This has important implications for mitigating risk and keeping clients in therapy, and at the same time can mean there is less time and space for other targets, such as stressors related to minority status (unless they were controlling variables or contributing factors to life-threatening or therapy-interfering behaviours). Therefore, while the treatment hierarchy can be a containing mechanism for working with high-risk behaviours, it may be helpful to spend time thinking with LGBQ+ clients in DBT about how they can negotiate and work towards LGBQ-associated targets (if relevant) to increase motivation and likelihood of progressing towards those goals (Camp, Morris et al., accepted). It may be that LGBQ-associated difficulties are more likely to be targeted as key controlling variables or links in the chain of events precipitating higher-order targets, such as self-harm, and thus that therapists may need to support their LGBQ+ clients to consider which variables/links are the most important to target in sessions in line with their goals and the aims of the treatment. Where there are important LGBQ-associated targets/variables outside of the aims of DBT, thought as to how to meet these needs via other means or in future ('stage 2') interventions may be beneficial. Similarly, the young people also indicated a preference for DBT therapists to invite, thoughtfully, space for thinking about sexuality diversity in all modes of DBT (that is, individual sessions, skills group, phone coaching, and team consultation meetings) as appropriate and even if this is not taken up, in a way that is conveys that this is optional and to communicate that they are accepting and willing to support (Camp, Morris et al., accepted). This includes specifically asking about sexual orientation and other aspects of diversity, in order to lower the burden of the individual in needing to come out and to demonstrate the providers'/therapists' willingness to support in this area (Camp, Morris et al., accepted).

Phone coaching, the third mode of DBT, supports the generalisation of skills into the person's everyday life. This, again, may support with the individualisation and generalisation for LGBQ+ individuals, especially when experiencing stigma-related experiences outside of sessions that would benefit from more immediate support rather than waiting for the next individual session.

The fourth mode of DBT is the therapist consultation team meetings, which supports therapists to maintain adherence to DBT, therapeutic skills, and their wellbeing. It is incumbent on DBT therapists to use consultation meetings (or similar) to reflect on and develop competencies in LGBQ-affirmative care when working with these clients, get support from the team to support LGBQ+ clients where needed, and maintain anti-oppressive and anti-discrimination practices (Camp, Morris, et al., accepted). Similar to recommendations for developing anti-racist competencies in DBT teams (Pierson et al., 2021), it may be useful to build in appropriate training and reflective spaces regarding LGBQ-specific issues and LGBQ-affirmative consultations agreements such as those that commit the team to maintaining accepting, affirming, anti-oppressive practice, and agreements that detail how environmental interventions (that is, interventions by clinicians in a person's environment) may be more necessary in situations that involve heterosexist oppression and stigma, in consultation with the client, as the environment is likely to be too powerful when it comes to heterosexism. Additionally, consultation agreements could extend to reminding DBT therapists of their need to search for their blind spots and educate themselves on important matters regarding LGBQ+ social equity, and that while LGBQ + individuals are likely best placed to educate heterosexual therapists about sexual-minority-related issues, at the same time it should not be their responsibility to do so unless they are opting to, and that over-relying on LGBQ+ individuals to do so may cause fatigue and increase the burden of minority stress.

A final development in the structure of DBT that aligns well with supporting LGBQ+ individuals is the integration of 'stage 2' treatments within 'stage 1' DBT programmes. The predominant DBT model (described above) delivered is considered a 'stage 1' treatment with the primary aims of stopping life-threatening behaviours and reducing therapy-interfering behaviours and severely destabilising quality-of-life-interfering behaviours (otherwise referred to as stabilisation), in order to allow the progression onto 'stage 2' therapies (Linehan, 1993). 'Stage 2' therapies are often inclusive of trauma reprocessing interventions (Linehan, 1993). However, recent developments have seen the successful integration of a 'stage 2' therapy, DBT-Prolonged Exposure Therapy

(DBT-PE) for Post-Traumatic Stress Disorder (PTSD) symptoms, into the 'stage 1' programme to increase accessibility to these treatments and to acknowledge the often-reciprocal relationship between traumatic experiences and dysregulation (Harned, 2022). While PTSD is but one type of response to traumatic events, it is unsurprisingly shown to be higher in LGBQ+ individuals, given their increased risk of exposure to trauma, therefore this may be particularly relevant for LGBQ+ individuals accessing DBT (Livingston et al., 2020). In addition, Melanie Harned (2022) integrated the notion of how PTSD symptoms can arise from more subtle and insidious experiences (termed 'traumatic invalidation'), which provides a helpful way to apply DBT-PE interventions to events that do not fit the traditional criterion of what is classified as a 'traumatic event' according to diagnostic criteria, and instead include events more akin to the minority stress that can result in PTSD symptoms (Livingston et al., 2020). Integration of 'stage 2' targets in 'stage 1' DBT may also suggest that other important issues that LGBQ+ groups experience, which may not entirely fit the remit of a 'stage 1' intervention, could also be successfully integrated within standard DBT, such as identity development processes and managing stigma-related experiences (Camp, Morris et al., accepted).

DBT for Sexual Minorities: Current Evidence

Recent meta-analytic evidence found that only 11% of DBT randomised-controlled trials (RCTs) collected data on sexual orientation, although none stratified results by sexual-orientation-based groups (Harned et al., 2022). This is not dissimilar to evidence cited elsewhere regarding RCTs of psychological interventions more generally (Pachankis, 2018), and represents an exclusion of consideration regarding the efficacy of standard psychological interventions for sexual minority individuals. A review of the current literature regarding the effectiveness of adapted and non-adapted psychological interventions for sexual minorities highlighted the paucity of research in this area, albeit the frequency of studies in this area is increasing in recent years (O'Shaughnessy & Speir, 2018).

No known study has explored the effectiveness of standard/comprehensive DBT (without adaptation) applied to LGBQ+ adults or compared outcomes to heterosexual samples, despite the high representation of sexual minorities in samples of DBT efficacy studies (Harned et al., 2022). However, one study investigated whether outcomes were similar for sexual minority adults ($n = 84$) compared to heterosexual adults ($n = 357$) in a partial-hospital programme which included a group with aspects of DBT (mainly interpersonal effectiveness skills) combined with cognitive behavioural therapy techniques (Beard et al., 2017). The authors found no significant difference between the sexual minority group overall and the heterosexual group in self-reported anxiety and depression symptoms, self-harm and suicidal thoughts, substance use, and perceived quality of care at the end of the intervention. However, when looking at subgroups of sexual minorities they found that individuals identifying as bisexual reported more self-harm and suicidal thoughts, and worse perceptions of care at post-treatment compared to all other sexual orientation groups. This may suggest that the bisexual group was less able to benefit from the intervention, however no further work was completed to explore the reasons for this. This research also does not likely generalise to comprehensive DBT programmes as it included a limited number of DBT principles/skills. Nonetheless, it is important to note that the poorer outcomes in the bisexual group, as this is found elsewhere in the literature in other psychological therapies (for example, Rimes et al., 2019), and may represent issues with approaches not optimally meeting the needs of this or similar sexual minority groups.

While no further studies have investigated non-adapted DBT for LGBQ+ adults, two have explored outcomes in comprehensive DBT for adolescents. One study using an adolescent sample investigated whether outcomes of DBT for adolescents (18-week programme) were similar for sexual minority ($n = 16$) compared to heterosexual adolescents ($n = 23$). They found that LGBQ+ young people had, on average, a significant reduction in self-reported emotion dysregulation, depression and BPD symptoms, and a significant increase in self-reported adaptive coping from the start to post-treatment (Poon et al., 2022). These changes were similar to those seen in the heterosexual sample, suggesting equality of improvement by the end of DBT for adolescents. Similar results have been replicated in a national DBT service for adolescents in the UK, with a large representation of sexual minorities and sexual-orientation-based groups further disaggregated (Camp, Durante, Cooper, Smith, & Rimes, submitted for publication). The findings from this study suggest similar improvements in self-reported BPD symptoms, emotion dysregu-lation, self-harm, depression and anxiety symptoms, alongside reductions in accident and emergency department and inpatient admissions, for individuals identifying as bisexual/pansexual ($n = 46$) and gay/lesbian ($n = 15$), compared to their heterosexual peers ($n = 36$), in an eight- to 12-month tier-four DBT programme. This study also found that retention rates were not significantly different for sexual minority young people compared to heterosexual young people, albeit the bisexual and gay/lesbian group had (non-significant) lower completion rates (62–65%) compared to the pansexual (81%) and heterosexual (74%) group. A lack of significant differences may possibly speaking to the acceptability of the DBT approach for these minority groups, however it is important to note the low statistical power in both of these studies among other limitations that preclude firm conclusions.

As referenced above, early work has been published providing recom-mendations for how to adapt aspects of DBT specifically for the needs of sexual-minority groups (Camp, Morris, et al., accepted; Cohen et al., 2021; Pantalone et al., 2019; Skerven et al., 2019, 2021), alongside gender minority groups (Camp, Morris, et al., accepted; Sloan et al., 2017; Tilley et al., 2022). Two authors have also piloted DBT skills training groups adapted for the specific needs of sexual minority groups. Both have been piloted in adult veteran populations. Firstly, Cohen and colleagues (2021) developed an 'Affirmative' DBT skills training group for sexual minorities. The 10-week group programme included an intro-duction to minority stress in the context of the biosocial theory, core mindfulness skills, and the emotion regulation module. In the intro-duction to the group, the facilitators introduced the idea of cultural stigma and rejection of sexual minorities, and discussed aspects of the minority stress model, including rejection sensitivity, internalised stigma, and identity concealment. They also used examples and content tailored to sexual minorities specifically, including the use of acting in line with values and opposite action skills to reduce unjustified shame and anxiety related to identity concealment. They found a reduction in emotion dysregulation and depression symptoms in the majority of the six participants by the end of the group and found evidence of acceptability. The second study developed a DBT skills training group targeting stigma management in sexual- and gender-minority adults (Skerven et al., 2021). This 16-session group programme included skills from core mindfulness, interpersonal effectiveness, emotion regulation and distress tolerance. Two sessions near the beginning were focused on types of stigma and stressors unique to sexual and gender minorities (the latter from Cohen et al., 2021), and examples and content were tailored to minority-specific experiences. The four participants provided positive feedback regarding the safety and meaningfulness of the group, and most showed improvements in self-reported emotion dysregulation, depression symptoms, coping skills and aspects of burden associated with stigma experiences. No further work has yet been published on the effectiveness of adapted versions of DBT modes, or on how these adaptations may work within comprehensive DBT programmes. However, this emerging evidence suggests some useful ways that DBT skills can be adapted to support LGBQ+ individuals to manage stress related to identity stigma as well as non-minority-specific stressors.

Conclusions

This chapter has detailed how DBT may be well suited to working with distress experienced by LGBQ+ individuals. In particular, the transaction biosocial model may support with an understanding of how stressors from invalidating and oppressive heterosexist environments result in difficulties in emotion dysregulation and thus dysregulation in other aspects of life, validating their experience and detracting from self-invalidation and -blame. This model may also compliment and add to existing minority stress models (for example, Meyer, 2003) via its transactional component illuminating reciprocal and changing relationships between factors over time. The DBT skillset is also highly adaptable to LGBQ-specific, as well as general, difficulties and dilemmas, especially those with difficulties with emotion dysregulation. This skillset is thought to be a useful preventative tool, even for those where emotion dysregulation has not emerged, for developing appropriate emotion regulation and associated competencies (for example, Flynn et al., 2018). Finally, the dialectical philosophy, particularly balancing acceptance and change techniques, and the multiple modes of DBT, may be well suited to supporting LGBQ+ individuals generally, with some reasonable adaptions. The principle-based nature of DBT suggests that this intervention and model may be easily adapted for the needs of LGBQ+ individuals, however it may be that the focus of any DBT intervention needs to be carefully considered with the client based on their needs and difficulties, alongside the hierarchy of targets in any standard DBT programme (Linehan, 1993). For example, while feedback from a national UK DBT service for adolescents has suggested that DBT and DBT therapists largely met the needs of LGBQ+ individuals, one aspect that is not experienced as being sufficiently covered is sexual—and gender-identity development, alongside managing stigma-related experiences, and how these interact with distress (Camp, Morris, et al., accepted in prep). This may highlight areas where DBT could be optimised to support this group of adolescent LGBQ-identifying clients, although it is not yet known if this finding is transferable in adult populations. Little research has explored the experiences of LGBQ+ clients who have undergone DBT to understand where there may be gaps for these clients, which represents an important avenue for future qualitative studies. Additionally, services and research should better seek to include demographic information on sexual minorities as standard (in line with NHS specifications; NHS England Equality and Health Inequalities Unit, 2017), to increase the understanding of how well interventions, such as DBT, meet the needs of sexual minorities and to allow for outcomes to be disaggregated across LGBQ+ groups. Nonetheless, DBT represents a potentially useful and adaptable intervention for clinical distress in LGBQ+ individuals.

References

Bahji, A., Pierce, M., Wong, J., Roberge, J. N., Ortega, I., & Patten, S. (2021). Comparative efficacy and acceptability of psychotherapies for self-harm and suicidal behaviour among children and adolescents: A Systematic review and network meta-analysis. *JAMA Network Open, 4*(4), e216614. https://doi.org/10.1001/jamanetworkopen.2021.6614

Balsam, K., & Hughes, T. (2013). Sexual orientation, victimization, and hate crimes. In C. J. Patterson & A. R. D'Augelli (Eds.), *Handbook of psychology and sexual orientation* (pp. 267–280). Oxford University Press.

Beard, C., Kirakosian, N., Silverman, A. L., Winer, J. P., Wadsworth, L. P., & Björgvinsson, T. (2017). Comparing treatment response between LGBQ and heterosexual individuals attending a CBT- and DBT-skills-based partial hospital. *Journal of Consulting and Clinical Psychology, 85*(12), 1171–1181. https://doi.org/10.1037/ccp0000251

Ben-Porath, D., Duthu, F., Luo, T., Gonidakis, F., Compte, E. J., & Wisniewski, L. (2020). Dialectical behavioral therapy: An update and review of the existing treatment models adapted for adults with eating disorders. *Eating Disorders, 28*(2), 101–121. https://doi.org/10.1080/10640266.2020.1723371

Bohus, M., Stoffers-Winterling, J., Sharp, C., Krause-Utz, A., Schmahl, C., & Lieb, K. (2021). Borderline personality disorder. *Lancet, 398*, 1528–1540. https://doi.org/10.1016/S0140-6736(21)00476-1

Camp, J., Durante, G., Cooper, A., Smith, P., & Rimes, K. A., (submitted). *Clinical outcomes for sexual and gender minority adolescents in a dialectical behaviour therapy programme.* Manuscript submitted for publication.

Camp, J., Morris, A., Wilde, H., Smith, P., & Rimes, K. A. (accepted). *gender and sexuality minoritised adolescents in DBT; A Reflexive thematic analysis of minority-specific treatment targets and experience.* accepted for publication.

Camp, J., Vitoratou, S., & Rimes, K. A. (2020). LGBQ+ Self-acceptance and its relationship with minority stressors and mental health: A Systematic literature review. *Archives of Sexual Behaviour, 49*, 2353–2373. https://doi.org/10.1007/s10508-020-01755-2

Ceatha, N., Koay, A. C. C., Buggy, C., James, O., Tully, L., Bustillo, M., & Crowley, D. (2021). Protective factors for LGBTI+ youth wellbeing: A scoping review underpinned by recognition theory. *International Journal of Environmental Research and Public Health, 18*(21), 11682. https://doi.org/10.3390/ijerph182111682

Chen, S. Y., Cheng, Y., Zhao, W. W., & Zhang, Y. H. (2021). Effects of dialectical behaviour therapy on reducing self-harming behaviours and negative emotions in patients with borderline personality disorder: A meta-analysis. *Journal of Psychiatric and Mental Health Nursing, 28*(6), 1128–1139. https://doi.org/10.1111/jpm.12797

Cohen, J. M., Norona, J. C., Yadavia, J. E., & Borsari, B. (2021). Affirmative dialectical behavior therapy skills training with sexual minority veterans. *Cognitive and Behavioral Practice, 28*(1), 77–91. https://doi.org/10.1016/j.cbpra.2020.05.008

DeCou, C. R., Comtois, K. A., & Landes, S. J. (2019). Dialectical behavior therapy is effective for the treatment of suicidal behavior: A meta-analysis. *Behavior Therapy, 50*(1), 60–72. https://doi.org/10.1016/j.beth.2018.03.009

Doyle, D. M., & Molix, L. (2015). Social stigma and sexual minorities' romantic relationship functioning: A meta-analytic review. *Personality and Social Psychology Bulletin, 41*(10), 1363–1381. https://doi.org/10.1177/0146167215594592

Eubanks-Carter, C., & Goldfried, M. R. (2006). The impact of client sexual orientation and gender on clinical judgments and diagnosis of borderline personality disorder. *Journal of Clinical Psychology, 62*(6), 751–770. https://doi.org/10.1002/jclp.20265

Feinstein, B. A., Xavier Hall, C. D., Dyar, C., & Davila, J. (2020). Motivations for sexual identity concealment and their associations with mental health among bisexual, pansexual, queer, and fluid (bi+) individuals. *Journal of Bisexuality, 20*(3), 324–341. https://doi.org/10.1080/15299716.2020.1743402

Flynn, D., Joyce, M., Weihrauch, M., & Corcoran, P. (2018). Innovations in practice: Dialectical behaviour therapy—skills training for emotional problem solving for adolescents (DBT STEPS-A): Evaluation of a pilot implementation in Irish post-primary schools. *Child and Adolescent Mental Health, 23*, 376–380. https://doi.org/10.1111/camh.12284

Fruzzetti, A. E., & Shenk, C. (2008). Fostering Validating responses in families. *Social Work in Mental Health, 6*, 215–227. https://doi.org/10.1300/J200v06n01_17

Fruzzetti, A. E., Shenk, C., & Hoffman, P. D. (2005). Family interaction and the development of borderline personality disorder: A transactional model. *Development and Psychopathology, 17*(4), 1007–1030. https://doi.org/10.1017/s0954579405050479

Gordon, A. R., & Meyer, I. H. (2007). Gender nonconformity as a target of prejudice, discrimination, and violence against LGB individuals. *Journal of LGBT Health Research, 3*(3), 55–71. https://doi.org/10.1080/155740908 02093562

Grove, J. L., & Crowell, S. E. (2019). Invalidating environments and the development of borderline personality disorder. In M. A. Swales (Ed.), *The Oxford handbook of dialectical behaviour therapy*. Oxford University Press. https://doi.org/10.1093/oxfordhb/9780198758723.013.47

Haktanır, A. & Callender, K. A. (2020). Meta-analysis of dialectical behavior therapy (DBT) for treating substance use. *Research on education and psychology*, Meta-Analysis Special Issue, 74–87.

Harned, M. S. (2022). *Treating Trauma in dialectical behavior therapy: The DBT Prolonged Exposure Protocol (DBT PE)*. Guilford Publications.

Harned, M. S., Coyle, T. N., & Garcia, N. M. (2022). The inclusion of ethno-racial, sexual, and gender minority groups in randomized controlled trials of dialectical behavior therapy: A systematic review of the literature. *Clinical Psychology: Science and Practice, 29*(2), 83–93. https://doi.org/10.1037/cps 0000059

Hatzenbuehler, M. L. (2009). How does sexual minority stigma 'get under the skin'? A psychological mediation framework. *Psychological Bulletin, 135*(5), 707–730. https://doi.org/10.1037/a0016441

Hatzenbuehler, M. L., McLaughlin, K. A., & Nolen-Hoeksema, S. (2008). Emotion regulation and internalizing symptoms in a longitudinal study of sexual minority and heterosexual adolescents. *Journal of Child Psychology and Psychiatry, 49*, 1270–1278. https://doi.org/10.1111/j.1469-7610.2008.019 24.x

Helminen, E. C., Ducar, D. M., Scheer, J. R., Parke, K. L., Morton, M. L., & Felver, J. C. (2022). *Self-compassion, minority stress, and mental health in sexual and gender minority populations: A meta-analysis and systematic review*. Science and Practice. Advance online publication. https://doi.org/10.1037/cps0000104

Jaspal, R., Lopes, B., & Breakwell, G. M. (2022). Minority stressors, protective factors and mental health outcomes in lesbian, gay and bisexual people in the UK. *Current Psychology, Advance Online Publication*. https://doi.org/10.1007/s12144-022-03631-9

Johnstone, O. K., Marshall, J. J., & McIntosh, L. G. (2022). A review comparing dialectical behavior therapy and mentalization for adolescents with borderline personality traits, suicide and self-harming behavior. *Adolescent Research Review, 7,* 187–209. https://doi.org/10.1007/s40894-020-001 47-w

Kapatais, A., Williams, A. J., & Townsend, E. (2022). The mediating role of emotion regulation on self-harm among gender identity and sexual orientation minority (LGBTQ+) individuals. *Archives of Suicide Research,* 1–14. Advance online publication. https://doi.org/10.1080/13811118.2022.206 4254

King, M., Semlyen, J., Tai, S. S., Killaspy, H., Osborn, D., Popelyuk, D., & Nazareth, I. (2008). A systematic review of mental disorder, suicide, and deliberate self-harm in lesbian, gay and bisexual people. *BMC Psychiatry, 8,* 70. https://doi.org/10.1186/1471-244X-8-70

Linehan, M. M. (1993). *Cognitive-behavioral treatment of borderline personality disorder.* Guilford Publications.

Linehan, M. M. (2015). *DBT skills training manual.* The Guilford Press.

Linehan, M. M., Korslund, K. E., Harned, M. S., Gallop, R. J., Lungu, A., Neacsiu, A. D., McDavid, J., Comtois, K. A., & Murray-Gregory, A. M. (2015). Dialectical behaviour therapy for high suicide risk in individuals with borderline personality disorder: A randomized clinical trial and component analysis. *JAMA Psychiatry, 72*(5), 475–482. https://doi.org/10.1001/jamapsychiatry.2014.3039

Livingston, N. A., Berke, D., Scholl, J., Ruben, M., & Shipherd, J. C. (2020). Addressing diversity in PTSD treatment: Clinical considerations and guidance for the treatment of PTSD in LGBTQ populations. *Current Treatment Options in Psychiatry, 7*(2), 53–69. https://doi.org/10.1007/s40501-020-00204-0

MacPherson, H. A., Cheavens, J. S., & Fristad, M. A. (2013). Dialectical behavior therapy for adolescents: Theory, treatment adaptations, and empirical outcomes. *Clinical Child and Family Psychology Review, 16*(1), 59–80. https://doi.org/10.1007/s10567-012-0126-7

Meyer, I. H. (2003). Prejudice, social stress, and mental health in lesbian, gay, and bisexual populations: Conceptual issues and research evidence. *Psychological Bulletin, 129*(5), 674–697. https://doi.org/10.1037/0033-2909.129.5.674

Morgan, E. M. (2013). Contemporary issues in sexual orientation and identity development in emerging adulthood. *Emerging Adulthood, 1*(1), 52–66. https://doi.org/10.1177/2167696812469187

Neacsiu, A. D., Eberle, J. W., Kramer, R., Wiesmann, T., & Linehan, M. M. (2014). Dialectical behavior therapy skills for transdiagnostic emotion dysregulation: A pilot randomized controlled trial. *Behaviour Research and Therapy, 59*, 40–51. https://doi.org/10.1016/j.brat.2014.05.005

National Health Service England Equality and Health Inequalities Unit. (2017). *Sexual orientation monitoring: Full specification.* Retrieved from (January 2023). https://www.england.nhs.uk/wp-content/uploads/2017/10/sexual-orientation-monitoring-full-specification.pdf

National Institute for Health and Care Excellence. (2009). *Borderline personality disorder: Recognition and management, clinical guidance [CG78].* Retrieved from (July 2022). https://www.nice.org.uk/guidance/cg78

National Institute for Health and Care Excellence. (2022). *Self-harm: Assessment, management and preventing recurrence.* Retrieved from (January 2023). https://www.nice.org.uk/guidance/ng225

Oginni, O. A., Jern, P., & Rijsdijk, F. V. (2020). Mental health disparities mediating increased risky sexual behavior in sexual minorities: A twin approach. *Archives of Sexual Behavior, 49*(7), 2497–2510. https://doi.org/10.1007/s10508-020-01696-w

O'Shaughnessy, T., & Speir, Z. (2018). The state of LGBQ affirmative therapy clinical research: A mixed-methods systematic synthesis. *Psychology of Sexual Orientation and Gender Diversity, 5*(1), 82–98. https://doi.org/10.1037/sgd0000259

Pachankis, J. E. (2018). The scientific pursuit of sexual and gender minority mental health treatments: Toward evidence-based affirmative practice. *American Psychologist, 73*(9), 1207–1219. https://doi.org/10.1037/amp0000357

Pachankis, J. E., Rendina, H. J., Restar, A., Ventuneac, A., Grov, C., & Parsons, J. T. (2015). A minority stress—emotion regulation model of sexual compulsivity among highly sexually active gay and bisexual men. *Health Psychology, 34*(8), 829–840. https://doi.org/10.1037/hea0000180

Pantalone, D. W., Sloan, C. A., & Carmel, A. (2019). Dialectical behavior therapy for borderline personality disorder and suicidality among sexual and gender minority individuals. In Pachankis, J. E. & Safren, S. A (Ed.), *Handbook of evidence-based mental health practice with sexual and gender minorities.* Oxford University Press.

Pierson, A. M., Arunagiri, V., & Bond, D. M. (2021). You didn't causes racism, and you have to solve it anyways: Antiracist adaptations to dialectical behaviour therapy for white therapies. *Cognitive and Behavioral Practice.* Advance online publication. https://doi.org/10.1016/j.cbpra.2021.11.001

Poon, J. A., Galione, J. N., Grocott, L. R., Horowitz, K. J., Kudinova, A., & Kim, K. L. (2022). Dialectical behavior therapy for adolescents (DBT-A):

Outcomes among sexual minorities at high risk for suicide. *Suicide and Life-Threatening Behavior, 52*, 383–391. https://doi.org/10.1111/sltb.12828

Rimes, K. A., Ion, D., Wingrove, J., & Carter, B. (2019). Sexual orientation differences in psychological treatment outcomes for depression and anxiety: National cohort study. *Journal of Consulting and Clinical Psychology, 87*(7), 577–589. https://doi.org/10.1037/ccp0000416

Rodriguez-Seijas, C., Eaton, N. R., & Pachankis, J. E. (2019). Prevalence of psychiatric disorders at the intersection of race and sexual orientation: Results from the national epidemiologic survey of alcohol and related Conditions-III. *Journal of Consulting and Clinical Psychology, 87*(4), 321–331. https://doi.org/10.1037/ccp0000377

Rodriguez-Seijas, C., Morgan, T. A., & Zimmerman, M. (2021). A population-based examination of criterion-level disparities in the diagnosis of borderline personality disorder among sexual minority adults. *Assessment, 28*(4), 1097–1109. https://doi.org/10.1177/1073191121991922

Semlyen, J., King, M., Varney, J., & Hagger-Johnson, G. (2016). Sexual orientation and symptoms of common mental disorder or low wellbeing: Combined meta-analysis of 12 UK population health surveys. *BMC Psychiatry, 16*, 67. https://doi.org/10.1186/s12888-016-0767-z

Skerven, K., Mirabito, L., Kirkman, M., & Shaw, B. (2021). Dialectical behaviour therapy skills group including stigma management: A pilot with sexual and gender minority veterans. *The Cognitive Behaviour Therapist, 14*, E33. https://doi.org/10.1017/S1754470X21000295

Skerven, K., Whicker, D., & LeMaire, K. (2019). Applying dialectical behaviour therapy to structural and internalized stigma with LGBTQ clients. *The Cognitive Behaviour Therapist, 12*, E9. https://doi.org/10.1017/S1754470X18000235

Sloan, C. A., Berke, D. S., & Shipherd, J. C. (2017). Utilizing a dialectical framework to inform conceptualization and treatment of clinical distress in transgender individuals. *Professional Psychology: Research and Practice, 48*(5), 301. https://doi.org/10.1037/pro0000146

Tilley, J. L., Molina, L., Luo, X., Natarajan, A., Casolaro, L., Gonzalez, A., & Mahaffey, B. (2022). Dialectical behaviour therapy (DBT XE "Dialectical behaviour therapy (DBT)") for high-risk transgender and gender diverse (TGD) youth: A qualitative study of youth and mental health providers' perspectives on intervention relevance. *Psychology and Psychotherapy: Theory, Research and Practice, 95*(4), 1056–1070. https://doi.org/10.1111/papt.12418

13

Psychodynamic Psychotherapies and Sexual Diversity

Poul Rohleder

Introduction

Sigmund Freud, the founder of psychoanalysis, developed a 'talking cure' for the treatment of mental health problems, which were previously treated medically. The influence of his theories on the development of modern talking therapies do not need elucidation. Freud's work involved not just the development of a treatment modality, but a theory of human development too. Freud made sexuality a central focus of his understanding of the development of personality and of our psychic life. Freud was revolutionary at the time, but was seen by many as subversive and even 'perverse' for giving such a central focus to sexuality in understanding human behaviour, some calling him "a dirty-minded pansexualist" (Gay, 1988, p. 194). One might say that Freud was a key figure in bringing sexuality out into the open, and acknowledged

P. Rohleder (✉)
Psychosocial and Psychoanalytic Studies, University of Essex, Colchester, UK
e-mail: p.rohleder@essex.ac.uk

© The Author(s), under exclusive license to Springer Nature
Switzerland AG 2023
J. Semlyen and P. Rohleder (eds.), *Sexual Minorities and Mental Health*,
https://doi.org/10.1007/978-3-031-37438-8_13

the various forms in which sexuality could be expressed. As we shall see below, Freud had somewhat of a humane stance to sexual diversity viewing homosexuality as 'normal' as heterosexuality (although there is some ambivalence in his language usage). However, it is fair to say that psychoanalysis over time took a very heteronormative stance, and actively pathologized homosexuality, which may leave some LGBTQ individuals feeling suspicious about the potential that psychoanalysis has in pathologizing their sexual lives. Contemporary psychoanalysis has acknowledged this troubled history, and offers an approach which recognises and offers a rich understanding of sexual fluidity and diversity.

This chapter will provide a brief consideration of what psychodynamic psychotherapy may offer in terms of working with sexual minority patients (I use the term "patient" as commonly used in psychoanalysis). The chapter will briefly outline psychoanalysis' troubled history of pathologizing homosexuality and set out some of the contemporary positions. The chapter will then outline some of the past formulations about homosexuality, and introduce some of the new reformulated theories and thinking that take a more affirming stance. This discussion will focus primarily on Freud's theory of sexuality, including what is known as the Oedipus Complex, and its contemporary revisions. The chapter will then offer a psychoanalytic lens for thinking about homophobia and internalised homophobia, key concepts that have been highlighted in all chapters of this book. Finally, the chapter will explore how psychodynamic psychotherapy can be used to work with sexual minority patients in understanding difficult interpersonal dynamics and experiences that may involve aspects of internalised homophobia and shame. In this chapter, I will use the term "homosexuality" as it is a term regularly used in the psychoanalytic literature, but acknowledge that there are other preferred terms which are more frequently used.

It is worth first noting that there are a wide range of approaches to working psychoanalytically, that encompass time-limited and open-ended work, and work at a range of frequencies. Different terms tend to be used to differentiate between different formats, with psychodynamic psychotherapy typically referring to once weekly sessions for a time-limited period, or open-ended. Psychoanalysis usually referring to open-ended psychotherapy at a frequency of three to five times weekly (according to criteria of the International Psychoanalytic Association). These different ways of working differ in terms of intensity of sustained focus, and depth of unconscious material worked with, and to what extent there is more exploration with the past, and more focus on the current context. For the purposes of this chapter, I will use the term 'psychodynamic psychotherapies' as this is the form of psychotherapy that is typically more available (i.e. once a week), but I also use it as referring to all forms of therapeutic work which has at its core a psycho-analytic theoretical framework, and I will use the term 'psychoanalysis' to refer to the body of theory.

What Is a Psychodynamic Approach?

As there are different ways of working psychoanalytically, there are also different theoretical approaches forming the field of psychoanalysis, usually named after the most influential theoretical figure that has shaped that school of thought. Most known is the work of Sigmund Freud and contemporary Freudian psychoanalytic theory, which emphasises the role of instinctual urges of sexuality and aggression. In the UK, there is Kleinian and contemporary Kleinian psychoanalysis, which has an emphasis on an internal psychic world of representations of self and others, and a Winnicottian approach, which emphasises the role of the maternal environment for psychic development. In the United States, as well as Freudian, Kleinian and Winnicottian traditions, there is also more dominant schools known as Ego Psychology, and the Intersubjective and Relational approaches. Self Psychology and Interpersonal Psychoanalysis also developed in the USA and has been influential in other parts of the world. There is also French psychoanalysis, influenced by figures such as Lacan and others. These are theories that have developed from original theories of Freud. In addition to these psychoanalytic theoretical schools, there is Jungian analysis, which is considered as a distinct, albeit related, approach, with its own theoretical bodies of work and different style of training. It is beyond the scope of this chapter to outline all these different theoretical schools (interested readers can look at Chapter 2 of Abrahams & Rohleder, 2021 for a brief summary of the different theoretical schools), but it is useful to point out that the psychoanalytic theoretical schools demonstrate a shift in focus from a mostly biological framework (Freud) to a more social and interpersonal framework for understanding psychic life and the development of self.

Psychoanalysis is a detailed theory of human subjectivity, perhaps the most extensive theory of human subjectivity that there is in psychology, and at its core is the idea that much of our subjective experience is influenced by unconscious mental processes. This has been increasingly supported by research in neuroscience, and in particular the growing discipline of neuropsychoanalysis (e.g. Solms & Turnbull, 2002, 2011). Fonagy and Target (2003) have highlighted six central theoretical principles that are common to all the different psychoanalytic theories. These are that:

1. we have an unconscious mind, and that much of our behaviour, motivation and experience occurs at an unconscious level;
2. our early childhood experiences and interpersonal attachments significantly impact on our adult functioning;
3. our minds and perceptions of ourselves and others are shaped by, and are influenced by, both internal (psychic) and external (environmental) processes;
4. our experience of relationships are shaped by unconscious mechanisms of introjection (that is internalising or taking things in from the 'outside' to form part of our perception of self and others) and projection (that is externalising disavowed aspects of our self which influences our perception of others);
5. we all experience internal psychic conflicts that create anxiety, which we manage and cope with through the utilisation of different defence mechanisms (for example, denial, is perhaps the most known defence mechanism); and
6. our past experience, including interpersonal attachment experiences, are 'transferred' onto new interpersonal experiences, including the psychotherapeutic context. That is, that our perception of and experience of others is partly shaped by our past, childhood interpersonal experience.

Psychoanalysis and Homosexuality: A Troubled History

Psychoanalysis, as with psychiatry and psychology, has had a troubled history of pathologizing homosexuality and understanding it as a form of mental disturbance or illness. Many psychoanalytic theorists and writers of the past understood and conceptualised homosexuality as a sexual "perversion" and viewing homosexual men and women as having a pathological character, most often regarded as part of what would have been called a narcissistic or borderline personality (see Lewes, 2009, for a comprehensive review of the historic literature). Such views were most explicitly stated by some American psychoanalysts who were also psychiatrists, such as Charles Socarides, Irving Bieber, Edmund Bergler and others, who were vociferous in their views about homosexuality as pathology, and advocated for conversion therapy. For example, Bergler (1956), with seemingly little sense of personal awareness and shame, writes:

> I have no bias against homosexuals; for me they are sick people requiring medical help … Still, though I have no bias, I would say: Homosexuals are essentially disagreeable people, regardless of their pleasant or unpleasant outward manner … [their] shell is a mixture of superciliousness, fake aggression, and whimpering. Like all psychic masochists, they are subservient when confronted with a stronger person, merciless when in power, unscrupulous about trampling on a weaker person. (pp. 28–29)

In the UK, there were more diverging views, with some psychoanalysts actively advocating for the decriminalisation of homosexuality in the UK in the Wolfensen report (as reported in Newbigin, 2013), while others spoke in support of Section 28 (as reported in Ellis, 2021), which prohibited the teaching of same-sex relationships at school, regarding it as the "'promotion'" of homosexuality, which was regarded as a perversion. In a lot of 'classic' British psychoanalytic theoretical papers, homosexuality is regularly formulated as perversion and psychopathology.

Contemporary psychoanalysis has moved on from this past. Lewes (2009) observes a shift in thinking from the 1990s. In recent years, more formalised positions have been taken by the psychoanalytic profession. For example, in 2011, the British Psychoanalytic Council (BPC), a regulatory body comprising of 24 psychoanalytic member institutions, issued a statement declaring that homosexuality is not a psychopathology, and opposing discrimination on the basis of sexual orientation. The BPC is also a signatory, along with many other professional organisations, to the Memorandum of Understanding Against Conversion Therapy. There has also been a flurry of new writing about sexual diversity and psychoanalysis (examples include Domenici & Lesser, 1995; Hertzmann & Newbigin, 2020; Lemma & Lynch, 2015; O'Connor & Ryan, 1993).

In the UK, the BPC has for several years had a Task Group for Sexual and Gender Diversity in Psychoanalysis, which among other activities, have compiled a comprehensive annotated bibliography of psychoanalytic writings (classic, but mostly contemporary) on sexual, gender and relationship diversity (Full, 2023), which is regularly updated. The International Psychoanalytic Association too has a Sexual and Gender Diversity Studies Committee.

Freud's Theory of Psychosexual Development

There are many psychoanalytic contributions made to understanding the development and experience of sexuality. I will focus here primarily on Freud's contribution and briefly outline contemporary developments on Freud's theory. Some readers might be surprised to learn that Freud demonstrated openness to thinking about sexual diversity and, although there is much that he did not understand about homosexuality, he did not consider it as inherently psychopathological. In his *Three Essays on the Theory of Sexuality* (1905), Freud argued that homosexuality could be seen in many well-adjusted individuals, and thus could not be considered in itself a psychopathology. In a now famous letter that Freud wrote to a mother who was concerned about her son's homosexuality, Freud states:

> Homosexuality is assuredly no advantage, but it is nothing to be ashamed of, no vice, no degradation, it cannot be classified as an illness; we consider it to be a variation of the sexual function produced by a certain

arrest of sexual development. Many highly respectable individuals of ancient and modern times have been homosexuals, several of the greatest men among them (Plato, Michelangelo, Leonardo da Vinci, etc.). It is a great injustice to persecute homosexuality as a crime, and cruelty too…. (Freud, 1935, reprinted in the American Journal of Psychiatry, 1951, 107, 786–787)

However, there are some contradictions in Freud's writings. As is suggested in the passage above, Freud described homosexuality as an "arrest of sexual development", suggesting it as normal development that has gone wrong. This is formulated around his theory of the Oedipus Complex, which in classical psychoanalysis, and to some extent still today, forms a cornerstone of psychoanalytic theory of sexuality. Before outlining his theory of the Oedipus Complex, we need to understand his model of the human mind.

As well as outlining a model of the mind that comprises of a conscious, preconscious and unconscious mind (Freud, 1900), Freud proposed a model of the mind which comprises of three separate psychic components of the personality: the id, the ego, and the superego (Freud, 1923). The id is the basic, 'animalistic' part of the mind, which operates at mostly the unconscious level, and contains what he determined to be two basic instincts or drives, the sexual (libidinal) and aggressive instincts, which dominate psychological processes. These instincts are experienced as a biological energy, an urge, that seeks release or gratification through engagement with the external environment. Freud understood the instincts as involving the body experiencing an accumulation of tension or 'unpleasure', and the seeking of pleasure to gratify such instinctual demands. In colloquial terms, we would speak, for example, of feeling 'horny' and this (instinctual) urge leads us to seek gratification (sex).

Freud conceptualised the superego as the component of our personality that we may refer to as our conscience, and include social and cultural norms, values and ideals that we internalise from our familial and community attachment figures. The term 'internalisation' refers to how we take in relational experiences and absorb them into our personality in the form of internal representations (I will return to discuss this further below when considering internalised homophobia). Aspects of the superego can be in our conscious mind or in our unconscious mind. Freud understood the superego as exerting internal psychic pressure (like the instincts) on the individual, which influences our behaviour. So, for example, if one is born to parents who live by what we might describe as a strict, rigid and conservative moral code, that person will internalise this representation of a strict authority figure which is experienced as their internal conscience. This may result in a 'harsh superego' with the individual experiencing intense feelings of guilt and moral conflict at times when they do something that they construe as being 'bad'.

The ego, which is mostly at a conscious level, is the rational, executive part of our personality. What we may in some ways refer to as the "I" (although the self really includes the ego, the id and the superego). The ego operates in the world, under the demands of the external environment as well as the internal psychic demands of the id and the superego.

Freud's psychoanalytic theory is also a theory of human development, and the development of the personality. He placed emphasis on the sexual instinct as the main driver of human development (after all it is the creative force, rather than the destructive force), and his theory is a psychosexual theory of development. He proposed human development from birth, through childhood, adolescence and into adulthood, as passing through five sequential stages: the oral stage, the anal stage, the phallic stage, the latency stage and the genital stage of psychosexual development (Freud, 1905). He named these stages as such, because he observed these stages as involving areas of the body where sexual (or libidinal) instinctual energy is primarily located. It is beyond the scope of this chapter to outline his theory of development in full, and I shall concentrate primarily on the Oedipus complex, which forms part of the phallic stage of development. Before that, it is important to note, that while Freud's theory of psychosexual development remains influential and an important aspect of psychoanalytic theory, it is the first work of psychoanalytic theory, and later schools of psychoanalytic thought have moved away from the notion of instincts, to a greater emphasis on the intersubjective and relational context, and the development of the personality as being dependent on relational experience, rather than biological drives (see Abrahams & Rohleder, 2021). It is also important to note that Freud, controversially for his time, introduced the notion of "infantile sexuality". Readers unfamiliar with psychoanalytic theory may feel uncomfortable about reference to the infant and child as sexual. However, we are not talking about adult sexuality and sexual behaviours here, we are talking about sexual instinct in the form of the experience of pleasure and excitement in the body, which as the body matures, also becomes experienced in the genitals in puberty and adulthood.

According to Freud (1905), the beginnings of sexual identity is formed during the phallic stage of psychosexual development between the ages of 4 and 6, where the child becomes more aware of their genitals and the differences between the sexes, typically the male-sexed body and female-sexed body. During the Oedipus Complex, which forms part of the phallic stage, the child also begins to form a sexual identity and develop a cohering sense of themselves in relation to others, primarily the parents, and deepening expressions of intimacy and closeness. What starts in this stage, comes together more strongly during puberty, where the adolescent experiences sexual desire, may seek romantic relationships with their peers, rather than just friendships, and develop a stronger sense of sexual identity and orientation, which matures in adulthood.

The Oedipus Complex

I will give a brief, simplified summary of Freud's theory of the Oedipus Complex. The Oedipus Complex is a formulation involving the "organised body of loving and hostile wishes which the child experiences towards its parents" and "plays a fundamental part in the structuring of personality, and in the orientation of human desire" (Laplanche & Pontalis, 1974, pp. 282–283). According to Freud (1905), the boy at an unconscious level has his mother as the primary object of his desire. That is, his libidinal (sexual instinct) desires are more strongly directed towards the mother. We may observe behavioural manifestations of this, for example, when we observe boys at this stage expressing their wish to one day "marry mommy" and have a baby with her. Their fathers are perceived as the rival for their mother's affections, and may at times have hostile feelings towards their fathers. For example, we may see the boy pushing their father away from their mother, so that he can be close to her.

However, the child, as they mature, is increasingly able to observe their parents as individuals with their own complex and personal lives, and becomes increasing aware that his parents have an adult, intimate relationship, which he is excluded from. As the father is bigger and stronger, he is perceived as a feared rival, and, according to Freud, the boy has to manage the unconscious fear that his father will punish him by means of castration (Freud's concept of castration anxiety). The castration anxiety arises out of the observation that he and father have a penis, whereas mother and girls do not have a penis (Freud's theory was very phallic-centric), and so the fantasy that the penis was taken away. The boy resolves the Oedipus conflict, by renouncing his desire for his mother, accepting that he is a child not an adult, and starts to identify with his father, becoming like him, so as to attract a partner 'like mommy' in future.

Freud's theory of female sexuality was less developed, and for the female child he conceptualised the Electra Complex. The girl, like the boy, has the mother as the primary object of her desire. The mother is the primary care-giver and with whom, typically, the infant has the closest attachment, and so for both the male and female child, the mother is the primary object of desire. However, according to Freud, during the phallic stage, the girl child, observing the differences in the sexes, becomes aware that she does not have a penis, and also that her mother does not have one either. Envying her father's penis, and disappointed in her mother's lack of a penis, the girl renounces her desire for her mother, and turns her affection to her father, with whom she hopes to have a baby. Realising the impossibility of this, she identifies with the mother and seeks a partner, 'like father', with whom she can have a baby.

As well as the heterosexual Oedipus Complex as outlined above, Freud acknowledge that homosexuality could also be an outcome of the Oedipus Complex. Freud seemed to have some difficulty in theorising homosexuality, and does not present a definitive formulation of male homosexuality (Lewes, 2009) or female homosexuality (O'Connor & Ryan, 1993). Freud referred to a 'negative' Oedipus

Complex that accounts for a homosexual orientation (the heterosexual Oedipus Complex outlined above being referred to as the 'positive Oedipus Complex').

In his writing on Leonardo de Vinci, Freud (1910) understood male homosexuality as a solution to the castration anxiety of the Oedipus Complex. The boy child develops a castration anxiety for his love of his mother, but observing the mother to have 'no penis', he is left "horrified and disgusted" (Lewes, 2009, p. 24) and perceives the mother with loathing as a castrated figure, and turns away from her as a desired figure, for fear of being castrated like her. He then turns to a compromise figure, an effeminate male partner; "a 'woman with a penis'" (Lewes, 2009, p. 24). In his other works, Freud (1905) presents a different formulation; one where the boy who later becomes homosexual, has a very close bond with his mother (with a more distant father), and rather than relinquish this libidinal tie to the mother, he identifies with her and seeks a partner who is like him (i.e. a male partner). In this way, the libidinal relationship to the mother is preserved at an unconscious level, while relinquished in reality. Lewes points out the complimentary aspects of these 2 formulations:

> In the first, the child rejects women to relieve his loathing and horror of the [castrated] mother, while in the second he flees them to ensure his fidelity to her. However these two mechanisms can be seen as complementary, leading to a complex compromise formation, as the child flees from castration anxiety, yet maintains the libidinally gratifying bond with the mother. (Lewes, 2009, p. 26)

Freud's formulation about female homosexuality is presented in a case study of a young woman (1920), where he understood the woman's same-sex object choice as involving a resentful turning away from the father and men, either adopting a masculine identification and finding a 'mother-substitute' in a feminine partner, or is attracted to a masculine woman as a way of satisfying bisexual tendencies (see below for further discussion on Freud's concept of psychic bisexuality).

While Freud did not regard homosexuality as pathology, his formulations of the 'negative' Oedipal Complex nevertheless is problematic.

Least of all due to the reliance on heteronormative constructions about gender pairing. I will return to some of his more nuanced ideas below. Following Freud's theory of the Oedipus Complex, later theorists adopted a pathologizing stance to homosexuality, where the 'normal', 'healthy' resolution of the Oedipus Complex was regarded as heterosexuality, based on Darwinian notion of sexuality being about procreation. Homosexuality was then understood as pathological, in that the Oedipus Complex could not be adequately resolved, and normal heterosexuality could not be achieved. Homosexuality thus represented a fixation or arrest of development to a pre-Oedipal stage of development, an immature personality (as reviewed in Lewes, 2009).

There have been numerous critiques of Freud's theory of the Oedipus Complex. Feminist psychoanalysts and social theorists have critiqued the centrality of the penis in Freud's theory and the notion of penis envy and castration anxiety, suggesting, for example, that for the male child there is envy for the mother's (female) capacity to bear children (see Mitchell, 1974). A feminist defence of Freud's theories about penis envy, involved reformulating the biological object of the 'penis' with the construction of the 'phallus' representing power and domination. Thus, for girls, it is not the penis itself that is envied, but rather patriarchal power (Mitchell, 1974).

Contemporary Readings of the Oedipus Complex and Same-Sex Desire

In other parts of his writings on sexuality, Freud (1905) had a much less heteronormative conceptualisation of sexuality, and indeed could be argued to understand sexuality as fluid, involving pleasure, rather than only desire (Van Haute & Westerink, 2021). He formulated the sexual drive as at first disorientated, becoming orientated through psychosexual development. He argued that the sexual drive did not have an innate, biological aim or object. He theorised that humans are innately psychically bisexual, and so one's sexual instincts and desires are directed to either sex. Heenan-Wolff (2011) points out how Freud formulated what is known as the 'complete' Oedipus complex, which involved the inter-action of both the so-called 'positive' and 'negative' Oedipus complex, and the potential for a bisexual orientation, which Freud did not view as 'structurally more pathological than another drive destiny' (Heenan-Wolff, 2011, p. 1216). Luepnitz (2021) too emphasises Freud's later conceptualisation of a 'complete' Oedipus Complex that we all pass through with both 'positive' and 'negative' sides. Freud (1923) writes:

> Closer study usually discloses the more complete Oedipus complex, which is twofold, positive and negative, and is due to the bisexuality originally present in children; that is to say that a boy has not merely an ambivalent attitude towards his father, and an affectionate object choice towards his mother, but at the same time he also behaves like a girl and displays an affectionate feminine attitude to his father and a corresponding jealousy and hostility towards his mother. (1923, p. 33)

Luepnitz rightly points out the gendered assumptions made by Freud in the quote above equating homosexual men with being 'like a girl', but nevertheless stresses the importance of Freud's apparent acknowledge-ment of same-sex desire as a normal variation of human sexuality. The terms 'positive' and negative' Oedipus Complex also creates the potential for pathologizing, and Luepnitz suggests the use of the terms "cross-sex" and "same-sex" for the two sides of the complete Oedipus Complex. Thus, we all have a tendency for both same-sex and opposite-sex desire.

Richard Isay (1986, 2010), a gay psychoanalyst from the USA, has reformulated Freud's theory of the Oedipus Complex for gay men. Drawing on considerable clinical experience and case study research, he observes an Oedipal Complex formulated around the father being experienced as a primary object of desire. Important to note here that with Freud's theory of psychic bisexuality, a child does have feelings of same-sex desire as well as opposite-sex desire, yet for the Oedipus Complex, Freud does not seem to consider this, even though for the Electra Complex, the female child's primary object of desire is of the same sex. Isay (1986, 2010) and Rose (2007) observe how for some gay men, there is an indication in their early history of their fathers turning away from the homoerotic desires of their sons. This challenges some of the psychoanalytic theory that formulated male homosexuality as 'caused by' the male child having a distant and unavailable father figure, and thus over-identifying with their mother. According to Isay, it is not that the child's father is distant, but rather than they become distant because of their discomfort and fear of their sons emerging homoerotic desires and sexuality.

Goldsmith (1995, 2001), drawing on the work of Isay, and through observations made in clinical work, reformulated an Oedipus complex (along Freudian) lines for the gay man, where the father is the primary object of desire (as discussed above, with Freud's concept of psychic bisexuality, this is not a new idea), and experiencing the mother as the rival, towards whom he may hold competitive and aggressive feelings. The resolution of the Oedipus complex involves his ability to master these feelings so as to not fear reprisal from her. Thus, for Goldsmith, the homosexual dynamics of the Oedipus complex are primary for homosexual boys, whereas for heterosexual boys, they are secondary.

Parental Responses to Sexuality

It is important to consider the parental response to the child's emotional experience, including emerging sexuality. Later psychoanalytic theorists (for example, Laplanche, 1997) emphasised that the development of sexuality also involves sensual experiences that are transmitted to the child by the parental other. Sexuality develops as a result, not only of desire, but also, the pleasure-giving experiences offered by the parent. We are not referring here to actual sexual seductions in the form of sexual abuse, but rather the maternal and paternal caressing, touching of the skin when bathing, holding, cuddling that typically occurs on a daily basis, which transmit a sensuous experience. The child, hopefully, experiences loving feelings from the primary caregiver(s) as well as having loving feelings of their own in return. In this intricate intersubjectivity the child's growing sense of themselves as someone who is loved and desired is realised. As the child's sexuality becomes more expressed, the caregiver, quite rightly, needs to install a boundary, and so there is always some experience of the parent turning away from the child's sexual expression (Target, 2007), or the introduction of acts being forbidden. For example, parents may start to tell their children not to play with their genitals in front of others, or to not play 'doctor-doctor' games with other children. The manner in which this is done is influential in how the child may experience feelings of shame in relation to sexuality. An empathic, understanding response versus an angry response or fear. Some parents may observe some homoerotic sexuality in their children (e.g. 2 boys playing 'doctor-doctor'), and respond with disgust or fear. For the child who will grow up to be gay, lesbian or bisexual, they may learn from early on from their parents' responses, comments and behaviours, and those of other significant adults, that their sexuality is "unsanctioned by others" (Lynch, 2015, p. 140) and thus may experience their sexuality as wrong or something to be ashamed about.

As Isay observes, for some gay boys, their fathers may turn away and become distant to their son's homosexuality. Isay and Rose observe how this 'oedipal rejection' may result in some gay men having difficulties with establishing and sustaining intimacy in their relationships, as the object of desire is internalised as a rejecting one. Some gay men may struggle to be intimate with a man, fearing and expecting rejection; having sex with another man is fine, but having an intimate, loving relationship may feel more precarious to navigate.

The Oedipus Complex as a Model of Triangulated Relationships

Contemporary psychoanalysis considers the Oedipus Complex as more than just involving the orientation of sexuality, but rather as a framework of triangulated relationships (Hartke, 2016) where the child is born into a structure of triangulated relationships with a, typically, mother-child bond and a father-child bond and an adult parental relationship that the child is excluded from (Britton, 1989). In a same-sex family there would be the child's individual bonds with each parent, and the adult parental relationship that the child is excluded from. The child has to learn their position in the family and navigate the rivalries and jealousies that this structure entails.

Furthermore, the Oedipus Complex is also about the growing independence of the child from their parents, which involves the diminishing libidinal-dependent bonds to the parents and the child taking on more responsibility for themselves (Loewald, 1979). Loewald states that the 'resolution' of the Oedipus Complex involves a

> dual activity in which aspects of oedipal relations are transformed into ego-superego relations (internalization), and other aspects are, qua relations with external objects, restructured in such a way that the incestuous character of object relations gives way to novel forms of object choice. These novel object choices are under the influence of those internalization. (1979, p. 758)

That is that we retain internalised representations of our parents and parent-child relationships, and we withdraw our libidinal-dependent bonds on them, enabling us to seek our own sexual partners in adulthood, aspects of such relationships being influenced by our internalised parental figures. For sexual minorities, such internalisations may include homophobic content.

Internalized Homophobia and Shame

In many of the chapters in this book, reference is made to the role of internalised homophobia and biphobia in the poor mental health of gay, lesbian and bisexual individuals. The term 'internalised homophobia', or biphobia, has become a frequently used concept but may not always be properly delineated. What is meant by 'internalised homophobia'?

Malyon (1982) is often cited for a definition of internalised homophobia, who described how "the empathic antipathy which distinguishes contemporary social attitudes toward homosexuality tends to bias the socialization process and, in turn, the intrapsychic development of gay men" (p. 59). The concept of internalised homophobia was first introduced by George Weinberg (1972), who created the term 'homophobia' to describe what he referred to as a fear of homosexuals and the expressed prejudicial attitudes are then internalised by the gay individual, resulting in self-loathing feelings.

As briefly mentioned earlier, internalisation is a psychoanalytic concept. From a psychoanalytic perspective, we are not born with a self, we develop a self through our interactions with the social world, and most importantly, with our primary adult figures in our life, our parent(s) or primary caregiver(s). Freud states that we are not born with an ego, we develop one. Although more contemporary theorists argue that we are born with a rudimentary ego or self (e.g. Bollas, 1992; Winnicott, 1965). Nevertheless, our ego or self, develops. During childhood, we make identifications with primary adult figures, we 'take in' (internalise) messages, attitudes, characteristics that we are exposed to and incorporate it into a developing psyche, becoming part of who we feel ourselves to be and how we experience ourselves in relation to others. This generally occurs at an unconscious level. It is not that we make a conscious decision to be *like* someone—this would be mimicking—but rather we unconsciously absorb aspects of others and they are incorporated into our developing selves. Readers may be familiar with the experience of suddenly catching yourself behaving or talking or thinking in a way that is similar to one of your parents ("Oh, I sound just like my father!"). We may make conscious choices to not be like someone, and thus resist possible identifications.

Thus, when we refer to internalised homophobia, we are referring to how one may be exposed to constant homophobic messages and attitudes, from an early age, which are internalised and become part of our sense of self. As Malyon (1982) describes:

> Internalized homophobic content becomes an aspect of the ego, functioning as both an unconscious introject, and as a conscious system of attitudes and accompanying affects. As a component of the ego, it influences identity formation, self-esteem, the elaboration of defenses, patterns of cognition, psychological integrity, and object relations. Homophobic incorporations also embellish superego functioning and, in this way, contribute to a propensity for guilt and intropunitiveness among homosexual males. (p. 60)

Malyon writes about internalised homophobia with reference to gay men, but the same can be said for lesbian and bisexual individuals. Malyon goes on to state that internalised homophobia precedes the conscious realisation and acceptance of same-sex desire, thus making it something unacceptable before it can be realised and accepted. If we go back to Freud, internalised homophobia may be internalised during the Oedipal stage, before same-sex desire can be actually realised in adolescence, and later accepted during the process of coming out. As many lesbian, gay and bisexual individuals state, they had, from an early age, a sense of being "different" and, more problematically, of "something being wrong" with them.

This internalised homophobia may generate a conflict around desire and intimacy. For example, writing about gay men, Moss (2002) describes how while some gay men have the experience of desiring another man, there is also the simultaneous hitting up against the internalised sense of shame and even disgust about same-sex desire, and so the experience of the relationship and intimacy becomes conflicted. Hertzmann (2011) similarly observes this in her work with some lesbian and gay couples, where internalised homophobia and shame may reside in the shared world of the couple, who may unconsciously (even consciously) struggle with a sense of conflict at simultaneously desiring each other, but feeling that something about them as a couple is 'wrong':

> it can generate punitive unconscious beliefs along the lines of – 'something about our coupling is bad, wrong, we shouldn't be like this or if only we weren't like this'. This can then prevent even the idea of a creative couple state of mind from fully emerging because something about the relationship itself is felt to be wrong. (Hertzmann, 2011, p. 352)

Other oppressed and marginalised individuals may also grow up in a hostile and prejudiced social context, leading to some internalisation of negative content. However, as Blum and Pfetzing (1997) point out, children of other oppressed and marginalised groups may typically have parents who also have these identities, and so may help the child by responding to their distress and conflicts in an affirming and containing way, helping them navigate these prejudices and offering alternative identifications. For many gay, lesbian and bisexual individuals, they may be alone, with straight parents, and few adults to turn to for help with homophobia. And indeed for some, such homophobic content may come from the parents themselves.

Elsewhere, I have discussed how underlying internalised homophobia may also be internalised misogyny (Rohleder, 2020), where much of the homophobic content that may be internalised revolve around constructions of 'normal' gender. Homophobic attitudes towards gay men, for example, typically include reference to notions of femininity and masculinity, with gay men being portrayed and demonised as being 'like women'. Gay men are hated not just for homosexuality, but for being feminine ("sissy", "pansy") and thus betraying masculinity. Such internalised content may then be expressed within the gay community, with "femme" gay men potentially being derided. In these instances, some gay men may project their own homophobia onto others, portraying gay men perceived as 'too effeminate' as the 'bad gays'. For example, research examining online ads for communities of men who have sex with men, demonstrate how masculinity is often promoted as the ideal, with effeminacy being marginalised (Miller, 2015). For some gay men living with HIV and struggling with internalised homophobia, they may perceive their HIV as a kind of 'punishment' for their homosexuality, and emphasise an internalised sense of themselves as 'dirty' and 'sinful' (Rohleder, 2016).

Moss (2002) argues how internalised homophobia is not just an issue for gay men, but can also be an important consideration for straight men, who may feel they have to deny themselves certain experiences or interests for fear of being perceived by others as gay. If we go back to Freud's notion of psychic bisexuality, straight men and women also have the possibility of having same-sex desire. Internalised homophobia may lead to an unhelpful overly-repressed same-sex desire, which may explain how for some men, having intimate, close male friendships feel threatening. Rubinstein (2003) observes how some bisexual individuals may split their lives into homosexual and heterosexual 'periods' as a way of coping with internalised homophobia, and prejudice from both communities, until such time as a more integrated experience can be reached.

What Psychodynamic Psychotherapy Can Offer

As it might, hopefully, be apparent in some of the discussion above, psychoanalysis is not only a 'one-person psychology', but has a specific focus of the self as it develops, and the individual experiences themselves in an interpersonal context. When it comes to sexual diverse individuals, there may be difficulties related to deep-seated traumatic experiences, anxieties and conflicts around exclusion and inclusion, and internalised homophobia and feelings of shame around same-sex desire. These are all areas that can be fruitfully worked with in a psychodynamic psychotherapy approach.

A key aim of psychodynamic psychotherapy is to expand self-knowledge, bringing unconscious conflicts and defensive strategies into consciousness, and, in doing so, expand insight and sense of autonomy and choice (Abrahams & Rohleder, 2021). Psychodynamic psychotherapy offers the patient a deep understanding of self, based on a detailed exploration of early personal family history and interpersonal dynamics. A key aspect of psychodynamic psychotherapy is the use of the relationship with the therapist as a focus of exploration and understanding, through the exploration of what is known as the 'transference', which refers to the various emotional and behavioural responses that the patient may have towards the therapist, which are based on internalised relational experiences with past significant others, most usually one's parents (Abrahams & Rohleder, 2021). Thus, during the course of psychotherapy, a patient who has had repeated past experiences of being rejected and abandoned, may perceive the therapist as a potentially rejecting and abandoning figure, and thus behave and respond to them on the basis of this 'transference'. For example, they may behave in an acquiescing manner, so as not to 'upset' the therapist and risk potential rejection. This then provides a 'live' opportunity to understand and work through this anxiety and interpersonal dynamic.

The psychodynamic psychotherapist adopts what is known as an 'analytic attitude' which involves principles of anonymity, abstinence and neutrality (Abrahams & Rohleder, 2021). That is, that the therapist aims to not bring their personal lives into the work, to abstain from giving advice and gratifying wishes and maintaining a neutral, non-judgemental position. The psychodynamic psychotherapist does not aim to help the patient by providing active acceptance and support, but rather facilitate the exploration and understanding of internal conflicts and emotional experiences, internalised homophobia, and challenging unhelpful defences. An aim is not to reassure, but to understand, share and work through anxieties and conflicts. For example, it would be considered unhelpful for the therapist to say to a patient "you have nothing to be ashamed of". Rather, the therapist would say "tell me about that shame", to explore these feelings in depth, their historical routes and how they may shape current interpersonal experiences. In this way, acceptance is gradually developed from within the self, rather than provided by the psychotherapist from without. It is important to note that what I am describing here is a contemporary Freudian analytic attitude of abstinence, most practiced in the UK. The question of the LGB psychotherapists' self-disclosure of their sexuality to the patient is contested and debated. More relational approaches, such as practiced in the USA, would accept that psychotherapists may need to self-disclosure their LGB identity to an LGB patient, recognising that the psychotherapists own subjectivity is influential in the work and what happens in the consulting room (Drescher, 1998).

Time-limited models of psychodynamic psychotherapy typically focus on current interpersonal difficulties, and unconscious dynamics that may be involved in these difficulties, such as defensive behaviour, projections of disavowed traits onto others, or internalised past experiences they may be distorting or influencing current relationships. One model of short-term psychodynamic psychotherapy that has recently been adopted by the NHS, is Dynamic Interpersonal Therapy (DIT) (Lemma et al., 2011), a 16-session model which is one of the recommended therapies for depression by the NICE guidelines.

In DIT, patients are encouraged to bring stories of their experiences with other people—family, friends, colleagues, partners—and the therapist will identify possible repeated experiences across different interpersonal contexts. In the assessment phase of the therapy (first 4 sessions) the focus is on the collaborative development of a working formulation of a recurring pattern of interpersonal difficulties, called the Interpersonal and Affective Focus (or IPAF). Using the IPAF, the therapist then aims, during the course of the remaining sessions, to facilitate a deeper exploration of this pattern of relating to self and others, and how some internalised past relational experiences affect this pattern of relating, to help the patient to become more aware of these repeating patterns and possible unconscious dynamics involved, so that the patient can consider possible ways in which to think and respond differently to interpersonal difficulties.

There are three dimensions of the IPAF. Firstly, there is the Self-representation, which refers to the way that the patient typically feels about themselves in relation to others, in particular the problematic aspects of this representation. Referring to discussions above about the ego and identifications, this may refer to problematic internalisations that we have incorporated into our sense of self. Secondly, there is the Other-representation, which refers to the way in which the patient may repeatedly experience and perceive other people. This may also represent internalised experiences of others and aspects of the superego. For example, experiencing and perceiving others as critical. Thirdly, there is the emotional dimension of this interpersonal self-other interaction, which may be, for example, depression, anxiety, frustration, despair, or shame. What we are looking for is a repeated pattern of interpersonal interactions, which may have roots in early attachment experiences.

In DIT, using the IPAF as a focus, the therapist can work with patients to understand the impact of internalised homophobia in relationship difficulties. I will use a case vignette to illustrate. I have created a composite case vignette drawing on some of the typical sorts of past and current experiences and relationship difficulties that I may find in my consulting room.

Charlie is a gay man in his early 40s who has come for therapy for depression and loneliness. Charlie has had a reasonably successful and steady career in sales, but feels he has not advanced his career and risen to more senior positions. He said he gets on well with some of his colleagues, particularly two female colleagues. He said there are a few guys in the company who he gets on with well enough, but describes them as "blokes" and they sometimes go together to football matches, but he is not interested in that. He describes his boss as a nice man, a bit of an "alpha male", but a good boss. He does well enough in sales and often goes over his sales targets, so earns well enough. However, he feels unsatisfied and stuck in his current job, and feels he should try and take on a more senior role, but feels he does not have the confidence to do so. He does not think that others will take him seriously enough if he had to take a more leadership role.

Charlie lives on his own, and at times gets quite lonely. He goes occasionally with some friends to one of the gay bars, but says that on the whole he does not really like the whole gay scene. When I asked why, he just said that he did not like what he described as a "culture of performance and drama". He likes to drink, and can get quite drunk at times; "a depressed drunk", he added. He says he has a friend, who he calls "a fuck buddy". He has used Grindr [a 'hook-up' App on his phone] fairly often and had some hook-ups. He said how he tends to be a "bottom" and likes to be dominated, which at the time he really enjoys, but then afterwards feels a little ashamed with himself, and he struggled to articulate why. He said his first relationship was with a guy called Mark when he was at university. His "first love" he said. Mark was older than him and very good looking and he felt very insecure with him, sure that he was cheating on him, and they had frequent arguments and break-ups. Eventually he did find out that Mark had slept with someone else, and he ended the relationship. He had a few other short relationships, and there was similar feeling of jealousies and mistrust. He says he would like to have a relationship, but added that he is not sure he is good at it. When people get close to him, he feels insecure and feels he does not have enough to offer.

When he described his childhood and family, he at first said he had an "okay" childhood, but later probing revealed some painful dynamics. He has an older brother and older sister and a younger brother. He said he was fairly close to his mother, and they talked regularly. She could get depressed sometimes and tended to turn to him for support. He did not get on very well with his father. His father is a policeman, and described him as very much a "bloke", who enjoys football. This was never something he was interested in, and was a pursuit that his father enjoyed with his 2 brothers more. He feels his father was frustrated with him as a child for being "soft". At school he did alright academically, but was not a popular boy. He was bullied a bit by some of the boys, who would call him "faggot" at times. When he came out *his mother was upset, but ultimately was accepting, while his father did not want to talk much about it, and asked him not to tell any of the extended family or friends that he was gay, he did not want others to know.*

In this short case vignette Charlie describes some of the overt homophobia he experienced at school, but also at home, particularly in relation to his father. It seems that from an early age his father had a closer relationship to his two other sons, seemingly noticing a difference in Charlie that he disapproved of. His homophobia more overtly expressed in his own shame at his son's sexuality when he came out. We get a picture of a boy that is not helped to feel good about himself, but gets on by fairly quietly, doing well enough at school and having some friends. His internalised homophobia is evident in his low self-esteem and sense of inferiority in relation to other men, and the feelings of shame that he experiences at times after sexual encounters, perhaps related to being "bottom" and internalised representations he may have associated with that about masculinity and being "soft" and a "faggot". He may also be projecting some of his shame onto others in the 'gay scene' which he alludes to describing as involving "drama". The Oedipal rejection of his father (as outlined earlier in the chapter) is repeated in interpersonal dynamics, particularly with men, where he has a sense of himself as not being good enough, or not having enough to offer, and other men being more "alpha" and potentially rejecting. This creates insecurities for him in a relationship context.

So, in terms of the IPAF, we may then represent this diagrammatically as shown in Fig. 13.1.

Some may criticise the psychodynamic model and a focus on internalised homophobia as focusing the problem as being 'in the mind' of the individual, as if to the exclusion of consideration of actual homophobia. This would be a misreading and misunderstanding of a psychodynamic approach. In the case of Charlie, for example, there is no denying the past and probably present experience of homophobia, but a psychodynamic model provides an understanding for the impact of this on the internal sense of self as an individual and in relation to others. Charlie struggles to advance in his career because he has concluded for himself that he would be rejected, and found lacking. He has not tested this to be true or not. When it comes to relationships, he seems to hold a part

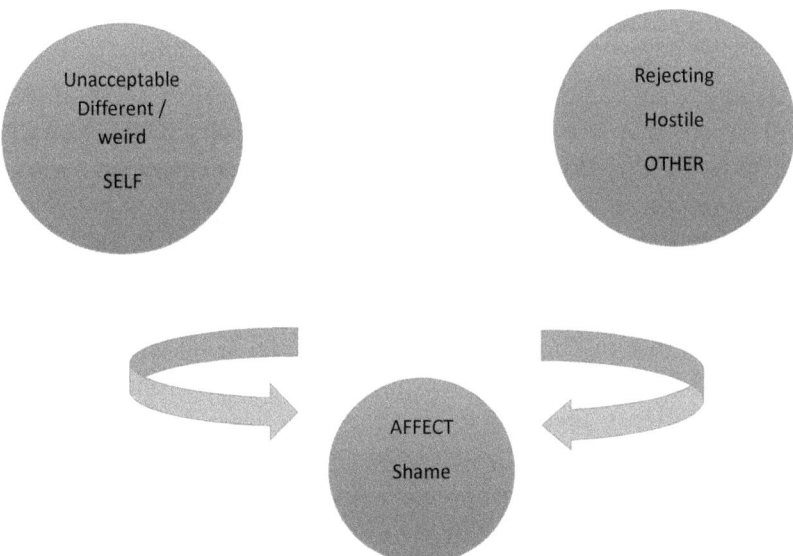

Fig. 13.1 An interpersonal affective focus formulation for "Charlie"

of him cautiously back, keeping a distance with others, in the expectation that they would inevitably be rejecting. There is also a rejecting part of him, denigrating others' behaviours, representing that which he is internally shamed about. Thus, the concept of internalised homophobia, does not negate actual homophobia, but it provides a means for understanding the psychological consequences of this for the individual and their sense of themselves. In individual psychotherapy it is this that can be worked with. An aim is to make unconscious anti-homosexuality conflicts conscious, so that they can then be modified. Through this process, the patient can come to challenge their own internalised homophobia and gradually develop more accepting and affirming self-representations and a broader range of other-representations, which include the possibility of non-rejecting figures.

Does Psychodynamic Therapy Work?

A critique that is sometimes levelled at psychodynamic psychotherapy is the claim that it does not have an evidence base. While it may be correct to say that there are far more studies that demonstrate cognitive behavioural therapy (CBT) to be effective, compared to psychodynamic psychotherapy, this does not mean that CBT is effective and psychodynamic psychotherapy is not. It just means there are more published studies! Recent reviews on the efficacy of psychodynamic psychotherapy have shown that psychodynamic psychotherapies are at least as effective as CBT (Fonagy, 2015; Leichsenring & Klein, 2014; Shedler, 2010). Dynamic Interpersonal Therapy is a newly developed semi-manualised therapy, and so does not have a large evidence base. Results from the first randomised control trial for DIT (Fonagy et al., 2019) found it to be as effective as CBT. In addition to findings showing efficacy, a meta-analysis of 23 randomised control trials (Abbass et al., 2006) suggests that psychodynamic psychotherapy may have a longer lasting effect post treatment, suggesting that psychodynamic psychotherapy "sets in motion psychological processes that lead to on-going change, even after therapy has ended" (Shedler, 2010, p. 101).

Conclusions

Some LGBTQ individuals may be suspicious of psychodynamic psychotherapies, suspecting it to be a psychotherapeutic approach that pathologizes non-heterosexual sexuality, and non-normative sexual practices. This would not be an entirely unfair criticism, given psychoanalysis' problematic views of homosexuality in the past. However, as I have tried to outline in this chapter, albeit only briefly, contemporary psychoanalysis recognises sexuality in much more fluid terms. Contrary to some beliefs, psychoanalysis is also not about arriving at some pre-established or determined truth, but rather the careful and deep exploration of the unique subjective experience of the individual. As Hodges (2011) states, "from a queer perspective psychoanalytic techniques do not constitute practices for revealing the truths of human nature but are rather techniques for the construction and reconstruction of selves and identities" (p. 35). For sexual minority individuals who have struggled with internalised homophobia and sense of self damaged by feelings of shame, psychodynamic psychotherapies may offer a different experience of emotional intimacy with another (therapist) where vulnerabilities can be understood and an internal sense of acceptance can be gradually developed.

References

Abbass, A. A., Hancock, J. T., Henderson, J., & Kisely, S. (2006). Short-term psychodynamic psychotherapies for common mental disorders. *Cochrane Database of Systematic Reviews,* Issue 4, Article No. CD004687. https://doi.org/10.1002/14651858.CD004687.pub3

Abrahams, D., & Rohleder, P. (2021). *A clinical guide to psychodynamic psychotherapy.* Routledge.

Bergler, E. (1956). *Homosexuality: Disease or way of life.* Hill & Wang.

Blum, A., & Pfetzing, V. (1997). Assaults to the self: The trauma of growing up gay. *Gender and Psychoanalysis, 2*(4), 427–442.

Bollas, C. (1992). *Being a character: Psychoanalysis and self experiences.* Routledge.

Britton, R. (1989). The missing link, parental sexuality in the Oedipus complex. In R. Britton, M. Feldman, & E. O'Shaughnessy (Eds.), *The Oedipus complex today.* Karnac.

Domenici, T., & Lesser, R. C. (Eds.). (1995). *Disorienting sexuality: Psychoanalytic reappraisals of sexual identities.* Routledge.

Drescher, J. (1998). *Psychoanalytic therapy and the gay man.* The Analytic Press.

Ellis, M. L. (2021). Challenging identities; lesbians, gay men, and psychoanalysis. *Psychodynamic Practice, 27*(3), 241–258.

Fonagy, P. (2015). The effectiveness of psychodynamic psychotherapies: An update. *World Psychiatry, 14*(2), 137–150.

Fonagy, P., Lemma, A., Target, M., O'Keeffe, S., Constantinou, M. P., Wurman, T. V., Luyten, P., Allison, E., Roth, A., Cape, J., & Pilling, S. (2019). Dynamic interpersonal therapy for moderate to severe depression: A pilot randomized controlled and feasibility trial. *Psychological Medicine, 50*(6), 1010–1019.

Fonagy, P., & Target, M. (2003). *Psychoanalytic theories: Perspectives from developmental psychopathology*. Whurr Publishers.

Freud, S. (1900). The interpretation of dreams. In J. Strachey (Ed.), *The standard edition of the complete psychological works of Sigmund Freud* (Vol. 4/5). Hogarth Press.

Freud, S. (1905). Three essays on the theory of sexuality. *The standard edition of the complete psychological works of Sigmund Freud* (J. Strachey, Trans., Vol. 7). Vintage Classics.

Freud, S. (1910). Leonardo da Vinci and a memory of his childhood. In J. Strachey (Ed.), *The standard edition of the complete psychological works of Sigmund Freud* (Vol. 11). Hogarth Press.

Freud, S. (1920). The psychogenesis of a case of female homosexuality. *The International Journal of Psycho-Analysis, 1*, 125–149.

Freud, S. (1923). The ego and the id. In J. Strachey (Ed.), *The standard edition of the complete psychological works of Sigmund Freud* (Vol. 19). Hogarth Press.

Freud, S. (1935|1951). Letter to an American mother. *American Journal of Psychiatry, 107*, 786.

Full, W. (2023). *BPC bibliography on gender, sexuality and relationship diversity*. https://www.bpc.org.uk/professionals/diversity

Gay, P. (1988). *Freud: A life for our time*. J. M. Dent & Sons.

Goldsmith, S. J. (1995). Oedipus or Orestes? Aspects of gender identity development in homosexual men. *Psychoanalytic Inquiry, 15*(1), 112–124.

Goldsmith, S. J. (2001). Oedipus or Orestes? Homosexual men, their mothers, and other women revisited. *Journal of the American Psychoanalytic Association, 49*(4), 1269–1287.

Hartke, R. (2016). The Oedipus complex: A confrontation at the central crossroads of psychoanalysis. *The International Journal of Psychoanalysis, 97*(3), 893–913.

Heenan-Wolff, S. (2011). Infantile bisexuality and the 'complete Oedipal complex': Freudian views on heterosexuality and homosexuality. *International Journal of Psychoanalysis, 92*, 1209–1220.

Hertzmann, L. (2011). Lesbian and gay couple relationships: When internalized homophobia gets in the way of couple creativity. *Psychoanalytic Psychotherapy, 25*(4), 346–360.

Hertzmann, L., & Newbigin, J. (Eds.). (2020). *Sexuality and gender now: Moving beyond heteronormativity*. Routledge.

Hodges, I. (2011). Queering psychoanalysis: Power, self and identity in psychoanalytic therapy with sexual minority clients. *Psychology & Sexuality, 2*(1), 29–44.

Isay, R. A. (1986). The development of sexual identity in homosexual men. *Psychoanalytic Study of the Child, 41,* 467–489.

Isay, R. (2010). *Being homosexual: Gay men and their development.* Vintage.

Laplanche, J. (1997). The theory of seduction and the problem of the other. *The International Journal of Psycho-Analysis, 78*(4), 653.

Laplanche, J., & Pontalis, J. B. (1974). *The language of psychoanalysis.* Karnac Books.

Leichsenring, F., & Klein, S. (2014). Evidence for psychodynamic psychotherapy in specific mental disorders: A systematic review. *Psychoanalytic Psychotherapy, 28*(1), 4–32.

Lemma, A., & Lynch, P. E. (Eds.). (2015). *Sexualities: Contemporary psychoanalytic perspectives.* Routledge.

Lemma, A., Target, M., & Fonagy, P. (2011). *Brief dynamic interpersonal therapy: A clinician's guide.* Oxford University Press.

Lewes, K. (2009). *Psychoanalysis and male homosexuality (20th anniversary ed.).* Jason Aronson.

Loewald, H. W. (1979). The waning of the Oedipus complex. *Journal of the American Psychoanalytic Association, 27*(4), 751–775.

Luepnitz, D. A. (2021). A return to Freud's "complete Oedipus complex": Reclaiming the negative. *American Imago, 78*(4), 619–630.

Lynch, P. E. (2015). Intimacy and shame in gay male sexuality. In A. Lemma & P. E. Lynch (Eds.), *Sexualities: Contemporary psychoanalytic perspectives* (pp. 138–155). Routledge.

Malyon, A. K. (1982). Psychotherapeutic implications of internalized homophobia in gay men. *Journal of Homosexuality, 7,* 59–69.

Miller, B. (2015). "Dude, where's your face?" Self-presentation, self-description, and partner preferences on a social networking application for men who have sex with men: A content analysis. *Sexuality & Culture, 19*(4), 637–658.

Mitchell, J. (1974). *Feminism and psychoanalysis.* Allen Lane.

Moss, D. (2002). Internalized homophobia in men: Wanting in the first person singular, hating in the first person plural. *The Psychoanalytic Quarterly, 71*(1), 21–50.

Newbigin, J. (2013). Psychoanalysis and homosexuality: Keeping the discussion moving. *British Journal of Psychotherapy, 29*(3), 276–291.

O'Connor, N., & Ryan, J. (1993). *Wild desires and mistaken identities: Lesbianism and psychoanalysis.* Virgo Press.

Rohleder, P. (2016). Othering, blame and shame when working with people living with HIV. *Psychoanalytic Psychotherapy, 30*(1), 62–78.

Rohleder, P. (2020). Homophobia, heteronormativity and shame. In L. Hertzmann & J. Newbigin (Eds.), *Sexuality and gender now: Moving beyond heteronormativity* (pp. 40–56). Routledge.

Rose, S. H. (2007). *Oedipal rejection: Echoes in the relationships of gay men.* Cambria Press.

Rubinstein, G. (2003). Does psychoanalysis really mean oppression? Harnessing psychodynamic approaches to affirmative therapy with gay men. *American Journal of Psychotherapy, 57*(2), 206–218.

Shedler, J. (2010). The efficacy of psychodynamic psychotherapy. *American Psychologist, 65*(2), 98–109.

Solms, M., & Turnbull, O. H. (2002). *The brain and the inner world: An introduction to the neuroscience of subjective experience.* Karnac Books.

Solms, M., & Turnbull, O. H. (2011). What is neuropsychoanalysis? *Neuropsychoanalysis, 13*(2), 133–145.

Target, M. (2007). Is our sexuality our own? A developmental model of sexuality based on early affect mirroring. *British Journal of Psychotherapy, 23*(4), 517–530.

Van Haute, P., & Westerink, H. (2021). *Reading Freud's three essays on the theory of sexuality: From pleasure to the object.* Routledge.

Weinberg, G. (1972). *Society and the healthy homosexual.* St Martin's.

Winnicott, D. W. (1965). *The maturational processes and the facilitating environment.* Hogarth Press.

14

Sex and Couples Therapy: Working with Same-Sex Intimate Relationships

Silva Neves and Jordan Dixon

Introduction

In this chapter, we are going to focus on gay male and lesbian couples. We recognise the many sexual and relationship diversities which live simultaneously side by side with gay and lesbian people. Lisa Diamond (2017) noted the majority of those with same-sex or gender attractions don't consider themselves to fall under the labels of lesbian, gay or bisexual (Igartua et al., 2009). Nevertheless, most literature on sexual minorities centre on those who identify as "lesbian or gay" (Diamond, 2017). A recalibration in which we term lesbian, gay, bisexual and other identities is therefore invited. This includes queer, pansexual, asexual, hetero-flexible identities to name just a few. 'Couples therapy' implies intimate relationships with two people. To work more inclusively with other relationship styles such as polyamory and consensual

S. Neves (✉) · J. Dixon
London, UK
e-mail: sntherapy@googlemail.com

J. Semlyen and P. Rohleder (eds.), *Sexual Minorities and Mental Health*,
https://doi.org/10.1007/978-3-031-37438-8_14

non- monogamy etc., we recommend using 'intimate partner relationship therapy'. Many of the themes and interventions discussed in this chapter are applicable to sexual and relationship orientations within the umbrella of gender, sex and relationship diversities (GSRD).

Until 1990, 'Homosexuality' was a term previously ascribed to mental health disorder in the International Classification of Diseases (ICD). Since many words are loaded with pathology, The LGBTQIA+ communities can be more acutely aware of language. The fluidity of language and its evolving nature mean it is vital for clinicians to be informed of adaptive changes. Doing so signals to clients that clinicians wish to be inclusive. Chapter 9 provides different areas for consideration for inclusive therapy, including language.

The term 'Queer' is favoured by some people within the LGBTQIA+ community. It's worthy to note some people don't like or ascribe to this identity. Some men prefer the term MSM (Men who have Sex with Men), others identify with 'gay man'. Similarly, some women prefer 'gay woman' or WSW (Women who have Sex with Women) rather than lesbian and some don't wish to be labelled at all. Therefore, it's crucial to listen to each clients' own experience and expression of self-identity and echo this, rather than rely on our own perceptions.

As therapists, it's imperative to be aware of the words we use. Words have the power to confirm or deny someone's very existence (Nelson, 2020). Part of practicing GSRD affirmative therapy is understanding the importance of language both verbal and non-verbal. When speaking and listening to our clients' experiences, the clinician's non-verbal cues such as eyes, tone of voice, body gestures, and so on, are just as important as the words that are said. A clinicians' body language and facial expressions can quickly penetrate a therapy space, either welcoming or excluding what is said with words. This is referred to as meta-communication and sadly it's often a neglected area of training (Watts-Jones, 2010).

The presenting issues gay and lesbian couples bring to therapy are similar to heterosexual couples. Themes of attachments, intimacy, money, household duties and sexual health principles are universally applicable to all sexual orientations but the psycho-socio context in which these themes live are different. A therapist employing common couple's therapy tools and interventions without a thorough awareness of specific LGBTQIA+ landscapes may miss the nuances when working with these populations.

Same-Sex Intimate Relationships

The psychological and psychosexual fields of same-sex intimate relationships are multi-layered, each overlapping, creating a unique terrain where the relationship resides. Clinicians are invited to consider:

1. The psychological field: childhood development, possible history of trauma of growing up gay or bisexual in a heteronormative world.
2. The psychosexual field: sexual and erotic orientation, relationship orientation and sexual development.
3. The range of responses in the here-and-now of each individual in the relationship to the heteronormative world, including minority stress.
4. The core beliefs people have about sex and relationships, including attachment styles and myths perpetuated by society, family, culture, religion etc.

The Psychological Field

Chapter 5 considered sexual orientation across the lifespan. We want to highlight a couple of psychological aspects of growing up gay or lesbian here. From early age, young people may not have the language to understand different sexual orientations and may experience a feeling-sense of difference ('*I'm not like the other boys/girls*'). In UK society, many young people are raised to be heterosexual by parents and schools, etc. In adolescence, there's a scarcity of support networks which endorse other possibilities of sexuality diversity. This is magnified by a lack of inclusive sex education that teaches the validation and pleasure of same-sex relationships. The expression of sexual orientations become important for sexual development and the process of attachments with peers.

The LGBTQIA+ teenager may compare themselves to their heterosexual counterparts and repress their own burgeoning sexuality. They may pretend to be straight to survive, fearing it's unwelcome (this is also in the context of continuing social prejudice and homophobic abuse) despite existing equality laws (see Chapter 3). As a result, repression of sexuality can foster a sense of defectiveness which becomes toxic over time.

The Psychosexual Field

Kinsey (1948), a pioneer in sexology, demonstrated sexuality being a spectrum rather than fixed into the binary of heterosexuality or homosexuality. Richards and Barker (2013) expanded our understanding of gender, sex and relationship diversities. Identifying as gay or lesbian does not only describe having sex with someone of the same sex; it also includes many other aspects.

1. Gender fluidity. Some gay men and lesbians enjoy their masculine or feminine side, some are predominantly attracted to masculinity (androsexual) or femininity (gynosexual). Gender fluidity is not a one-size fits all. Many embrace more fluid ways of being where they can choose to express their gender in a variety of ways that don't conform to heteronormative expectations (see Chapter 7).
2. The linkage between sexual/romantic relationship experience and sexual identification may not always be obvious. Same-sex intimate relationships among non-lesbian women and non-gay men do exist (whether they identify as bisexual, heterosexual, or whether they decline to label their sexuality at all).
3. Erotic orientation. Like in heterosexual relationships, some gay men and lesbians are oriented in Vanilla erotic expressions, and some lean towards kink, including BDSM. Sprott and Williams (2019) define BDSM (Bondage/Discipline, Dominance/Submission, Sadism/Masochism) as a sexual orientation for some and a *"serious leisure activity"* for others. Some gay men and lesbians may find it difficult to embrace their kink because of feeling shame about it. As a therapist working with the GSRD population, it's important to be

kink-affirmative, this also extends to heterosexual people (Shahbaz & Chirinos, 2017).
4. Relationship orientation. Like heterosexual people, some gay men and lesbians identify as monogamous, some polyamorous, and some within a wide range in-between, including what author Dan Savage (2005) calls "*monogamish*".

These are slices of the multiple intersections of how gay men, lesbians, and all people can self-identify. Some aspects may be fixed for some people and some fluid for others. It's worthwhile remembering that people's self-identity is a statement in the here-and-now.

Another psychosexual aspect to consider is the sexual development of each person in the relationship. The enquiries of sexual development include:

1. HIV-related sexual anxiety: although we're no longer in the AIDS epidemic the stigma of HIV prevails. Still today, HIV is mostly considered a 'gay disease'. Amongst gay men, there is a hierarchy of worth as the common language used is 'clean' to mean 'HIV-negative', implying that being HIV-positive is 'dirty'. Despite much campaign such as $U = U$ (an undetectable viral load means the virus is untransmittable), gay men's perception of attractiveness is associated with an absence of sexually transmitted infections (Sarno & Mohr, 2020).
2. First coming out. The first experience of coming out is usually pivotal. Depending on how it happened, it may still be an unhealed wound or it may not; it's important not to assume. Coming out for many LGBTQ+ people can mean enduring a lifelong process of continuously coming out in their everyday lives. See Chapter 4 for more considerations about coming out.
3. First sexual experience. If the first sexual experience didn't go well, it's common for anxiety to linger into future sexual experiences, perpetuating the original sexual discomfort. Unfortunately, first sexual experiences are often filled with anxiety because of a lack of sex education. However, some lesbians report less sexual difficulties as a result of anxiety compared to heterosexual women (Beaber & Werner, 2009).

4. History of relationships. Many people often conduct their present relationships based on what they learnt from past relationships including the ones from their parents. For LGBTQIA+ it's especially useful to be curious about what these are as they can often be compounded by unhelpful narratives such as: 'relationships are to be endured', 'I'm hard to live with' and more homophobic ones such as 'nobody can really understand me' and 'I'm not lovable enough'.

The Here-and-Now Protective Response of Heteronormativity

As highlighted in previous chapters, UK society is still geared towards heteronormativity, therefore many people within the LGBTQIA+ community can feel minority stress for not adhering to this way of being. Belonging as part of a collective whole plays a crucial part in overall well-being and minority stress can be detrimental towards mental health. Some LGBTQIA+ people consciously and sometimes subconsciously feel they need to remain on alert to survive, often scanning their environment for danger. This can put the nervous system in a constant state of hyper-vigilance, which may cause difficulties with sexual function and impact the quality of intimate relationships. Referring to Sexual and Gender Minority (SGM) people, Skinta (2021) highlights:

> Sexual and Gender Minority Stress is a model that elucidates how societal bias harms SGM people, and does not reflect any inherent shortcomings among SGM individuals. (p. 17)

This is an important lens to use when working with LGBTQIA+ people because it helps to understand how some seemingly maladaptive behaviours, such as sabotaging relationships, may in fact be a creative adaptive response to living with minority stress. Meyer (2003) proposes minority stress contributes to the mental health difficulties of the LGBTQIA+ populations. One of the components is 'internalised homophobia', which is a set of homo-negative ideas (conscious and unconscious) that LGBTQIA+ people believe about themselves. People who struggle to start or maintain romantic relationships, and, sometimes, even friendships, may be due to a core belief they 'should not' love someone of the same gender and/or do not deserve to be loved. Despite the increased visibility and acceptance of LGBTQIA+ relationships in media, it appears minority stress is still relevant and felt by the LGBTQIA+ communities (Frost et al., 2022).

Core Beliefs, Attachment Styles and Sex Myths

We won't do justice to the vast field of attachment theories pioneered by John Bowlby, yet we feel it's important to have a grasp of them when working with intimate relationships. Our attachment styles are influenced by how we attached to our primary care givers as well as attachment ruptures in childhood, and throughout life. Many people in the LGBTQIA+ communities may experience attachment ruptures because of homophobia, biphobia, and transphobia.

Here is a brief and simplistic summary of the common core beliefs associated with different attachment styles which affect how people conduct their relationships (Bowlby, 1969, 1973, 1980):

1. Secure attachment: *'No matter what happens to me, I know there are people around me who love me'*
2. Anxious attachment: *'I have to work hard at being loved. I'm pretty sure people won't like me if they know who I truly am. My partner will probably leave me, unless I am perfect'*
3. Avoidant attachment: *'Love is a myth. I'm alone in the world and I have to fend for myself'*.
4. Disorganised attachment: *'Why would anyone trust anyone. The world is a bad place'*

Fern (2020) highlights the fluidity of attachment styles not being fixed and how they can shift from insecure to secure: "Your attachment styles are survival adaptations to your environment and since they were learned, they can also be unlearned" (p. 26).

The knowledge of attachement styles can bring clarity to couples in understanding their dynamics, particularly if their attachement styles are different or cause conflicts. For example, using a fictional case, the more Patrick (avoidant attachment) needs some distance to regulate himself, the more David (anxious attachment) believes the distance created is because he's done something wrong or because Patrick stopped loving him. David responds to his anxiety by wanting to grab Patrick's attention to keep him close. Patrick's space is denied which creates more frustration for him, therefore he demands more distance, to which David interprets as confirmation Patrick doesn't love him. This intensely polluted and emotive cycle can be explosive, often leaving the people in the relationship miserable.

When couples become aware of their attachment styles, they can navigate their romantic relationships with better maps. Erotic maps are also an important guide for couples sexual adventuring. Unfortunately, sex education is generally poor and is not inclusive of diverse sexual orientations (although this is slowly changing). The lack of inclusive sex education allows for the absorption of heteronormative sex myths, which are often unchallenged. Some of them are:

'Monogamy is gold standard'
'HIV is a gay disease'
'If you're bottom, you're the 'feminine one'
'Sex without penetration is not real sex'
'Couples have an orgasm at the same time'
'Making love' is more desirable than 'fucking'
'Bisexual men are gay men in the closet'
'Bisexuality is greedy, they have their cake and eat it, they can't make their mind up, they will leave for the other'
'Polyamory is a sign of unhealthy relationship'
'It's not ok to have children if you're a same-sex couple'
'Women should want children'

These myths can feed shame, re-inforce internalised homophobia and interact with individual's attachment styles.

Now that we've explored some of what the GSRD populations battle with in terms of conscious and subconscious core beliefs, minority stress, disrupted childhood, homophobia, biphobia, transphobia, and sex myths, we can now better understand how multi-layered it is to work with a gay male couple, or a lesbian couple. Now we will consider this further in detail.

Working with Gay Male Couples and Intimate Relationships

In our experience of working with gay male couples, it appears many can hold strong assumptions that '*the grass is greener on the other side of the fence*', an idea that is reinforced by hook-up apps offering the illusion of something '*better*' around the corner. Pachankis et al. (2020) highlight "intra-minority stress" within the gay male population, which means that they tend to compete with each other, with a high likelihood of rejection. This directly taps into the core beliefs of the people with anxious and avoidant attachment styles, internalised homophobia and shame.

These obstacles are likely to affect how gay men relate to each other precipitating communication problems, frequent conflicts, resentment, as well as sexual problems. We will now illustrate common difficulties with clinical vignettes. These vignettes are anonymised composite cases to ensure the maintenance of our clients' confidentiality.

Sexual Desire Discrepancy: 'Charlie and Robert'

Robert complained that Charlie didn't want sex with him. Charlie was irritated by how Robert kept pestering him for sex. Charlie believed they had 'enough sex' and thought Robert was 'too sexual'; Robert thought Charlie hardly wanted sex and felt unimportant. Finding themselves in headlock, they both battled with this issue for over a year. They blindly carried on and further arguments ensued as a result.

The therapist (he/him) noticed they were both eloquent enough to express their needs, so he wondered if their communication problem was not the one on the surface but the implicit one. The therapist was curious about the meanings they each assigned to sex, intimacy, and relationships. Robert was the one bringing the complaint and Charlie was the one reacting to it. The therapist decided to start the conversation with Robert. He invited Robert to delve towards the layers underneath the surface, asking him to explain to Charlie what was so important about seeing and hearing Charlie wanting to have sex with him. Robert explained his meaning of sex was about intimacy and safety, which led him to connect with past emotional pain. As a young boy, Robert was the victim of severe homophobic bullying at school only to come home to a homophobic family. For much of his childhood, he needed to hide and edit himself in order to survive the inhospitable environment. As a result, he carried a core belief of '*I'm unlovable*'. Although he knew that Charlie loved him, his deep internal wounds made him doubt it. Robert's consistent demand for sex was his way to seek reassurance that Charlie loved him because, for Robert, connecting sexually with another man was his antidote to his own homophobic trauma, therefore his consistent demand for sex with Charlie was to seek reassurance Charlie loved him and he was loveable. When Charlie was able to hear Robert's vulnerability and the deep-seated meaning behind Robert's requests for sex, he was able to transmute his irritation to a more empathetic response. '*When Robert asks for sex, he is wanting to heal from his homophobic trauma*'.

The therapist then turned his attention to Charlie, asking him to explain to Robert what was underneath his reaction of being annoyed by his demand for sex. Charlie explained he thought his sex life with Robert was good but because Robert wanted more than Charlie could give, he translated it as '*I'm not good enough for Robert*'. The therapist asked Charlie if the thought '*I'm not good enough*' was a familiar terrain for him. With tears, Charlie nodded. It reminded him of painful childhood memories. He recounted his father clearly preferring the company of his straight brother because he liked playing football and how he perceived Charlie as the 'odd son' because he didn't like football. Charlie never felt good enough to meet his father's expectations. When Robert heard the vulnerability behind Charlie's irritation, he understood more. When Robert asked for sex, it reminded Charlie of his father's conditional love.

It now made more sense to them why they'd both been in head-lock. Their emotional worlds were never seen by each other before. They realised in their own way that they were both wounded by the homophobic events of their past, and that they were both subconsciously asking the other to heal those wounds (Hendrix, 2001). With their new understanding of each other's inner worlds, Charlie and Robert learnt their sexual desire discrepancy was not a personal attack on each other but more an invitation for a deeper connection. Charlie became more conscious to use a sexual language with Robert, swapping words like "*you look good in those jeans*" with "*you look sexy in those jeans*". Changing one word transformed the whole sentence and energy that came with it. Deep down, it was all Robert needed to hear when Charlie was not ready for sex. Robert was now able to alter his language too, making softer requests for sex rather than demands, which made the space warmer for Charlie to engage in. This actually increased Charlie's desire to have sex with Robert.

Anodyspareunia (Pain During Receptive Anal Sex): 'Philip and Peter'

Philip and Peter had been together for 5 years and struggled with sex throughout their relationship. Although they enjoyed oral sex with each other they were unable to have anal sex because Peter felt pain during intercourse. Philip identified as 'top', for him anal penetration played an important part of sexual satisfaction, he felt oral sex was only a 'second best'. Peter described himself as 'versatile', he'd always had painful anal sex and wanted to resolve this issue. Peter also experienced sexual anxiety because he was aware that Philip was disappointed by his 'problem'. It had become such a distressing issue, they considered separation.

A study by Damon and Simon Rosser (2005) finds:

> Men with anodyspareunia reported that psychological factors were the primary contributing cause of their pain. The findings contradict the myth that pain is a necessary consequence of receptive anal sex and show that anodyspareunia is similar to dyspareunia in women in terms

of prevalence, mental health consequences, and contributing factors. (p. 129)

Moreover, Grabski and Kasparek (2020) assert that "Clinicians addressing sexual anal pain should consider performance anxiety, internalized homophobia, and younger age as possible operating factors" (p. 716).

Although Philip and Peter expressed their desperation to 'fix' their problem, the therapist avoided jumping at their rescue. First, the therapist was more interested in challenging some of their ideas and meaning behind anal sex and penetration. These enquiries challenged Philip more than Peter on two levels: first, rather than a relationship issue he thought he was in couples therapy to fix Peter's problem. Second, he had to examine his thoughts around the value of penetration, which he'd not thought about before. Could it be the importance of penetration is a heteronormative value that he had somehow internalised as 'the proper way to have sex'?

Opening the erotic discussions about why penetration had become a 'gold standard' in their relationship and offering the options that non-penetrative sex can be just as valid as opposed to 'second best' was a rocky road for both of them. When the therapist sensed they were upset with him, he brought his rationale to them: the less there was pressure on penetration, the easier it might be. This is not to discount the pleasure of penetration and how some people enjoy it. This intervention is designed to take penetration off its pedestal, to create a more playful erotic space with no demands and expectations. Sex therapy is a modality which sometimes integrates 'homework' for couples (Campbell, 2020). The first 'homework' was to experiment with being pleasure-focused rather than performance-focused centred on penetration.

Having had medical examinations done, this cleared any possible organic issues of anodyspareunia. The psychological factors which maintained the problem started to change. Putting less pressure on themselves about 'doing' penetration reduced their anxiety about it. Indeed, a sexual problem is not one person's problem, it's shared between the people involved in the sexual activities. Although Peter was dealing with anodyspareunia, he responded to Philip's heightened emotions and energy about penetration, which increased his own anxiety and thoughts of defectiveness. Reversely, when Philip became more relaxed Peter responded accordingly.

During the course of therapy, the therapist suggested Peter to create 'alone time' with his anus: brushing a finger at the entrance whilst paying attention to the pleasure of it. When he felt ready, then to insert a finger gently using plenty of lubricant (Morin, 2010). Some people like to experiment with sex toys too. This 'alone time' was important for Peter to examine his own anxieties with anal sex, including the heteronormative taboo ('*sodomy is wrong*'). After a few weeks of 'alone time' with his anus, Peter felt relaxed enough to have some 'partnered time'.

With less demands and feeling comfortable about their sexual pleasure, they both became excited about re-discovering penetration. They found a new way to prepare for sex, to warm each other up and be empathically responsive to each other's bodies. There was no more pain, anodyspareunia was resolved.

Phillip and Peter's sexual problem was a reflection of the non-existent sex education on anal pleasure which was magnified by internalised homonegativity associated with it. A psychosexual treatment employing a behavioural, cognitive and gay-affirmative approach is usually successful.

Unreliable Erections: 'Alex and Ben'

Ben's unreliable erections were so frequent that it impacted on their sex lives significantly. His erection problems started three months after they first met, Alex was worried it might be because Ben didn't find him attractive enough.

The therapist was curious about what happened in the first three months into their relationship. When he asked questions, a heavy silence settled in. When Ben and Alex met, it was instant sexual chemistry and they had great sex. After three months, the relationship deepened, and at that point Ben disclosed to Alex that he was HIV-positive and undetectable. Alex, who is HIV-negative, took great offence at the delay of the disclosure. Ben didn't feel it was important to disclose since he was undetectable. Alex, on the other hand felt he should have had all the facts in order to make an informed choice about having sex with Ben.

The therapist asked Alex if he would have had sex differently with Ben if he had known about his HIV status? The answer was 'no' because they had used protection anyway. Alex's answer revealed a deeper problem: if Alex had known Ben's HIV status at the beginning he would not have pursued a relationship with him. It became apparent not only did Alex feel righteous for being 'duped' by Ben, he also felt uncomfortable admitting his judgmental thoughts about HIV. Ben felt anger towards Alex and his perceived narrow mindedness, this re-opened Ben's internal wounds and negative thoughts of 'not good enough' and 'damaged goods'.

For Ben, there was also a parallel story. Ten years before meeting Alex, he acquired the virus from a past boyfriend whom he was in love with. By not disclosing his HIV status, the past partner betrayed him and knowingly infected Ben in an attempt to 'own him'. This marked the end of their relationship. Witnessing Alex's reaction to his HIV disclosure, reignited the past causing him to fear he'd become like his abusive ex-boyfriend.

Since Ben's HIV-status disclosure, the unreliable erections started. This communicated there were unresolved issues around Ben's HIV status, Alex's ongoing resentment and Ben's negative thoughts about himself. Alex's disappointment in Ben's erections reinforced both the resentment and negative thoughts. Since the disclosure, they hadn't spoken much, barely at all on what this meant for each of them until now in the therapist's consulting room. They realised not talking about it didn't make the problems go away, it had the opposite effect, exasperating them.

Through guided conversations, Ben learnt that behind Alex's judgmental ideas about HIV was fear. Alex was young when the AIDS epidemic hit Britain in the 80's, nevertheless he remembered his parents sending a consistent message to him that sex was dangerous. When he came out his mother panicked and told him that 'wanting to be gay was a death sentence'. Alex realised he'd made all his sexual decisions based on his mother's fear. He admitted choosing partners who looked 'clean' and behaved well.

Listening to Ben's story, Alex learnt he had been the victim of an abusive ex-partner and was wounded by homophobia in his childhood. Both his parents punished him for being 'too sensitive like a girl'. He felt 'abnormal' as a child, a feeling that persisted in his adult life. Ben explained hearing Alex say he wouldn't have chosen to be with him if he'd known about his HIV-positive status, reinforced that painful core belief.

In therapy, Ben and Alex could hear that behind their conflicts was emotional pain and fear. With increased empathy towards each other, their relationship which previously felt icy became warmer. They both understood now that Ben's unreliable erections were not his sole problem but a relationship problem.

Once the resentment was cleared, Sensate Focus exercises could begin. The Sensate Focus process is a typical and effective psychosexual intervention (Singer Kaplan, 1974). By guiding the couple in a slow process of re-discovering their bodies, it's a programme designed to reduce anxiety around sexual functioning and erections. It centres on sexual pleasure without the pressure of 'performance' or anxiety of 'success'. However, it's important to adapt it to suit the couple's presentations. Nichols (2021) reminds us that although presentations of couple difficulties are similar across all sexual orientations, there are some specific factors that need to be considered when working with gay male couples.

> You need to understand that the men probably treat each other as equals in day-to-day live, no matter what their roles in the bedroom. You must appreciate the role of sexuality in the gay male ethos, and understand something about consensual nonmonogamy and BDSM. It is helpful to gain some knowledge of HIV, PrEP, and the medications used to keep the virus under control, and you will need to find out how HIV has impacted your gay male clients. (p. 113)

The typical Sensate Focus process comprises five phases: (1) sensual touch without touching erogenous zones, (2) sensual touch including erogenous zones, (3) moving sensual touch to sexual touch, including sexual arousal and perhaps mutual masturbation, (4) introducing 'play' and 'experimenting', (5) 'containment' which means penetration (for gay men who don't want penetration the 'containment' may be oral sex).

In phase one, Alex and Ben reconnected with each other through eye contact which brought tears because they missed the meaningful connection they had experienced when they first met. Alex and Ben also reconnected with their eroticism but without the pressure of 'performance'.

In Phase two, they both noticed anxiety-provoking thoughts like: '*is my penis big enough?*', '*does my partner like my body?*', '*what does my partner think of me?*'. In the therapy session, the therapist guided them to discuss all of these anxieties: asking the questions to their partner, seeking clarification and reassurance.

In Phase three, Alex and Ben learnt each to take responsibility for their own arousal (pleasure and erections). This can be a tricky process because many couples can hold myths their arousal depends on their partner. Paradoxically, the less focused they were on erections, the easier they happened. Gay male couples might sometimes compare each other's erections. Alex's erections occurred much quicker than Ben's erections, which produced a return of anxiety for him ('*I'm not fixed yet*'). Alex assigned meaning on Ben's erections not being so quick ('*Doesn't he like what we're doing?*'), which was addressed in the therapy session, informing the couple that it was 'normal' for erections to be different and to come at different times.

In Phase four, Ben and Alex learnt to celebrate their eroticism in the here-and-now rather than focusing on the problems that occurred in the past.

In Phase five, penetration remained daunting for Ben so the therapist suggested they might want to try 'containment' with oral sex. Ben was anxious to have his penis in Alex's mouth because of the fear of losing his erection. When they discussed the fear in their therapy session, it was an opportunity for Alex to reassure Ben that even if his penis became soft, they could still 'play' and have a 'good quality sexy time'. This reduced Ben's anxiety enough to make oral sex enjoyable. In fact, they decided to go past containment and have oral sex until ejaculation. Ben was shocked Alex wanted to swallow his semen. In their next therapy session, Alex discussed it was important for him to show Ben he no longer had anxiety about Ben's HIV status, he learnt he was safe with Ben, having challenged his judgmental thoughts. It was an immense pivotal and reparative moment for both Ben and Alex.

Working with Lesbian Couples and Intimate Relationships

The body of research on female same-gender sexuality is largely under-represented in comparison to what is available on gay men. Integrating contemporary voices in the field will best prepare clinicians on how to conduct effective therapy sessions when working with lesbian couples.

Walby (1990) argues that heterosexuality presents as a patriarchal institution for men to dominate and oppress women by silencing female sexual desires. Simply existing as a woman within a societal system influenced by hegemonic patriarchal structures of heteronormativity and cisnormativity requires lesbian couples to continuously consider the degree to which they will be open (or out) about their relationship with others.

Sexless Relationship: 'Grace and Emma'

Grace and Emma came to therapy because they were no longer having sex. They feared they fell in the stereotype category of the ghastly term 'lesbian bed death'. This is a term that assumes the narrative that when women commit to a romantic relationship they automatically stop wanting to have sex with each other, which erases same-sex female sexuality. The therapist (she/her) asked couples to tell their story of how their relationship began. It has the dual purpose of both understanding their journey that led them to therapy and also to remind them of the initial romantic and sexual desires that they might have forgotten.

Grace was in an unhappy relationship when she met Emma. Spending time with her was exciting. They first connected on Instagram, via direct messaging they engaged in thrilling conversations before deciding to meet each other. Their encounters were always secret liaisons, happening only behind closed doors. Their passion was ignited in the forbidden. Perel (2006) discusses how the illicit is a potent source for the erotic. Their most erotic times with one another were spent in hotel rooms away from the rest of the world. They were a team in creating their own havens. They spoke of the longing and anticipation they felt planning for their next encounters. Both choosing their outfits carefully and sending pictures to tease the other. There was a lot of erotic play at the beginning of their relationship. As they both recounted their stories in the therapy room, there was a sense of erotic aliveness. Morin (1995) writes that longing and anticipation are some of the cornerstones of eroticism. Together they enjoyed experimenting with sexual practices they hadn't dared to explore before. Grace discovered she had a 'sub' (submissive) side and liked Emma to take charge. Sex was orgasmic for both of them. An echo of such eroticism resurfaced briefly in therapy as they told their story, but it was accompanied by sadness at the loss of it.

When Grace decided to leave her partner, they decided to move in together because they were in love, it was during the COVID-19 pandemic, and it made better financial sense. Their focus quickly shifted on making a home together, working hard to develop their careers and they threw themselves in the mundane 'functional' tasks of life. Gradually, their sex life became undernourished which they both perceived as a failure. Emma's erotic role of 'dom' (dominant) turned into resentment for being the only one initiating sex, and Grace's penchant for being 'sub' became the 'autopilot'. For both of them, sex descended into a repetitive and boring chore, it was no longer orgasmic.

As the therapy progressed, both Emma and Grace shared with each other why their sexless relationship felt so painful. Emma was a black woman who grew up in a local area where there were frequent racial attacks. When she was young, her older brother came out as gay and was rejected by the family. Because of these two crucial elements, Emma was good at hiding in order to survive her childhood. For Emma, being in charge and being a 'dom' was one way she could take her power back to embrace her sexuality fully and be seen. She described feeling like she mattered in that role, but it came at the cost of feeling like she was 'dragging' Grace into sexual play. She perceived Grace as being less and less willing, which then reinforced her childhood fear of not being accepted.

Grace grew up in a white middle-class family. Both her parents were doctors and they expected her to excel in medicine too. Grace was sent to boarding school when she was 7 years old, which was a serious attachment rupture for her. Although Grace was a high achiever academically, she enjoyed playing sports more. She had felt othered by her peers because she wasn't the 'typical girl'. At her parent's dismay, Grace later dropped out of medical school to pursue her passion in fitness as a personal trainer. Grace described having a submissive erotic orientation for as long as she can remember, but she never felt safe enough to explore it until she met Emma. When Grace came out to her parents, they perceived it as yet another disappointment. When they met Emma, they were also covertly disappointed that she'd chosen a black person. Emma was never referred to as Grace's partner, only 'a good friend'.

Grace and Emma held intersecting identities, Nichols (2021) assert that many WSW relationships are multi-ethnic, nearly double the rate of heterosexual relationships. It is crucial for clinicians to use an intersectional lens with working with WSW couples. Intersectionality can be applied as a prism to see the way in which various forms of inequality often operate together and exacerbate each other. This approach helps to explore the ways that race, ethnicity, gender, sexuality, class, religion, ability, and other experiences can overlap to form unique identities and oppressions that can impact the relationship (Parks et al., 2004). See Chapter 6 for further discussion about sexual diversity and intersecting minority ethnic identities.

In therapy, both Grace and Emma realised that they bypassed their early stages of seduction, from a secret affair in hotel rooms to a committed home life. Grace's family erasing her sexuality and Emma's not feeling safe to come out to hers meant they shared the emotional turmoil of being isolated. Their sense of belonging was reliant on the other, compounded by the fact neither of them had made mutual friends outside of the relationship. Community is a great need for lesbians where they can best locate supportive networks and for connecting with others with similar experiences especially for LGBTQIA+ people (Carastathis et al., 2017). Enquiring further into their relationship, outside of the roles they played in the household both Grace and Emma had not created any time to be with the other. Indeed, there was no more play of any kind.

In the therapy sessions the therapist explored with Grace and Emma the dreaded stereotype of 'bed death' and how this idea had been ingrained by a society who failed to recognise lesbian relationships as sexual ones. The therapist reminded each of them that neither society nor their families had given them the possibility of thinking that a same-sex relationship could be successful. Grace and Emma were both constantly exposed to minority stress: questions around getting married to men, micro-invalidations at work and exclusions within their family. However, the therapist informed them that according to Blair et al. (2018) women in same-sex relationships reported more frequent orgasms resulting from their partners' stimulation of their clitoris and from oral sex than women in heterosexual relationships. This was an important information to counter the 'bed death' myth.

Lesbian and bisexual women experience greater prevalence of generalized anxiety compared to their heterosexual counterparts (Cochran et al., 2003). The therapist suggested to both Grace and Emma to create more time for themselves every day for their own personal self-care rather than relying on the other for it. They experimented with various methods such as breathing exercises and mindfulness, to help regulate their emotions. They also explored pursuing personal hobbies and activities to increase their sense of independence whilst regrouping together meeting at locations outside of the home to encourage a new sense of curiosity about the other.

It was reassuring for Grace and Emma (as well as many couples) to know that experiencing fluctuations or ebbs and flow in sexual desire is a normative feature of relationships rather than defective. When Grace and Emma were ready to talk about sex, the therapist offered a discussion on the binary thinking of 'all or nothing sex script': either it had to be perfect, connected and orgasmic, or it was a failure. Inviting the couple to veer towards a middle ground of pleasure, it was encouraging for both of them to give up the goal of orgasm. Embracing a new fluidity of eroticism gave them the freedom to enter into a new play state, different from the one they had enjoyed when they first met. Collaboratively, the therapist and the couple came up with creative ideas to develop new ways of individualisation, prioritising a space of curiosity about the other. This fostered a sense that even though they lived together, they had yet to discover more things about each other.

The therapist equipped them with new knowledge: both 'spontaneous' and 'responsive' desire works (Nagoski, 2015), and the conditions for 'good sex' proposed by Gurney (2020): Psychological arousal, physical touch and being in the moment. Grace and Emma were able to become a team again. This time rather than plan illicit encounters in hotel rooms, they were invited to create what Iasenza (2020) calls their own '*Sexual Menu*'. By positively communicating what they both liked, wanted and needed, this took away the pressure on specific physical acts. This gave them room to enjoy walks in the parks whilst holding hands, simultaneously gifting them on how to communicate to one another about their desires to re-enter in the consensual play of dom/sub in a more authentic way.

Sex After Trauma: 'Cass and Gill'

The Office for National Statistics reports that 618,000 women were sexually assaulted in one year: "Of sexual offences recorded by the police in the year ending March 2020, the victim was female in 84% of cases" (ons.gov.uk). Unfortunately, it is common for psychosexual therapists to see female clients complaining about sexual problems which have roots in past sexual trauma.

Cass and Gill had been in a relationship with each other for ten years. They described their relationship as 'happy' but they struggled with their sex life for the duration of their relationship. Cass didn't like to be touched and pushed Gill away each time she tried to come close. Although Cass liked being hugged, she feared that a hug could be an invitation for sex so she avoided all physical closeness. Gill was understanding but over time the physical distance created an emotional one.

Cass was raped by a group of young men when she was sixteen. It was her first sexual experience. She blamed herself for it because she was drunk at the time. Those young men were peers at high school, they spread rumours that she was 'a slut'. Cass never reported the assault because of shame. After that, she hadn't had sex until she met her first girlfriend whom she fell in love with. This is when she noticed that she had some post-traumatic stress symptoms. Her body would go into a 'freeze' state each time her girlfriend tried to touch her. Occasionally, she would have a flashback (vivid memories of the young men raping her) as though it was happening in the here-and-now, which was very distressing. Her girlfriend wasn't sympathetic and called her 'weird' then broke up with her. Cass was devastated and she believed she was 'broken'.

When she met Gill, she was honest about her sexual problems. Gill reassured her that they could work something out. Unfortunately, after ten years, they realised they didn't manage to improve their sex life. Now, as an adult, she consciously understood that what had happened to her was wrong and it was not her fault but her body continued to react with post-trauma stress symptoms. Van Der Kolk (2014) informs us that although we might intellectually understand what had happened, it is not sufficient to resolve trauma because it is often a somatic response rather than an intellectual one.

One of the important considerations for therapists working with traumatised clients is not to re-traumatise them by moving therapy too fast. Although they were both desperate to have a sex life together, pacing them was key. Rothschild (2021) tells us to *'put on the brake'* and taking plenty of time helping clients learn emotional regulation skills before discussing trauma. In order to help Cass feel safer with her body, she needed to understand that she had control with consent in the here-and-now.

The therapist proposed Betty Martin's (n.d.) Wheel of Consent exercises. They are gentle short exercises helping couples to experiment with *'taking'*, *'allowing'*, *'giving'* and *'receiving'*, and most importantly done with explicit language of the intentions before actions. This helped Cass regulate her nervous system to a calmer state as she had a controlled experience of Gill's good intentional and careful touch. Over time, she was able to tolerate a longer hug from Gill, with the explicit invitation that the hug was not going to be an invitation for sex.

Later, the therapist suggested that they could try a hug lying in bed. Cass was reluctant at first because the flashback of the abusers usually happened when she was in a lying position. The therapist asked her if there was a particular lying position she would feel more comfortable with. She identified she didn't like lying on her back but she might be fine on her side. When she was ready, she tried it and it was successful. The same exercise was repeated accompanied with a kiss. Over time, slowly, Cass could feel that her body became more relaxed, she could breathe more deeply and there was no more flashbacks or freeze, but it wasn't the end.

Cass and Gill never had the chance to explore a sex life together because the trauma got in the way, but now that there was more space, the therapist proposed that they could slowly invite eroticism into their space. First, they agreed that they would read an erotica story to each other. This was successful in awakening their mutual eroticism. They then felt comfortable moving on with sharing one of their sexual fantasies. When the space between them was warmer, the next step was to enter a gentle version of Sensate Focus (without the 'containment'/penetration phase as neither of them were interested in it), but focused on the various ways to massage and stimulate their clitorises. With patience, love and perseverance, they eventually discovered a satisfying sex life together which flourished and thrived over time.

Conclusion

Clinicians working with intimate relationships of the GSRD populations need to adopt a pluralistic view of psychotherapeutic practices because each individual in the relationship may bring a complex intersection of psychological, psychosexual, relational and emotional elements which often shapes the unique landscape of the relational space between them. Utilising the common theories and interventions from the psychosexual and relationship field, trauma therapy and general psychotherapy framed with a robust knowledge of GSRD-specific knowledge, such as minority stress, intra-community minority stress, micro-aggression, intersectionality, the impact of heteronormativity, societal oppression and strengths-focused affirmative practices, will equip clinicians well to help LGBTQIA+ people struggling with their intimate relationships. As we all know, what works for some people doesn't work for others. Rather than being solely dependent on what 'should work', practicing curiosity and irreverence with all clients, as Iantaffi (2020) highlights, can gift therapists more diversified ways of thinking. Remaining more connected to a clients' subjective experiences, therapists can forge stronger therapeutic alliances as a result.

References

Beaber, T. E., & Werner, P. D. (2009). The relationship between anxiety and sexual functioning in lesbians and heterosexual women. *Journal of Homosexuality, 56*(5), 639–654. https://doi.org/10.1080/00918360903005303. PMID: 19591037.

Blair, et al. (2018). Not all orgasms were created equal: Differences in frequency and satisfaction of orgasm experiences by sexual activity in same-sex versus mixed-sex relationships. *The Journal of Sex Research, 55*(6), 719–733. https://doi.org/10.1080/00224499.2017.1303437

Bowlby, J. (1969). *Attachment and loss, Volume 1: Attachment.* Pimlico.

Bowlby, J. (1973). *Attachment and loss, Volume 2: Separation.* Pimlico.

Bowlby, J. (1980). *Attachment and loss, Volume 3. Loss.* Pimlico.

Campbell, C. (2020). *Contemporary sex therapy: Skills in managing sexual problems.* Routledge.

Carastathis, G., Cohen, L., Kaczmarek, E., & Chang, P. (2017). Rejected by family for being Gay or Lesbian: Portrayals, perceptions, and resilience. *Journal of Homosexuality, 64*(3), 289–320.

Cochran, et al. (2003). Prevalence of mental disorders, psychological distress, and mental health services use among lesbian, gay, and bisexual adults in the United States. *Journal of Consulting and Clinical Psychology, 71*(1), 53–61. https://doi.org/10.1037/0022-006X.71.1.53

Damon, W., & Simon Rosser, B. R. (2005). Anodyspareunia in men who have sex with men. *Journal of Sex & Marital Therapy, 31*(2), 129–141. https://doi.org/10.1080/00926230590477989

Diamond, L. M. (2017). Three critical questions for future research on lesbian relationships. *Journal of Lesbian Studies, 21*(1), 106–119. https://doi.org/10.1080/10894160.2016.1143756

Fern, J. (2020). *Polysecure: Attachment, trauma and consensual nonmonogamy.* Thorntree Press.

Frost, D. M., Fingerhut, A. W., & Meyer, I. H. (2022). Social change and relationship quality among sexual minority individuals: Does minority stress still matter? *Journal of Marriage and Family, 84*(3), 920–933. https://doi.org/10.1111/jomf.12827

Grabski, B., & Kasparek, K. (2020). Sexual anal pain in gay and bisexual men: In search of explanatory factors. *The Journal of Sexual Medicine, 17*(4), 716–730. https://doi.org/10.1016/j.jsxm.2020.01.020

Gurney, K. (2020). *Mind the gap: The truth about desire and how to futureproof your sex life.* Headline Publishing Group.

Hendrix, H. (2001). *Getting the love you want: A guide for couples.* Pocket Books.

Iantaffi, A. (2020). *Gender trauma.* Jessica Kingsley.

Iasenza, S. (2020). *Transforming sexual narratives: A relational approach to sex therapy.* Routledge.

Igartua, K., Thombs, B. D., Burgos, G., & Montoro, R. (2009). Concordance and discrepancy in sexual identity, attraction, and behavior among adolescents. *Journal of Adolescent Health, 45*, 602–608.

Kinsey, A. C. (1948/1998). *Sexual behavior in the human male.* Indiana University Press.

Martin, B. (n.d.). *Wheel of consent.* https://bettymartin.org

Meyer, I. H. (2003). Prejudice, social stress, and mental health in lesbian, gay, and bisexual populations: Conceptual issues and research evidence. *Psychological Bulletin, 129*(5), 674. https://doi.org/10.1037/0033-2909.129.5.674

Morin, J. (1995). *The erotic mind.* HarperCollins.

Morin, J. (2010). *Anal pleasure & health: A guide for men, women, and couples* (4th revised ed.). Down There Press.

Nagoski, E. (2015). *Come as you are: The surprising new science that will transform your sex life.* Simon & Schuster.

Nelson, T. (2020). *Integrative sex & couples therapy: A therapist's guide to new and innovative approaches.* PESI Publishing & Media.

Nichols, M. (2021). *The modern clinician's guide to working with LGBTQ+ clients: The inclusive psychotherapist.* Routledge.

Office of National Statistics. *Sexual offence.* https://www.ons.gov.uk/peoplepopulationandcommunity/crimeandjustice/articles/sexualoffencesvictimcharacteristicsenglandandwales/latest

Pachankis, J. E., Clark, K. A., Burton, C. L., Hughto, J., Bränström, R., & Keene, D. E. (2020). Sex, status, competition, and exclusion: Intraminority stress from within the gay community and gay and bisexual men's mental health. *Journal of Personality and Social Psychology, 119*(3), 713–740.

Parks, et al. (2004). Race/ethnicity and sexual orientation: Intersecting identities. *Cultural Diversity and Ethnic Minority Psychology, 10*(3), 241–254. https://doi.org/10.1037/1099-9809.10.3.241

Perel, E. (2006). *Mating in captivity: Unlocking erotic intelligence.* Harper-Collins.

Richards, C., & Barker, M. (2013). *Sexuality and gender for mental health professionals: A practical guide.* Sage.

Rothschild, B. (2021). *Revolutionizing trauma treatment: Stabilization, safety & nervous system balance.* Norton.

Sarno, E. L., & Mohr, J. J. (2020). Partner attractiveness and perceived sexually transmitted infection risk among sexual minority men. *The Journal of Sex Research, 57*(5), 559–569. https://doi.org/10.1080/00224499.2019.159 1335

Savage, D. (2005). *The commitment.* Penguin Group.

Shahbaz, C., & Chirinos, P. (2017). *Becoming a kink aware therapist.* Routledge.

Singer Kaplan, H. (1974). *The new sex therapy: Active treatment of sexual dysfunctions.* Brunner/Mazel, Inc.

Skinta, M. D. (2021). *Contextual behavior therapy for sexual and gender minority clients: A practical guide to treatment.* Routledge.

Sprott, R. A., & Williams, D. J. (2019). Is BDSM a sexual orientation or serious leisure? *Current sexual health reports.* Springer.

Van Der Kolk, B. (2014). *The body keeps the score.* Allen Lane. Penguin Books.

Walby, S. (1990). *Theorizing patriarchy.* Basil Blackwell.

Watts-Jones, D. (2010). Location of self: Opening the door to dialogue on intersectionality in the therapy process. *Family Process, 49*, 405–420. https://doi.org/10.1111/j.1545-5300.2010.01330.x

15

Addressing Substance Abuse

Michael Rolt and Alexander Margetts

Introduction

In this chapter, we explore the use of substances amongst sexual minorities and the interplay with their mental health for those for whom it becomes problematic. After considering the nomenclature and prevalence of such use, and possible influences within this, we discuss the importance of culturally sensitive practice and specific therapeutic and ethical considerations we must take within this work.

M. Rolt
Royal Holloway, University of London, London, UK

A. Margetts (✉)
University of Leicester, Leicester, UK
e-mail: am1131@le.ac.uk

© The Author(s), under exclusive license to Springer Nature   **359**
Switzerland AG 2023
J. Semlyen and P. Rohleder (eds.), *Sexual Minorities and Mental Health*,
https://doi.org/10.1007/978-3-031-37438-8_15

Defining Substance Abuse

Drug use encompasses an increasingly broad range of substances (European Monitoring Centre for Drugs & Drug Addiction, 2018). Whilst there has been a 20-year downward trend in the consumption of legal drugs such as alcohol and tobacco, a growing proportion of people consume illicit drugs (Seitz et al., 2019). In the UK, there were 275,896 adults in contact with drug and alcohol services between April 2020 and March 2021, a small rise compared to the previous year (270,705), and in the context of the Covid-19 pandemic (Office for Health Improvement & Disparities, 2021).

The legal status of a drug does not necessarily directly correspond to the potential harms of the drug (Nutt et al., 2010), and, as a social construct, legality can vary between and even within countries. However, legality does impact the societal and political responses to illicit drug use. There is a complex interplay between stigma, discrimination, criminalisation and healthcare provision (Global Commission on Drug Policy, 2017), with negative social and political representations of illicit drug users directly influencing clinical care (Schlag, 2020); research indicates that users of illegal drugs (c.f. legal) have fewer harm reduction and intervention opportunities made available to them (Schlag, 2020).

Patterns of substance use exist on a continuum from non-problematic to problematic (Global Commission on Drug Policy, 2017). Non-problematic substance use is defined as taking a substance for its intended purpose, including legal or illegal substances. This use could be under medical direction (e.g. for pain control) or taken recreationally for desired biopsychosocial effects (e.g. relaxation) with limited adverse consequences. Of those who consume illicit drugs, only a minority of people misuse them or use them in a problematic manner (Schlag, 2020). However, media representations of substance use are often sensationalist and damaging, focusing on the negative impact of problematic engagement (Aldridge, 2020). This has had the effect of creating 'moral panic' (the problematising of all substance use regardless of the level of consumption, Santoro et al., 2020), pathologising all users. For already stigmatised sexual minorities this complicates the development of appropriate public health responses (Pienaar et al., 2018).

Thus, whilst it is common to view the substance use experience through a lens of health risks to inform health care planning, it is important to note that many within the sexual minority community rarely see themselves as having difficulties with drugs. For example, many men who have sex with men (MSM) who engage with sexualised drug sex ('chemsex', see below) do not consider themselves drug users or relate to other drug users' experiences (Evans, 2019). The majority of MSM feel in control of their chemsex engagement and derive pleasure from it with few negative consequences (Platteau et al., 2019). However, substance use can become problematic, although this is not consistently defined, and the mechanisms for change are currently unknown (Platteau et al., 2019).

Problematic use is loosely defined as when individuals experience one or more unwanted outcomes (Platteau et al., 2020). A continuum approach to substance use suggests that there may be opportunities to support people at earlier stages of drug use to prevent or reduce problems at later stages. If a substance *is* used problematically, there is an increased risk that it may cause long-term physical and mental health difficulties for the user (Global Commission on Drug Policy, 2017). So how might those who need it get help and support?

A problem facing substance use services is that drug use is a complex and often relapsing, chronic condition (West & Brown, 2013). It requires multi-faceted and coordinated care and intervention approaches, needing co-operation between the criminal justice, social care, physical and mental health services. However, commissioning and delivering targeted and relevant services is challenging as the landscape of substance use is continuously changing. There are also many barriers to individuals accessing services. Whilst this includes users de-prioritising their own medical care (e.g. preferring to ignore the problem, or not perceiving the harms to warrant intervention), for those who do seek support they may fear, and in some cases sadly encounter, negative judgment from clinicians (Miller-Lloyd et al., 2020).

Researchers investigating the development of harm reduction interventions for individuals with substance misuse difficulties are also met with barriers. Substance users, problematic or otherwise, are generally under-represented in surveys, especially those with intensive use patterns

(Seitz et al., 2019). Researchers must also navigate the complex and changing political and social context in which their work is conducted (United Nations Office on Drugs and Crime [UNODC], 2019). Also, recent research suggests that the type of substance being used is an important factor to consider in providing interventions. For example, predictors of craving have been shown to vary significantly between alcohol, tobacco and illicit drugs (Enkema et al., 2020), potentially impacting relapse prevention support. With the broadening landscape of substances being used, research needs to keep pace with the proliferation of novel drugs and new polysubstance use combinations.

Chemsex

Sexualised drug use (SDU) refers to drug use before or during sex to enhance and prolong the sexual experience (Rosińska et al., 2018). A subset of SDU, 'chemsex', is a relatively recent phenomenon (e.g. Stuart, 2013) and is considered distinct from traditional sexual and substance misuse difficulties due to the drugs' specificity and the context of its use. There is no global consensus on the definition of chemsex (Torres et al., 2020), as it is subject to the availability of illicit drugs among subcultures within countries (Maxwell et al., 2019). In the UK, the drugs most commonly associated with chemsex are methamphetamine (crystal meth), gamma-hydroxybutyric acid (GHB) and methylmeth-cathinone (mephedrone) (Bourne et al., 2014). The drugs, often taken in combination, facilitate the sexual experience by increasing arousal and lowering inhibitions whilst inducing an immediate sense of connection and intimacy with sexual partners (Smith & Tasker, 2018). Chemsex events, also known as "chill out parties", may last several days involving multiple partners (Platteau et al., 2020).

Unintended consequences and harms of problematic use varies by substance and user, but can include agitation, anxiety, paranoia, aggression, and psychoses. If use is pronounced and sustained, physical dependency can occur, and if dosage misjudged, unconsciousness and death. There are also notable and serious interactions that can occur with alcohol and HIV antiretroviral medications (the latter also being impacted by impaired adherence). Beyond the direct physiological impact of the substance, further behavioural harms can include increased sexual risk behaviours from hypersexuality and disinhibition, such as STI and HIV transmission, sexual regret, genital trauma and sexual assault (Ma & Perera, 2016).

Chemsex is predominately associated with men who have sex with men (MSM). In the UK, chemsex amongst MSM is more prevalent than in the general population, with research suggesting that 6.6% of MSM in England had engaged in chemsex in the last four weeks, rising to 21.9% for those living with HIV (Bourne et al., 2014). However, as with other substance use, media representations of chemsex are often sensationalist and damaging, focusing on the negative impact of problematic chemsex engagement among MSM (Aldridge, 2020).

Many MSM who engage in chemsex consider sober sexual intimacy to be 'normal' or more authentic (Aldridge, 2020) and often report dissatisfaction with their reliance on drugs to enjoy sex. Individuals are increasingly seeking support to re-engage in 'sober sex', whereby they be 'present' during sex without drugs being involved, and the connection between body and mind is maintained. Relapse is common (Kunelaki, 2019) with the prevalence of chemsex among MSM, and the heightened pleasures associated with it, meaning that sexualised drug use can be challenging to disengage from (Moncrief, 2014).

There is no sophisticated understanding of the prevalence of drivers for chemsex (ACON, 2013). NHS Trusts do not consistently collect chemsex prevalence data among MSM in any UK national surveillance systems, with most available data being almost exclusively sourced from sexual health and drug clinics in metropolitan areas (Edmundson et al., 2018). Qualitative evidence consistently suggests that MSM engaged in chemsex initially access services when there is an urgent sexual health need, such as testing for sexually transmitted infections (STI) or post-exposure prophylaxis (PEP) following potential exposure to HIV. Most MSM engaged in chemsex do not initially seek support for drug-related difficulties (Hegazi et al., 2017). Some anecdotal reports indicate that engagement in chemsex, alongside an increasing demand for help, is becoming more common across the UK, resulting in calls for a national targeted sexual health response (Moncrief, 2014).

Unfortunately there is a lack of evidence about good practice in drug treatment for MSM service users, with limited studies measuring outcomes or evaluating service use by sexual orientation or gender identity (Williams et al., 2010). Part of the challenge of understanding chemsex use and ultimately developing treatments is that illicit drug users are often labelled as "hard-to-reach" populations, impacting recruitment into research studies (Cave et al., 2009). Such language however places blame and responsibility upon the users, rather than clinicians and researchers, with innovation and paradigm shift being required.

Without specific theory-driven or data-driven interventions for chemsex, many services support those seeking treatment by employing traditional substance misuse interventions to address substance use and sexual risk jointly (e.g., motivational interviewing and brief short-term structured behavioural change interventions; Moncrief, 2014). Some third-sector organisations also offer group psychosocial treatments such as mindfulness interventions (e.g., 'Spectra', Hoff et al., 2020).

It should be noted that chemsex research conducted with lesbian and bisexual women is very limited, with also almost nothing written about trans people (Abdulrahim et al., 2016). It, therefore, cannot be assumed that the already limited guidance developed from research into chemsex in MSM populations applies to these other groups. For example, research into alcohol and substance use indicates that bisexual women have higher use compared to other sexual minority women; 'binegativity' (the specific abuse, discrimination or erasure of bisexual people over and above that of lesbian/gay people, such as questioning of the legitimacy of their sexual identity) is highlighted as possible mediator (Schulz et al., 2022).

Prevalence

Chapter 2 of this book explored the prevalence of mental health problems, including addictions, in the sexual minority population. We return to look in more detail at the issue of problematic substance use here. As described in Chapter 2, illicit drug use amongst sexual minorities is more prevalent than in the general population (Medley et al., 2015, Fig. 15.1).

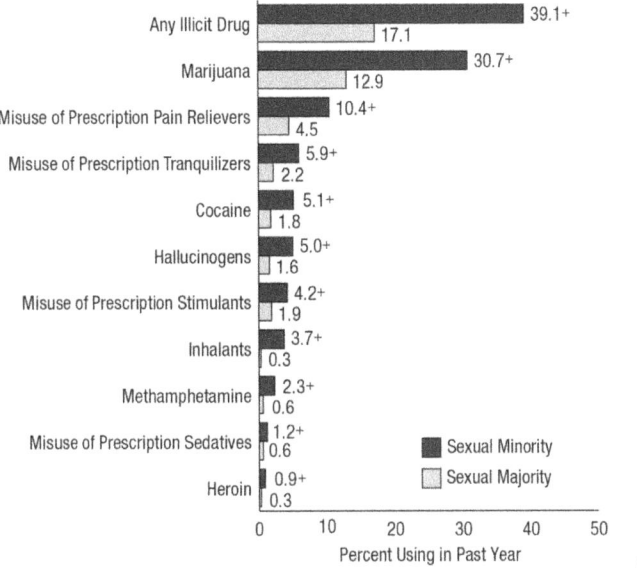

+ Difference between this estimate and the sexual majority estimate is statistically significant at the .05 level.
Note: Sexual minority adults identified as being lesbian, gay, or bisexual. Sexual majority adults identified as being heterosexual or straight.

Fig. 15.1 Past year illicit drug use among Sexual Minority and Sexual Majority adults aged 18 or older by drug type, percentages (figure reproduced with permission from the Center for Substance Abuse Treatment; available from: https://www.samhsa.gov/data/report/sexual-orientation-and-estimates-adult-substance-use-and-mental-health-results-2015-national)

The findings in illicit drug use are replicated amongst alcohol misuse also, with this being higher amongst lesbian, gay and bisexual people compared to their heterosexual counterparts (Pitman et al., 2021).

Such disparities in rates of substance use exist between sexual minority and heterosexual populations across the lifespan. Sexual minority youth report earlier initiation of substance use and increased substance use at younger ages (Corliss et al., 2010). The trajectory of substance use also appears to grow more rapidly for sexual minority youth compared with those young people who self-identify as heterosexual.

In addition to sexual minority status, research suggests a complex relationship between gender and substance usage. Historically men are much more likely than women to use illegal drugs recreationally (Becker et al.,

2017). There are likely to be many reasons for this; one being related to social roles, whereby more stigma is attached to substance usage in woman who are engaged in societally perceived 'traditional' roles (i.e., mother and caregiver; Kandall, 1999). Given those who identify as sexual minorities may be less likely to fit such heteronormative ascribed models, more specific research is required. For example lesbian women are nine times less likely to become pregnant than their heterosexual counterparts, and bisexual women twice less likely (Hodson et al., 2017).

Research suggests that whilst men are more likely to use illicit drugs, women are more likely to use prescribed drugs problematically (McCellan, 2017; Office of National Statistics [ONS], 2018). A recent study of lesbian, gay and bisexual men and women found higher rates of problematic alcohol use within these communities, compared to their heterosexual counterparts (Shahab et al., 2017). In the UK, problematic alcohol use was found to be significantly more prevalent for lesbian/gay (women: 19%; men: 30%) and bisexual participants (women: 24%; men: 24%) compared with heterosexual (women: 8%; men: 18%). Interestingly, this study's findings reported that the association of problematic alcohol use with being a sexual minority persisted after controlling for major sociodemographic confounders, but only amongst women. This suggests that there may exist specific influences that put lesbian and bisexual women at greater risk.

Being male is a significant but negative predictor of help-seeking behaviours (Gonzalez et al., 2011), with men being shown to be negatively associated with a willingness to actively seek substance use support (Sagar-Ouriaghli et al., 2019). As such, low mental health service use by males is observed across Western countries, where women are 1.6 times more likely to seek mental health treatment than men (Wang et al., 2005).Thus not only is the overall rate of illicit substance use higher in men, the length of time between first substance use and seeking treatment is longer, with men more reluctant to seek support (Elmquist et al., 2017).

Alongside higher use, it has been consistently reported that there is a greater likelihood of sexual minority adults having substance use *issues* compared with their sexual majority counterparts. This has been observed across subgroups of adults defined by sex and by age group with sexual minority adults more likely than their sexual majority counterparts to need substance use treatment (Medley et al., 2015).

Influences

Various theories have been suggested regarding the substance use disparities in sexual minorities; this chapter will focus on social influences and minority stress models.

The social environment of many sexual minority service users may facilitate the use of substances (Anderson, 2009; Hicks, 2000). Peer substance use patterns, use of substances at social gatherings, as well as attendance in "safe spaces" such as gay bars and gay clubs have historically served as social reinforcers for the use of drugs and alcohol for sexual minority individuals (Senreich, 2012). Non-heteronormative gender roles have also been suggested to be influential. For example, it has been suggested that lesbian and bisexual women are not as affected by the usual social restraints that limit the use of alcohol and drugs among heterosexual women (Senreich, 2012).

In addition to non-heteronormative social influences, many researchers have suggested that sexual minority individuals use substances to cope with 'minority stress', in this instance internalised homophobia (the discrimination faced by many sexual minorities, and the subsequent shame; Senreich, 2012). As outlined in earlier chapters, minority stress is described as the relationship between minority and dominant societal values and the conflict with the prevailing social-cultural climate experienced by minority group members (Meyer, 2003). Many sexual minority individuals internalise prevalent negative social attitudes in response to direct and implicit prejudice (Todd, 2016). Many sexual minorities develop negative feelings about themselves that originate from experiencing others as critical and rejecting. They may experience high levels of shame, a desire to escape, hide or conceal perceived deficiencies (Irons & Lad, 2014). High levels of shame are also associated with increased distress and other psychopathological symptoms (Gilbert, 1998). Young sexual minority individuals, in particular, often lack effective coping skills for such experiences, and consume alcohol and other substances in direct response to internalised homophobia (Dorn-Medeiros & Doyle, 2018).

It is also important to consider the multiple social identities of sexual minority individuals, including their membership of religious and racialised groups, which may have their own minority stress attributes (see Chapter 6). This perspective encourages practitioners to look at tensions between racialised sexual minority groups and the dominant White group culture (Brooks et al., 2009). It also acknowledges the inter-sectional tensions within sexual minority groups. However, there are few research studies exploring the experiences of racialised sexual minority service users in substance abuse programs, despite concerns about this population in the treatment literature (Senreich, 2012). Racially minori-tised sexual minority substance users are hypothesised to be using substances not only to cope with internalised homophobia but also to cope with societal racism (SAMHSA, 2001). In addition, they may face further racial discrimination from within the sexual minority community itself, whilst experiencing rejection by members of their own racialised community due to their sexual orientation (Senreich, 2012).

Intersectional approaches are based on the premise that individual identities are complex—the confluence of many personal characteris-tics. Therefore the health status of sexual minority individuals should not be examined in terms of a one-dimensional sexual minority cate-gory but must be informed by an individual's multiple identities and the simultaneous intersection of many characteristics (Institute of Medicine, 2011). The primacy of any identity characteristic cannot be assumed, and, as such, a culturally sensitive individual formulation approach is recommended.

Culturally Sensitive Practice

As noted and in keeping with their higher rate of substance use, sexual minority individuals actively seek support for substance use at higher rates than heterosexuals (Flentje et al., 2015). However, much of the support they receive is at best not culturally sensitive (Senreich, 2012), or worse deemed unsafe. Service experiences of sexual minority clients are impacted by:

(a) workforce issues, such as whether staff have sufficient knowledge and hold affirming beliefs and attitudes, and;
(b) organizational factors, such as non-heterosexist organisational climate and inclusive language (Drabble & Eliason, 2012).

In the UK, a recent survey of 108,000 LGBT individuals found that 13% of LGB people and 40% of transgender people have had negative experiences when accessing healthcare (Women & Equalities Committee, 2019). The negative experiences included staff demonstrating inappropriate curiosity, service users having their specific needs ignored, and avoiding treatment for fear of having a negative reaction. Other examples of an unsafe treatment environment includes professionals with inadequate awareness or training and service users experiencing direct homophobic comments (Smalley et al., 2018). Another issue is that many frontline staff do not consider sexual orientation or gender identity to be relevant to an individual's care (Women & Equalities Committee, 2019).

Without a feeling of safety, sexual minority individuals are less likely to fully explore some of the potentially crucial components underlying their substance use. Whilst some efforts have been made to foster cultural sensitivities in substance use services, these have largely ignored sexual minorities, or have merged the subgroups of this population, despite distinctly different needs (Drabble & Eliason, 2012; Mayer et al., 2008). When distinct psychosocial processes disadvantage a particular population, or that population experiences barriers to engaging in support, they fail to access the full benefit of the interventions (Pachankis et al., 2015).

To accommodate the distinct needs of sexual minority individuals the following ideas are proposed to tailor substance use services and interventions (McGeough, 2021):

1. *Service-level policies and procedures*
2. *Clinician cultural competence and cultural humility*
3. *Affirmation, validation, and discussion of sexual minority identities*

4. *Adaptation to interventions to incorporate minority stress risk factors*

These will now be explored below in more depth to allow reflection on our current practice and services and how these might be further enhanced. Chapter 9 presented important aspects of inclusive practice. We touch on some of these again here, in relation to thinking about substance use services.

Service-Level Policies and Procedures

Local community organisations have a responsibility to provide a safe therapeutic environment (Drabble & Eliason, 2012). Service-level policies and procedures should be adapted to recognise sexual minority clients and make them feel included and welcome and avoid reproducing the experiences of societal minority stress.

A pragmatic and meaningful engagement of 'experts by experience' (i.e. those with lived experience of the issues) is critical throughout all the processes of service development (Harm Reduction International, 2021). This begins with designing and implementation through to service evaluation. Peer involvement can help reduce known barriers to accessing services, such as shame and stigma (feared or actualised). Such discrimination is commonly experienced when service users access other services in the healthcare and social welfare system, and can contribute to an unsafe environment.

Improving the physical environment of a service can use a range of subtle approaches to affirm sexual minority identities. Waiting rooms can be made more welcoming through displaying rainbow stickers or flags, or displaying information of LGBT-specific support services (Mericle et al., 2018). To avoid risks of tokenism by such actions alone, this should be matched by the use of inclusive language in all forms of communication. For example amending all written forms and documents to make sexual minority individuals more visible and providing options to indicate their sexual identity should they choose to do so.

Individuals should also be able to designate who their family is, rather than it be presumed this is based upon biology. All staff, clinical and non-clinical, should verbalise inclusive language in every interaction with service users. Staff should ensure that their language and practice does not inadvertently exclude sexual minority service users as they may not be aware that the people they are engaging identify as a sexual minority. For example, the word 'partner' is preferred to husband/wife if the nature of the relationship to a single person is unknown. Similarly asking if the client has 'any partners' (not 'a partner') if it is not known if the client ascribes to monogamous relationships. Similar care should be taken that forms, signs, questionnaires, websites and waiting room literature reflect diversity.

Staff should be curious about, and be mindful to, use the client's preferred terminology (British Psychological Society, 2019). Clients may use many different terms to refer to their identities and practices, and staff are advised to use those that are used by clients themselves or to ask which terms are preferred. Some people choose not to use sexual minority category labels (lesbian, gay, bisexual and transgender), but may be comfortable with, for example, MSM (men who have sex with men), WSW (women who have sex with women), men loving men (Beam, 2008), or reclaimed terms like 'queer'.

A client's preferred name and pronoun should be used in person and in documentation. These may be gendered (he or she) or if the client prefers, gender-neutral (they, or the client's preferred gender-neutral term). Staff, who are comfortable doing so, can also include the choice of their own personal pronouns in communications (e.g. letters and emails). The prominence of a staff member's personal pronoun choice can help facilitate this conversation with service users about their own pronoun usage. However, it should be noted, that the declaration of personal pronouns is not neutral. The move towards declaration of pronouns presupposes that everyone "has pronouns"; which is to say that everyone has an inner gender identity, and being described by the pronouns he/him, she/her, they/them, zie/zem etc., as an expression of that identity. Some individuals choose not to associate pronouns with their lived experience as they may find themselves subject to stereotype threat.

As there are differences in sexual minority substance use practices across geographical locations (e.g., substance using venues and access to preferred substances), and access to appropriate services varies, local services should develop connections to regional and national sexual minority-specific substance use support resources (McGeough, 2021). This can include services having an awareness of, and connecting service users to, community support networks, and other substance specific clinics with specific specialisations should they not be locally available.

As social context is related to increased harmful alcohol use amongst LGBTQ+ people (Emslie et al., 2015), within this social context that there may be an opportunity to work alongside LGBTQ+ communities to begin the work of reducing alcohol and other drug-related health inequalities. A whole community approach may be of value in reducing the disproportionate alcohol and drug-related harms experienced both directly and indirectly by LGBTQ+ individuals, families, and communities. In terms of general approaches to reducing problematic drinking and substance use, these can include harm reduction poster campaigns at local LGBT venues, outreach work on the commercial gay scene, and community-led services such as alcohol-free cafes.

Clinician Cultural Competence and Cultural Humility

Sexual minority identities and practices should never be considered to be pathological, and these identities and practices should be accommodated and facilitated (British Psychological Society, 2019). The discomfort of others is an insufficient reason not to accommodate or facilitate an identity or practice. However, historically, medical and mental health services have not been so receptive, and older clients especially may have experienced discrimination, diagnostic labels and treatment that would be now rightly considered abusive and illegal, when these were categorised as 'mental illnesses' (e.g. Drescher, 2015). Research suggests that both cultural competence and cultural humility now are important in making substance use interventions more responsive to the needs of sexual minority individuals (McGeough, 2021).

'Cultural competence' involves increasing staff knowledge about the challenges sexual minority individuals commonly experience, especially issues unique to those with intersecting identities (Brooks et al., 2009).

Cultural competence also includes skilling up, and encouraging, clinicians to ask about sexual minority status during assessment in a way that facilitates a healthy and supportive dialogue (see below). This is particularly important for those individuals with high sexual minority identity salience (Pennay et al., 2018).

Whilst cultural competence is encouraged to build services that prioritise trust and establish a safe and supportive environment, clinicians themselves are encouraged to be aware of what they bring into the therapeutic space, and how this may impact the therapeutic alliance. Such 'cultural humility' is defined as an ongoing commitment to self-evaluation and self-critique, awareness of the influence of power imbalances, and developing "mutually beneficial and non-paternalistic clinical and advocacy partnerships with communities on behalf of individuals and defined populations" (Tervalon & Murray-García, 1998, p. 123).

Affirmation, Validation, and Discussion of Sexual Minority Identities

The intake and assessment of people who identify as sexual minorities who present at substance use services should occur in an affirming, non-judgmental manner (Smalley et al., 2018). In-depth assessment as well as subsequent treatment and care plans should address the following elements (adapted from Cabaj, 2014):

- *The degree and impact of internalized homophobia*
- *The stage in the coming out process and the experience of coming out*
- *Strength of support network (particularly a non-substance using one)*
- *Current relationship status and history of past relationships*
- *Relationships with family of origin as well as family of creation*
- *Degree of comfort with sexual/gender identity, and expression of sexual feelings and gender-affirming behaviours*
- *Vocational/educational/socioeconomic status*
- *Current and past health factors*
- *Current and past substance use behaviours*

Services should also be aware of an individual's desire (or lack thereof) for their sexual minority status to be known within the wider system (e.g. communication with a referrer, other healthcare practitioner, family, employer etc.).

An affirmative and validating dialogue with service users should aim to create a safe environment where they can freely discuss their experiences as sexual minority individuals, and how these experiences may have influenced their substance use. However, equally it should not be assumed that the difficulties the service users wish to discuss are associated with their sexual or gender identity. Overall, a clinician should provide a sense of acceptance and support that may provide a positive modelling experience for sexual minority clients, as opposed to the stigma they may have experienced elsewhere (see also Chapter 9).

Adaptation to Interventions to Incorporate Minority Stress Risk Factors

Recent studies have shown sexual minorities have better treatment outcomes in LGBT-adapted interventions than "traditional" (heteronormative) programs, and so culturally sensitive intervention approaches are recommended to support sexual minority individuals presenting with substance use difficulties (Pachankis & Safren, 2019). The following are an important range of minority sexuality specific facets to consider in substance use care provision:

(a) *Community Insight*

One adaptation to heteronormative practice is to support service users with identifying the source of both risk and resilience within sexual minority communities that are relevant to their recovery. Some sexual minority individuals struggle to build social relationships with other members of the community that are also consistent with their recovery. For example, LGB community involvement can revolve around social and sexual contexts in which alcohol and other substances are used (e.g.

bars, nightclubs, sex clubs) which can trigger a relapse. However, engagement in different facets of the LGB community may be a vital social resource for recovery; i.e. non-substance related LGB groups, activities and venues connected to a client's identity, values, hobbies and interests (e.g. a boardgame café queer meetup night, an MSM tennis group, an LBGT choir etc.). A critical goal of culturally informed treatment approaches is to support the sexual and gender identity development and community involvement of sexual minority service users in a way that minimises the risk of relapse. This is not to ghettoise or assume that sexual minority clients will exclusively, or at all, wish to use such spaces, but rather consider them as an option that can be sensitively explored.

(b) Sexuality Minority Specific Trauma

Sexual minority populations are more likely to experience traumatic experiences such as childhood sexual abuse, victimisation, and discrimination across the life course compared to their heterosexual peers. Current and/or past homophobia, biphobia and transphobia can serve as potent triggers for drinking and substance use, as clients seek to numb or distract from these painful experiences and their legacy. Culturally tailored treatment approaches must be trauma-informed by acknowledging these events' powerful and often enduring impact as critical triggers (including memories and images). It is often the case that sexual minority service users require referrals to trauma treatment and other mental health treatment to alleviate mental health symptoms that serve as triggers for problematic drinking and substance use.

(c) Service User Self-Disclosure

An early challenge that sexual minority service users will face is if to share their non-heterosexuality status with staff or other clients in treatment (Drabble & Eliason, 2012). This decision will often be made only if the service user feels safe to do so. Without disclosure, treatment plans may fail to consider many of the factors associated with the onset and maintenance of substance use (e.g. family and cultural pressures, internalised oppression, shame, and recent experiences of harassment from within the wider community). Although racialised sexual minorities report lower levels of "outness" compared to White peers, concerns about disclosure are salient across all racial groups (Drabble & Eliason, 2012).

(d) *Clinician Self-Disclosure*

Similarly, clinician's must navigate the usefulness of disclosure of their status, minority or otherwise. Whilst gay affirmative therapy can be provided by well-informed therapists regardless of their sexual orientation (Jeffery & Tweed, 2014), evidence suggests that matching sexual orientation when possible may be beneficial (Burckell & Goldfried, 2006). Sexual minority services users rated sexual minority clinicians, where available, as more helpful than their heterosexual counterparts. Sexual minority clinicians must negotiate the tensions between self and client welfare and do so in an ethical and therapeutically beneficial manner (for example using their own supervision to navigate any dilemmas or concerns). Within substance use there is also the consideration of self-disclosure of substance use (or lack thereof) itself. This is something for example that peer support workers may be more familiar and comfortable, or able, to do than healthcare professionals.

(e) *Minority Stress Responses*

A promising approach for adapting substance use interventions for the LGBT community recognises the impact of minorities stressors on individuals (McGeough, 2021). The response to these stressors is theoretically modifiable, with Pachankis et al. (2015) finding reductions in problematic substance use behaviours in gay and bisexual men when supporting adaptive coping in response to these stressors. Cognitive behavioural therapy (CBT) approaches are argued to be particularly well-suited to improve cognitive, affective, and behavioural minority stress processes (Balsam et al., 2006; Pachankis, 2014). This is because CBT:

1. locates present unhelpful/undesired states (e.g., low mood and substance use) as understandable and previously adaptive responses to minority stress
2. empowers clients to cope with adverse individually unchangeable environmental circumstances such as minority stress by promoting coping and self-efficacy
3. targets universal risk factors disproportionately affecting sexual minorities

Resulting interventions encourage adaptive reactions to stigma, such as locating the source of one's mental health difficulties in minority stress, drawing on personal resilience as a gay, bisexual or lesbian person, and learning strategies for reducing maladaptive minority stress reactions such as internalised homophobia or rejection sensitivity (Pachankis, 2014). The effectiveness of CBT interventions as applied to sexual minorities and substance use remains largely to be determined, and it should not be caricatured as 'blaming' of an individual or removing the responsibility and change required of those in wider sexual majority systems. More on sexual minorities and CBT is covered in Chapter 11.

(f) Religion and Service Provision

Group interventions are commonly utilised in the support for individuals with substance use difficulties. What little is known about the experiences of sexual minority individuals in traditional 12-step programs, such as Alcoholics/Narcotics Anonymous (AA/NA) suggests some ambivalence towards the spirituality underlying these approaches. Drabble and Eliason (2012) found that many sexual minority women do not connect with AA/NA groups due to negative, heterosexist experiences with religion. Similarly, some substance use programmes are either partly or wholly funded or located in religious organisations and buildings which could be problematic for those that have experienced or perceive that faith as being negative towards their sexuality.

Concerningly, recent research in the UK suggests that some LGBT service users experienced some faith-based substance use programmes as remaining conversion-orientated (Jayne & Williams, 2020). This study highlighted that some service users have experienced transferred gratitude and reciprocity whereby positive psychological experiences of alcohol recovery are attributed to God and/or the organisation. In turn, this can increase engagement with the faith-based organisation and conversion conversations with support workers. Understandably, some members of the LGBT community will be wary of engaging with support organisations historically associated with 'conversion therapy' (against which there is a Memorandum of Understanding on Conversion Therapy in the UK amongst various public and professional bodies).

(g) Group Work Challenges

Groups are often offered within substance abuse work, with benefits both of economy of scale for services and normalisation and peer support for clients. However specialised group programs can also be problematic for sexual minority individuals beyond those related to faith-based organisations, as identified above. LGBT service users have reported not feeling safe revealing their sexual orientation in a mixed group for fear of being exposed to homophobic attitudes (Senreich, 2012). However, if LGBT clients do not reveal their sexual orientation in group therapy, they may not be able to engage in the necessary therapeutic work to prevent relapse (Barbara, 2002; Cabaj, 2014). Therefore, it is crucial that group guidelines are discussed and agreed upon to ensure the safety of all participating individuals. Introducing sexual minority issues into mixed groups fosters communication between LGBT and heterosexual clients, educates heterosexual clients about LGBT issues, and could reduce phobic comments and reactions in the program.

An alternative is for specialised groups for sexual minority individuals (Cochran et al., 2007; Hicks, 2000; Neisen, 1997). Whilst there is little UK data, Cochran et al. (2007) found that of 7691 treatment programmes in the USA, only 62 offered specific LGBT services (0.8%). Particularly outside of major urban centres, sexual minority service users often lack access to substance use disorder treatment programs that deliver culturally tailored services, and a substantial minority of substance use disorder treatment staff may hold negative attitudes about sexuality minority clients, resulting in a 'don't ask, don't tell' approach

(Eliason & Schope, 2001). Innovative treatment models, potentially utilising technology-based interventions, are needed to expand the reach of culturally tailored substance use disorder treatment to LGBT populations. Services without the capacity to develop their programs should establish links to sexual community outreach programs or specialised LGBT online groups to help facilitate this challenge.

Furthermore, whilst the overwhelming majority of service users supported the idea of specialist LGBT groups, not all sexual minority service users will wish to access these (encountering current or past sexual, romantic or social contacts being a common concern). Therefore, the service user's individual needs should be formulated and respected as far as possible.

A further consideration is when a substance abuse program has a large White majority population. Racial and sexual minority service users may feel alienated from the group or experience racism (Senreich, 2010). Service users may also encounter homophobic attitudes from others within their own racial group, which may reinforce feelings that they 'do not fit in anywhere', and impede the recovery process (Senreich, 2012).

Despite concerns regarding the treatment needs of racial minority LGBT clients in substance abuse treatment programs, no differences in programs completions rates were found between White, Black, and Hispanic LGBT former clients of such programs (Senreich, 2010). In fact, this study found that Black and Hispanic clients of substance abuse programs each reported significantly higher levels of satisfaction with treatment than did White former clients.

(h) *Sexual Minority Therapists*

Sexual minority therapists may be favoured by some clients, and self-disclosure within this professional role would be required to necessitate this. Such therapists and their supervisors should also be cognisant to other unique challenges for sexual minority therapists working with sexual minority clients, namely the impact of their own minority stress, and the possibility of dual relationships.

Sexual minority therapists, like all sexual minority people, will have had their own experiences and possible challenges relating to their sexuality and substance use, be they current and/or historic. If working with sexual minority clients and with sexuality minority stress, there is an increased chance of identification of the therapist with the client, and reactivation of emotions and the possibility of self-disclosure within this. Reflections upon the ongoing impact of such work (and decisions around benefit and disadvantages of self-disclosure depending on the therapeutic frame) should be supported by regular supervision.

All clinicians are prohibited from engaging in sexual or romantic relationships with current clients due to the intimate nature of these therapeutic relationships and the power differentials that exist. Whilst this is relevant to all therapists regardless of sexual minority status, a greater challenge is that clinicians are also advised to refrain from working with clients with whom they have had previous relationships. This is particularly important when working in smaller communities (be they geographical, sexual, or both), where opportunities to meet sexual minority partners are more limited, and the chances of meeting clients or potential clients are increased. For example, a sexual minority therapist may like to attend a venue that is socially and/or sexually popular with a specific group within which their clients may also ascribe.

Furthermore, in recent years there has been a shift from finding sexual and romantic partners from "bricks and mortar" social venues to online sites and geolocation applications. Clinicians are not exempt from such popular means of dating and pleasure seeking, but have little guidance for how they should be utilising these and still remain ethical in their practice (Unhjem et al., 2021). It is not suggested that therapists should not use dating apps. But navigating the ethical considerations as a clinician is complex and unclear. Consideration (and potentially caution) should be given to what to include on one's profile, and the level of anonymity *vs.* identification and self-disclosure within this. This includes photographs and/or text, and language and descriptions within this. Likewise, there should be boundary anticipation and preparation for how to respond to any contact by a previous or current client (who may or may not even know they are messaging their therapist depending on what has been disclosed), or how we might respond to discovery of their profile on the same platform.

There is limited research in this area. One study (Stevens, 2016) found some everyday experiences when social workers encounter clients or other significant individuals in their clients' lives. Social workers found clients' or their relatives' profiles, clients or clients' relatives saw participants, and clients messaged clinicians. Multiple responses to these online encounters were reported, including blocking the client, deleting their account, discussing with supervisors, discussing the occurrence with the client in session, or taking no action (Stevens, 2016). The variety of responses may reflect that the social workers considered the best course of action based on the context of the situation and/or a lack of consensus on how to address such encounters. This further reinforces the importance of supervision for feedback, suggestions and support to avoid potential ethical, moral, or legal violations.

Conclusion

This chapter has considered various aspects relevant to assessing and intervening with sexual minority clients with substance abuse difficulties, and the design of such services to provide optimum care. Some of these adaptations will be relevant beyond sexual minority clients and substance use respectively, whereas others are borne from the unique interaction of the two. On behalf of any future clients you support who will now benefit from you engaging with this chapter, we thank you.

References

Abdulrahim, D., Whitely, C., & Bowden-Jones, O. (2016). *Club drug use among Lesbian, Gay, Bisexual and Trans (LGBT) people*. Novel Psychoactive Treatment UK Network (NEPTUNE)

ACON. (2013). *Health outcomes strategy 2013–2018: Alcohol and other drugs*.

Anderson, S. C. (2009). *Substance use disorders in lesbian, gay, bisexual, and transgender clients: Assessment and treatment*. Columbia University Press.

Aldridge, A. (2020). Intoxicating the 'charmed circle': Constructions of deviance and normativity by people who combine drugs and sex. *Criminology & Criminal Justice, 20*(5), 564–576. https://doi.org/10.1177/174889 5820937332

Balsam, K. F., Martell, C. R., & Safren, S. A. (2006). Affirmative cognitive-behavioral therapy with lesbian, gay, and bisexual people. In P. A. Hays & G. Y. Iwamasa (Eds.), *Culturally responsive cognitive-behavioral therapy: Assessment, practice, and supervision* (pp. 223–243). American Psychological Association.

Beam, J. (2008). *In the life: A black gay anthology*. RedBone Press.

Becker, J. B., McClellan, M. L., & Reed, B. G. (2017). Sex differences, gender and addiction: Sex, Gender, and Addiction. *Journal of Neuroscience Research, 95*(1–2), 136–147. https://doi.org/10.1002/jnr.23963

Barbara, A. M. (2002). Substance abuse treatment with lesbian, gay and bisexual people: A qualitative study of service providers. *Journal of Gay & Lesbian Social Services, 14*(4), 1–17.

Bourne, A., Reid, D., Hickson, F., Rueda, S. T., & Weatherburn, P. (2014). *Drug use in sexual settings among study: Gay and bisexual men in Lambeth, Southwark & Lewisham* (p. 3). Sigma Research, London School of Hygiene & Tropical Medicine.

British Psychological Society. (2019). *Guidelines for psychologists working with gender, sexuality and relationship diversity*. https://www.bps.org.uk/news-and-policy/guidelines-psychologists-working-gender-sexuality-and-relations hip-diversity

Brooks, K. D., Bowleg, L., & Quina, K. (2009). Minority sexual status among minorities. In S. Loue (Ed.), *Sexualities and identities of minority women* (pp. 41–63). Springer. https://doi.org/10.1007/978-0-387-75657-8_3

Burckell, L. A., & Goldfried, M. R. (2006). Therapist qualities preferred by sexual-minority individuals. *Psychotherapy: Theory, Research, Practice, Training, 43*(1), 32–49. https://doi.org/10.1037/0033-3204.43.1.32

Cabaj, R. P. (2014). Substance use issues among gay, lesbian, bisexual, and transgender people . In *Textbook of substance abuse treatment* (pp. 707–721). American Psychiatric Association.

Cave, J., Ismail, S., Liccardo, R., Rabinovich, L., Rubin, J., & Weed, K. (2009). *Tackling problem drug use* (TR-795-NAO; p. 76). UK National Audit Office. www.nao.org.uk/wp-content/uploads/2010/03/0910297_reviews.pdf

Cochran, B. N., Peavy, K. M., & Robohm, J. S. (2007). Do specialized services exist for LGBT individuals seeking treatment for substance misuse? A study of available treatment programs. *Substance Use & Misuse, 42*(1), 161–176.

Corliss, H. L., Rosario, M., Wypij, D., Wylie, S. A., Frazier, A. L., & Austin, S. B. (2010). Sexual orientation and drug use in a longitudinal cohort study of U.S. adolescents. *Addictive Behaviors, 35*(5), 517–521. https://doi.org/10.1016/j.addbeh.2009.12.019

Dorn-Medeiros, C. M., & Doyle, C. (2018). Alcohol as coping: Internalized homophobia and heterosexism's role in alcohol use among lesbians. *Journal of LGBT Issues in Counseling, 12*(3), 142–157. https://doi.org/10.1080/15538605.2018.1488230

Drabble, L., & Eliason, M. J. (2012). Substance use disorders treatment for sexual minority women. *Journal of LGBT Issues in Counseling, 6*(4), 274–292. https://doi.org/10.1080/15538605.2012.726150

Drescher, J. (2015). Out of DSM: Depathologizing homosexuality. *Behavioral Sciences, 5*(4), 565–575.

Edmundson, C., Heinsbroek, E., Glass, R., Hope, V., Mohammed, H., White, M., & Desai, M. (2018). Sexualised drug use in the United Kingdom (UK): A review of the literature. *International Journal of Drug Policy, 55*, 131–148. https://doi.org/10.1016/j.drugpo.2018.02.002

Eliason, M. J., & Schope, R. (2001). Does "don't ask don't tell" apply to health care? Lesbian, gay, and bisexual people's disclosure to health care providers. *Journal of the Gay and Lesbian Medical Association, 5*(4), 125–134.

Elmquist, J., Shorey, R. C., Anderson, S. E., & Stuart, G. L. (2017). A preliminary investigation of the relationship between dispositional mindfulness and eating disorder symptoms among men in residential substance use treatment. *Addiction Research & Theory, 25*(1), 67–73. https://doi.org/10.1080/16066359.2016.1198475

Emslie, C., Lennox, J., & Ireland, L. (2015). *The social context of LGBT people's drinking in Scotland* (p. 28). Glasgow Caledonian University.

Enkema, M. C., Hallgren, K. A., Neilson, E. C., Bowen, S., Bird, E. R., & Larimer, M. E. (2020). Disrupting the path to craving: Acting without awareness mediates the link between negative affect and craving. *Psychology of Addictive Behaviors, 34*(5), 620–627. https://doi.org/10.1037/adb0000565

European Monitoring Centre for Drugs and Drug Addiction. (2018). *European drug report 2018: Trends and developments*. Publications Office. https://doi.org/10.2810/800331

Evans, K. (2019). The psychological roots of chemsex and how understanding the full picture can help us create meaningful support. *Drugs and Alcohol Today, 19*(1), 36–41. https://doi.org/10.1108/DAT-10-2018-0062

Flentje, A., Livingston, N. A., Roley, J., & Sorensen, J. L. (2015). Mental and physical health needs of lesbian, gay, and bisexual clients in substance abuse treatment. *Journal of Substance Abuse Treatment, 58*, 78–83. https://doi.org/10.1016/j.jsat.2015.06.022

Gilbert, P. (1998). What is shame? Some core issues and controversies. In *Shame: Interpersonal behavior, psychopathology, and culture* (pp. 3–38). Oxford University Press.

Global Commission on Drug Policy. (2017). *The world drug perception problem: Countering prejudices about people who use drugs* (Report 2017).

Gonzalez, J. M., Alegría, M., Prihoda, T. J., Copeland, L. A., & Zeber, J. E. (2011). How the relationship of attitudes toward mental health treatment and service use differs by age, gender, ethnicity/race and education. *Social Psychiatry and Psychiatric Epidemiology, 46*(1), 45–57. https://doi.org/10.1007/s00127-009-0168-4

Harm Reduction International. (2021). *Chemsex and harm reduction for gay men and other men who have sex with men* (p. 8) [Briefing Note]. Harm Reduction International.

Hegazi, A., Lee, M., Whittaker, W., Green, S., Simms, R., Cutts, R., Nagington, M., Nathan, B., & Pakianathan, M. (2017). Chemsex and the city: Sexualised substance use in gay bisexual and other men who have sex with men attending sexual health clinics. *International Journal of STD & AIDS, 28*(4), 362–366. https://doi.org/10.1177/0956462416651229

Hicks, D. (2000). The importance of specialized treatment programs for lesbian and gay patients. *Journal of Gay & Lesbian Psychotherapy, 3*(3–4), 81–94.

Hodson, K., Meads, C., & Bewley, S. (2017). Lesbian and bisexual women's likelihood of becoming pregnant: a systematic review and meta-analysis. *BJOG: An International Journal of Obstetrics & Gynaecology, 124*(3), 393–402.

Hoff, B., Freeman, D., & Wang, D. (2020). *Mindfulness-based chemsex recovery* (Annual Report). Spectra.

Institute of Medicine. (2011). *The health of lesbian, gay, bisexual, and transgender people: Building a foundation for better understanding* (Vol. 49). The National Academies Press. https://doi.org/10.5860/CHOICE.49-2699

Irons, C., & Lad, S. (2014). Using compassion focused therapy to work with shame and self-criticism in complex trauma. *Australian Clinical Psychologist, 3*(1), 47–54.

Jayne, M., & Williams, A. (2020). Faith-based alcohol treatment in England and Wales: New evidence for policy and practice. *Health & Place, 66,* 102457. https://doi.org/10.1016/j.healthplace.2020.102457

Jeffery, M. K., & Tweed, A. E. (2014). Clinician self-disclosure or clinician self-concealment? Lesbian, gay and bisexual mental health practitioners' experiences of disclosure in therapeutic relationships. *Counselling and Psychotherapy Research,* 1–8. https://doi.org/10.1080/14733145.2013.871307

Kandall, S. (1999). *Substance and Shadow: Women and Addiction in the United States.* Harvard University Press.

Kunelaki, R. (2019). What is sober sex and how to achieve it? *Drugs and Alcohol Today, 19*(1), 29–35. https://doi.org/10.1108/DAT-11-2018-0064

Ma, R., & Perera, S. (2016). Safer 'chemsex': GPs' role in harm reduction for emerging forms of recreational drug use. *British Journal of General Practice, 66*(642), 4–5.

Maxwell, S., Shahmanesh, M., & Gafos, M. (2019). Chemsex behaviours among men who have sex with men: A systematic review of the literature. *International Journal of Drug Policy, 63,* 74–89. https://doi.org/10.1016/j.drugpo.2018.11.014

Mayer, K. H., Bradford, J. B., Makadon, H. J., Stall, R., Goldhammer, H., & Landers, S. (2008). Sexual and gender minority health: What we know and what needs to be done. *American Journal of Public Health, 98*(6), 989–995. https://doi.org/10.2105/AJPH.2007.127811

McCellan, M. (2017). *Lady lushes: Gender, alcoholism, and medicine in modern America.* Rutgers University Press.

McGeough, B. (2021). A systematic review of substance use treatments for sexual minority women. *Journal of Gay & Lesbian Social Services, 33*(2), 180–210. https://doi.org/10.1080/10538720.2021.1875346

Medley, G., Lipari, R. N., Bose, J., Cribb, D. S., Kroutil, L. A., & McHenry, G. (2015). *Sexual orientation and estimates of adult substance use and mental health: results from the 2015 National Survey on Drug Use and Health.* 54.

Mericle, A. A., de Guzman, R., Hemberg, J., Yette, E., Drabble, L., & Trocki, K. (2018). Delivering LGBT-sensitive substance use treatment to sexual minority women. *Journal of Gay & Lesbian Social Services, 30*(4), 393–408. https://doi.org/10.1080/10538720.2018.1512435

Meyer, I. H. (2003). Minority stress and mental health in gay men. In L. D. Garnets & D. C. Kimmel (Eds.), *Psychological perspectives on lesbian, gay, and bisexual experiences* (2nd ed.). (2003-00760-026; pp. 699–731). Columbia University Press. http://search.ebscohost.com/login.aspx?direct= true&db=psyh&AN=2003-00760-026&site=ehost-live

Miller-Lloyd, L., Landry, J., Macmadu, A., Allard, I., & Waxman, M. (2020). Barriers to healthcare for people who inject drugs: A survey at a syringe exchange program. *Substance Use & Misuse, 55*(6), 896–899. https://doi. org/10.1080/10826084.2019.1710207

Moncrief, M. (2014). *Out of your mind: Improving provision of drug & alcohol treatment for lesbian, gay, bisexual & trans people.* London Friend.

Neisen, J. H. (1997). An inpatient psychoeducational group model for gay men and lesbians with alcohol and drug abuse problems. In *Chemical dependency treatment: Innovative group approaches* (pp. 37–51). Routledge

Nutt, D. J., King, L. A., & Phillips, L. D. (2010). Drug harms in the UK: A multicriteria decision analysis. *The Lancet, 376*(9752), 1558–1565. https:// doi.org/10.1016/S0140-6736(10)61462-6

Office for Health Improvement & Disparities. (2021). *Adult substance misuse treatment statistics 2020 to 2021: Report.* Office for Health Improvement & Disparities. https://www.gov.uk/government/statistics/substance-misuse-tre atment-for-adults-statistics-2020-to-2021/adult-substance-misuse-treatm ent-statistics-2020-to-2021-report

Office of National Statistics (ONS). (2018). *Adult drinking habits in Great Britain: 2017.* Office of National Statistics (ONS). https://www.ons.gov. uk/peoplepopulationandcommunity/healthandsocialcare/drugusealcoholα ndsmoking/bulletins/opinionsandlifestylesurveyadultdrinkinghabitsingrea tbritain/2017

Pachankis, J. E. (2014). Uncovering clinical principles and techniques to address minority stress, mental health, and related health risks among gay and bisexual men. *Clinical Psychology: Science and Practice, 21*(4), 313.

Pachankis, J. E., Hatzenbuehler, M. L., Rendina, H. J., Safren, S. A., & Parsons, J. T. (2015). LGB-affirmative cognitive-behavioral therapy for young adult gay and bisexual men: A randomized controlled trial of a transdiagnostic minority stress approach. *Journal of Consulting and Clinical Psychology, 83*(5), 875–889. https://doi.org/10.1037/ccp0000037

Pachankis, J. E., & Safren, S. A. (2019). Handbook of evidence-based mental health practice with sexual and gender minorities. *Oxford University Press.* https://doi.org/10.1093/med-psych/9780190669300.001.0001

Pennay, A., McNair, R., Hughes, T. L., Leonard, W., Brown, R., & Lubman, D. I. (2018). Improving alcohol and mental health treatment for lesbian, bisexual and queer women: Identity matters. *Australian and New Zealand*

Journal of Public Health, 42(1), 35–42. https://doi.org/10.1111/1753-6405. 12739

Pienaar, K., Murphy, D. A., Race, K., & Lea, T. (2018). Problematising LGBTIQ drug use, governing sexuality and gender: A critical analysis of LGBTIQ health policy in Australia. *International Journal of Drug Policy, 55*, 187–194. https://doi.org/10.1016/j.drugpo.2018.01.008

Pitman, A., Marston, L., Lewis, G., Semlyen, J., McManus, S., & King, M. (2021). The mental health of lesbian, gay, and bisexual adults compared with heterosexual adults: Results of two nationally representative English household probability samples. *Psychological Medicine, 1–10.*

Platteau, T., Herrijgers, C., & de Wit, J. (2020). Digital chemsex support and care: The potential of just-in-time adaptive interventions. *International Journal of Drug Policy, 85*, 102927. https://doi.org/10.1016/j.drugpo.2020. 102927

Platteau, T., Pebody, R., Dunbar, N., Lebacq, T., & Collins, B. (2019). The problematic chemsex journey: A resource for prevention and harm reduction. *Drugs and Alcohol Today, 19*(1), 49–54.

Rosińska, M., Gios, L., Nöstlinger, C., Vanden Berghe, W., Marcus, U., Schink, S., Sherriff, N., Jones, A.-M., Folch, C., Dias, S., Velicko, I., & Mirandola, M. (2018). Prevalence of drug use during sex amongst MSM in Europe: Results from a multi-site bio-behavioural survey. *International Journal of Drug Policy, 55*, 231–241. https://doi.org/10.1016/j.drugpo.2018. 01.002

Sagar-Ouriaghli, I., Godfrey, E., Bridge, L., Meade, L., & Brown, J. S. L. (2019). Improving mental health service utilization among men: A systematic review and synthesis of behavior change techniques within interventions targeting help-seeking. *American Journal of Men's Health, 13*(3), 155798831985700. https://doi.org/10.1177/1557988319857009

SAMHSA: Substance Abuse and Mental Health Services Administration. (2001). *Summary of findings from the 2000 National Household Survey on Drug Abuse. NHSDA Series H-13, DHHS Publication No (SMA) 01-3549.* Office of Applied Studies.

Santoro, P., Rodríguez, R., Morales, P., Morano, A., & Morán, M. (2020). One "chemsex" or many? Types of chemsex sessions among gay and other men who have sex with men in Madrid, Spain: Findings from a qualitative study. *International Journal of Drug Policy, 82*, 102790. https://doi.org/10.1016/j. drugpo.2020.102790

Schlag, A. K. (2020). Percentages of problem drug use and their implications for policy making: A review of the literature. *Drug Science, Policy and Law, 6*, 205032452090454. https://doi.org/10.1177/2050324520904540

Schulz, C. T., Glatt, E. M., & Stamates, A. L. (2022). Risk factors associated with alcohol and drug use among bisexual women: A literature review. *Experimental and Clinical Psychopharmacology, 30*(5), 740–749. https://doi.org/10.1037/pha0000480

Seitz, N.-N., Lochbühler, K., Atzendorf, J., Rauschert, C., Pfeiffer-Gerschel, T., & Kraus, L. (2019). Trends in substance use and related disorders. *Deutsches Aerzteblatt Online.* https://doi.org/10.3238/arztebl.2019.0585

Senreich, E. (2010). Differences in outcomes, completion rates, and perceptions of treatment between white, black, and Hispanic LGBT clients in substance abuse programs. *Journal of Gay & Lesbian Mental Health, 14*(3), 176–200. https://doi.org/10.1080/19359701003784675

Senreich, E. (2012). Lesbian, gay, and bisexual clients in a substance abuse treatment program serving a mostly black and Hispanic population. *Journal of LGBT Issues in Counseling, 6*(4), 310–336. https://doi.org/10.1080/15538605.2012.730474

Shahab, L., Brown, J., Hagger-Johnson, G., Michie, S., Semlyen, J., West, R., & Meads, C. (2017). Sexual orientation identity and tobacco and hazardous alcohol use: Findings from a cross-sectional English population survey. *BMJ Open, 7*(10), e015058. https://doi.org/10.1136/bmjopen-2016-015058

Smalley, K. B., Warren, J. C., & Barefoot, K. N. (2018). *LGBT health: Meeting the needs of gender and sexual minorities.* Springer Publishing Company. http://0-search.ebscohost.com.catalogue.libraries.london.ac.uk/login.aspx?direct=true&db=psyh&AN=2017-36752-000&site=ehost-live

Smith, V., & Tasker, F. (2018). Gay men's chemsex survival stories. *Sexual Health, 15*(2), 116–122. https://doi.org/10.1071/SH17122

Stevens, M. B. (2016). *Social workers' experiences related to online dating: A descriptive study* (Masters Thesis). Smith College, Northampton, MA.

Stuart, D. (2013). Sexualised drug use by MSM: Background, current status and response. *HIV Nursing, 13*(1), 6–10.

Tervalon, M., & Murray-García, J. (1998). Cultural humility versus cultural competence: A critical distinction in defining physician training outcomes in multicultural education. *Journal of Health Care for the Poor and Underserved, 9*(2), 117–125. https://doi.org/10.1353/hpu.2010.0233

Todd, M. (2016). *Straight jacket—How to be gay and happy.* Transworld Digital.

Torres, T. S., Bastos, L. S., Kamel, L., Bezerra, D. R. B., Fernandes, N. M., Moreira, R. I., Garner, A., Veloso, V. G., Grinsztejn, B., & De Boni, R. B. (2020). Do men who have sex with men who report alcohol and illicit drug use before/during sex (chemsex) present moderate/high risk for substance use disorders? *Drug and Alcohol Dependence, 209*, 107908. https://doi.org/10.1016/j.drugalcdep.2020.107908

Unhjem, L., Hoss, L., Roberts, B., & VanderTuin, S. (2021). Swipe right for... my therapist? Ethical considerations for therapists using dating apps. *Contemporary Family Therapy, 43*(2), 177–188. https://doi.org/10.1007/s10591-020-09561-7

United Nations Office on Drugs and Crime [UNODC]. (2019). *World Drug Report 2019* (pp. 1–56).

Wang, P. S., Lane, M., Olfson, M., Pincus, H. A., Wells, K. B., & Kessler, R. C. (2005). Twelve-month use of mental health services in the United States: Results from the national comorbidity survey replication. *Archives of General Psychiatry, 62*(6), 629. https://doi.org/10.1001/archpsyc.62.6.629

West, R., & Brown, J. (2013). *Theory of addiction* (2nd ed.). Wiley.

Williams, H., Varney, D. J., Taylor, J., Durr, P., & Elan-Cane, C. (2010). *The lesbian, gay, bisexual and trans public health outcomes framework companion document* (p. 57). Public Health England.

Women and Equalities Committee. (2019). *Health and social care and LGBT communities*. House of Commons.

16

Preventing LGBTQ+ Youth Suicide: A Queer Critical and Human Rights Approach

Elizabeth McDermott and Hazel Marzetti

Introduction

In this chapter we address the established problem of the heightened risk of suicide amongst LGBTQ+ young people. While this book focuses primarily on sexual diversity, we, as do many of the chapters in the book, adopt an intersectional approach to include gender diversity. We do not intend to list the risk and resilience factors associated with this phenomena because the international evidence base that demonstrates the higher risk of suicidality in LGBTQ+ youth compared to their cis-heterosexual counterparts is substantial (Marshal et al., 2011; Surace et al., 2021). A brief literature search will reveal a raft of systematic

E. McDermott (✉)
University of Birmingham, Birmingham, UK
e-mail: e.mcdermott.1@bham.ac.uk

H. Marzetti
University of Edinburgh, Edinburgh, UK
e-mail: Hazel.Marzetti@ed.ac.uk

© The Author(s), under exclusive license to Springer Nature
Switzerland AG 2023
J. Semlyen and P. Rohleder (eds.), *Sexual Minorities and Mental Health*,
https://doi.org/10.1007/978-3-031-37438-8_16

reviews, meta-analysis and literature reviews examining the topic from a variety of perspectives—emergency care, nursing, psychology, psychiatry, social work (Ancheta et al., 2021; de Lange et al., 2022; Gorse, 2022; Hatchel et al., 2021; Marchi et al., 2022; Marraccini et al., 2022; Poštuvan et al., 2019; Russon et al., 2022; Schultz et al., 2022). In this chapter, we will develop a critically queer approach to suicidology in order to ask some key questions of this literature, as we seek to broaden understandings of LGBTQ+ young people's suicidal distress. Most crucially, we are asking *why* there are so few attempts internationally to intervene and prevent LGBTQ+ young people from feeling they no longer want to live.

We start by examining how LGBTQ+ suicide is conceptualised: the different theories and concepts used across a variety of disciplines to explain why there is a heightened risk of suicidal thoughts, feelings and attempts in this group of young people. Pathology is the key concept around which these theories orientate and we group the theories into 3 broad approaches: those that pathologize, seeing suicide as a mental health problem; those that focus on homophobia, biphobia and transphobia (taken together queerphobia [Marzetti, 2018]) as the sole causes of suicidal distress; and those that aim to use an intersectional lens to look more holistically at suicide both incorporating queerphobia and mental health problems, whilst also going beyond to consider the whole individual situated within their socio-political context, which we have termed a queer critical suicidology perspective. The ways one explains the link between suicidal distress, LGBTQ+ people and youth is fundamental because it guides how to tackle the problem and intervene to prevent suicide. In our view there is a clear link between pathology and the low priority given to LGBTQ+ young people's suicidality in international policy-making.

Secondly, we use a queer critical suicidology lens to examine what might work to prevent suicide amongst LGBTQ+ young people. The literature on this topic is under-developed and remains focussed on individual psycho-medical approaches. However, increasingly, scholars and practitioners are articulating alternative approaches using socio-ecological, systems and human rights framings of the problem. Lastly, we return to the question of why national policies and practices remain resistant to developing suicide prevention for LGBTQ+ young people despite the increasing acknowledgement of the elevated risk by national governments and global organisations like WHO and the UN. We conclude by arguing for a human rights approach to suicide prevention for LGBTQ+ young people. We suggest that framing LGBTQ+ youth suicide as a human rights issue may focus global attention on the matter and persuade those in seats of power to act.

Understanding LGBTQ+ Suicide

Psycho-Medicalised Approaches to Understanding and Preventing Suicide

Suicide is a complex, biopsychosocial issue (O'Connor & Kirtley, 2018), which can be theorised as an attempt to escape unbearable pain. How this pain develops and why suicide is seen as the most accessible way of escaping it however, has been subject to enormous debate. One suggestion from Thomas Joiner's (2007) *Interpersonal Theory of Suicide* (IPTS), which has dominated twenty-first century understandings of suicide behaviours, is that suicidal thoughts occur when an individual experiences a sense of (i) thwarted belonging in which they lack reciprocally caring relationships; and (ii) perceived burdensomeness, in which they believe their loved ones would be better off without them. An alternative theory, O'Connor's (2023) *Integrated Motivational-Volitional (IMV) model* offer defeat, humiliation and entrapment as the key steps in developing suicidal distress. Bringing them together, both the IMV model and the IPTS propose that to act on these thoughts and attempt suicide, individuals increase their tolerance for pain and reduce their fear of death; with self-harm often positioned in response to this, as a risk factor for suicide (Owens et al., 2002).

Although such theoretical positions do recognise that the roots of suicidal distress are formed in both the fabric of society through socioeconomic inequalities and through interpersonal difficulties such as adverse childhood experiences (both of which are widely associated with increased risk of suicide (Dube et al., 2001; Platt, 2016), ultimately suicide prevention is usually conceptualised in an individualised way, understanding that suicidal feelings are something located *within* the individual and can therefore be healed by working *with* that individual, rather than engaging with the socio-political and economic contexts they are situated within (Button, 2016; Marzetti, Oaten et al., 2022b). Interventions targeting young people are often school-based as an efficient method of engaging with a large number of youths (Robinson et al., 2013), and tend to focus on raising awareness of suicidal feelings and encouraging them to reach out to a trusted adult either if they are feeling suicidal or if they have concerns about their peers (Gould & Kramer, 2001). Once a young person has then been identified, they might be referred on for therapeutic support, with studies showing that Cognitive Behavioural Therapy (CBT) and Dialectic Behavioural Therapy (DBT) can have some positive effects on reducing suicidal distress (Gould & Kramer, 2001; King et al., 2018; Robinson et al., 2011), whilst innovative work from Australia has been piloting the use of online support for young people thinking about suicide (Bailey et al., 2020).

Although youth suicide is a major public health concern globally and there is a huge desire to find effective prevention methods, the evaluation of therapeutic support can be limited as young people experiencing suicidal distress are often deemed ineligible for clinical trials due to concerns about vulnerabilities (Bailey et al., 2018; Calear et al., 2016; King et al., 2018). In addition to this, it has also been noted that for a variety of reasons, young people at greatest risk of suicide may not feel able to engage with such support (LeCloux et al., 2017) and this can particularly be the case for LGBTQ+ young people who have reported challenges accessing therapeutic support due to concerns about dismissive or discriminatory attitudes both about their LGBTQ+ identity and about their suicidal feelings (McDermott & Roen, 2016; McDermott et al., 2018a). As a result, LGBTQ+ young people instead expressed a preference to try and cope with suicidal feelings independently, until at crisis point (McDermott, 2015; McDermott et al., 2008; Scourfield et al., 2008). One such method of independent coping used by LGBTQ+ young people is self-harm (McDermott et al., 2016), which has historically been understood as a 'risk factor' for suicide. However, recent work has challenged this conventional wisdom, suggesting that whilst self-harm may precede a suicide attempt, correlation is not causation and there may be other explanations of the relationship between self-harm and suicide (Marzetti et al., 2023). Indeed, it is suggested that self-harming practices can be used to de-escalate suicidal distress and self-soothe during times of crisis (Chandler & Simopoulou, 2020). Alternatively, many LGBTQ+ young people reach out through informal support channels such as friends, online spaces or LGBTQ+ groups (McDermott et al., 2016).

This presents some clear challenges for practitioners who wish to make their services accessible to LGBTQ+ young people, which perhaps requires a different kind of thinking beyond conventional psychological methods. Indeed instead of focussing on individuals' thoughts, feelings and behaviours as mental health problems that invite treatment and prevention, throughout the rest of this chapter we will propose a broader lens of understanding to more holistically account for the complexity of this issue and a broader theoretical framework within which to conceptualise supporting LGBTQ+ youths living with suicidal distress.

Minority Stress Theory

Although both in historic and contemporary times, tensions have existed between LGBTQ+ people and professionals working in psychology and psychiatry alike (for a detailed exploration on this topic please see: Davy, 2015; Davy & Toze, 2018; Hubbard & Griffiths, 2019; Jowett, 2017; Riggs et al., 2019), today LGBTQ+ suicide is generally considered a consequence of queerphobia. Primarily this has been explained using Meyer's *Minority Stress Theory* (Meyer, 1995, 2003), which proposes that in addition to the day-to-day stresses that everyone experiences, LGBTQ+ people face additional stresses specific to their LGBTQ+ identity, due to both individual and community-level expectations, experiences and negotiations of queerphobia, which in turn can have negative impacts on both their physical and mental health (see Chapter 3 for more detailed discussion of stigmatisation and

social prejudice). Applying Minority Stress Theory to suicide necessarily complexifies understandings of suicidal distress, encouraging us to
understand how suicide impacts LGBTQ+ young people as *people experiencing suicidal distress*; as *young* people experiencing suicidal distress; and
as *LGBTQ+* young people experiencing suicidal distress (Marzetti, 2020)
(Fig. 16.1). Furthermore, it also encourages us to think beyond ideas
such as Joiner's 'perceived burdensomeness', to consider whether understandings of distorted perceptions are helpful, or whether this is for some,
an accurate understanding of the way in which they are being treated by
their family, peers or wider society; which may have consequences for
treatment in practice

Using Minority Stress Theory we can see how experiences related
to being young and ageism; being LGBTQ+ and queerphobia; and
feeling suicidal and sanism; can interact with one another to create
the specific experiences of LGBTQ+ young people experiencing suicidal
distress. Furthermore, how these experiences intersect with other forms
of marginalisation and oppression such as ableism, racism, sexism and
classism which exist both within and out with LGBTQ+ communities (Formby, 2017), should be considered where relevant. In doing so
however, we do not wish to suggest that these experiences are additive,
and instead use Crenshaw's (1989) theory of intersectionality, to argue
that whilst each set of experiences should be taken into account, the
ways that they intersect and interact with one another mean that an individual's experience will be different from the individual experiences that
comprise it.

Avoiding Individualisation, De-politicisation and De-contextualisation

Although *Minority Stress Theory* encourages us to think about the ways
in which minority stresses interact with the types of stresses that the
whole population experiences, the application of this theory in suicide
research has tended to focus on minority stresses *in isolation*. Such explanations also tend to focus on *experiences* of minority stress, finding that
peer and family rejection can contribute, either directly or indirectly, to

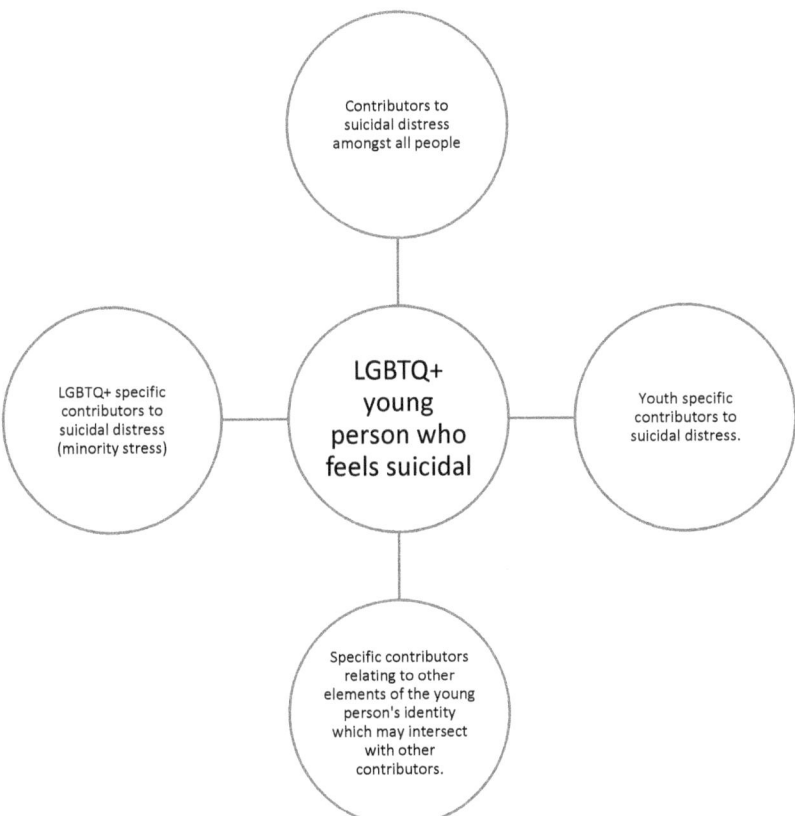

Fig. 16.1 Contributors to LGBTQ+ young people's suicidal distress

suicidal distress (Poštuvan et al., 2019; Puckett et al., 2017; Williams et al., 2021). Often absent within such analysis however, is the ways in which community level experiences of stigmatisation and victimisation may impact on individual LGBTQ+ people's *expectations* of how they will be treated, regardless of whether they themselves have had personal experiences of queerphobia, and the ways in which they behave in order to avoid them, which were emphasised as equally important within Meyer's (2003) theoretical development. As a result, queerphobic victimisation is often reduced to the individual actions and interactions between 'victims' and 'perpetrators', decontextualized from the broader cis-heteronormative social and political landscapes that make these individual acts of queerphobia possible (Marzetti, Chandler et al., 2023). Thus, rendering the perhaps more subtle, yet nonetheless damaging, normative social relations that sustain and circulate minority stresses within societies invisible (Formby, 2015; Wozolek et al., 2017). Consequently, some of the rich nuances of Minority Stress Theory are missed: primarily that minority stress is not an individual, but instead a community experience, that cannot be depoliticised and decontextualized, due to the fundamental and deep-seated entanglement between everyday queerphobic acts and both the contemporary and historic contexts in which they take place.

A further drawback of such narrow conceptualisations of minority stress is the lack of consideration of how experiences of queerphobia can interact with other challenges faced by all people, and particularly all young people, living with suicidal distress. There is a wide and established literature that seeks to understand youth suicide (Cash & Bridge, 2009; Evans et al., 2004), which is often left out when we talk about LGBTQ+ youth suicide. Some contributory factors are shared between youth and adult populations such as the detrimental impact of experiencing 'adverse childhood experiences'[1] (Dube et al., 2001), lower socio-economic status (Miller & Eckert, 2009), and living with mental health problems or previously having attempted suicide (Gould & Kramer, 2001) although they may have different effects related to age; whilst others, such as educational difficulties are specific to youths (Hawton et al., 2012). Bringing the findings of such research into conversation with Minority Stress Theory can then help us to complicate the picture further and understand how suicide specifically comes to be amongst LGBTQ+ youth. For example, both adverse childhood experiences and bullying which are found to be significantly associated with suicide in the wider youth population, are also thought to disproportionately affect LGBTQ+ youths (Almeida et al., 2009; Clements-Nolle et al., 2018; Schnarrs et al., 2019; Ybarra et al., 2015).

---

[1] Abuse (sexual, physical, emotional); witnessing domestic violence against their mother; household substance use; household mental illness; parental separation or divorce; and having a member of their household incarcerated.

The Pipeline Problem: Troubling the 'Suicide Consensus'

The willingness to individualise LGBTQ+ people's suicidal distress, is possibly facilitated by a social readiness to accept and indeed amplify the idea of LGBTQ+ people as *at risk* of suicide (Bryan & Mayock, 2017). Although it has been widely demonstrated that LGBTQ+ people are more likely than their cisgender, heterosexual peers to think about and attempt suicide (di Giacomo et al., 2018; Marshal et al., 2011; Miranda-Mendizábal et al., 2017), termed the 'suicide consensus' (Eliason, 2010), there is a limited appetite for questioning *why* this disparity existed in the first place or what can be done to improve the lives of LGBTQ+ youths, creating a society in which it is easier for them to continue living. McDermott and Roen (2016) have argued that such a readiness to accept LGBTQ+ people as suicidal is perhaps one of the many legacy effects of the history of pathologisation (previously discussed), in which being LGBTQ+ was itself seen as a mental illness, forging a "dangerous association" (p. 1) still witnessed today between *being LGBTQ+* and *being suicidal*.

As part of the critique of the acceptance of the suicide consensus, further questions have been raised by queer critical suicidologists about the impacts that such cultural scripts can have on LGBTQ+ youths' suicidal distress (Canetto et al., 2021; Cover, 2012). It has been argued that the almost linear relationship projected between queerphobic victimisation and suicide could create looping effects (Hacking, 2006; Waidzunas, 2012) or cultural scripts (Canetto et al., 2021; Savin-Williams, 2001) that normalise and consolidate suicide as a response to queerphobic victimisation, in turn increasing LGBTQ+ youths' risk of suicide (Cover, 2012). To begin to understand such normative regimes impacting on LGBTQ+ suicidal distress it has been suggested that we need not only to explore the proliferation of exacting normative standards that LGBTQ+ young people are subject to (such as cis-heternormativity and norms of emotional regulation and maturation (Marzetti, McDaid et al., 2022a; McDermott & Roen, 2016)), but also the ways in which this is made sense of by LGBTQ+ young people (Hatzenbuehler, 2009).

Our queer, critical suicidology perspective attempts, like others, to connect suicidal distress with social, cultural, political and economic environment, and specifically social norms of gender and sexuality that make life in general difficult for some young people because they cannot fit with the acceptable boundaries of cis-heteronorms. This theoretical approach attempts to move beyond pathology and the focus on individual, psychological risk factors such as victimization and discrimination. In doing so it seeks to reconceptualise suicide prevention, which often focusses on what has been termed 'death prevention' methods (Marzetti, Oaten et al., 2022b), rather than considering how society could be transformed to ensure that more LGBTQ+ young people want to live.

LGBTQ+ Youth Suicide Prevention

We have suggested that there are 3 broad theoretical approaches to understanding the relationship between LGBTQ+ suicide: individual pathology; minority stress; and queer critical suicidology. In this last section, we want to consider what we know about ways of preventing LGBTQ+ youth suicide. The literature on this topic is much less well developed and predominantly focuses on individual psycho-medical approaches. Increasingly, alternative approaches are being developed using socioecological, systems and human rights framings. We will explore these, whilst considering why national policies and practices often remain resistant to developing suicide prevention practices that are tailored for LGBTQ+ young people, despite the increasing acknowledgement of the elevated risk by national governments and global organisations like WHO and the UN.

What Prevents LGBTQ+ Youth Suicide?

Despite the large body of international research evidence that has accumulated over the last few decades focussed on the prevalence of LGBTQ+ suicide, and the associated contributory and protective factors, there is very limited research on effective approaches to preventing suicide in this population group. In part, perhaps, because there have been very few interventions to address LGBTQ+ young people's suicidal thoughts and feelings (we will return to why later in the chapter) (Marshall, 2016; McDermott & Roen, 2016). Thus empirical evaluations of large-scale interventions that attempt to prevent or reduce LGBTQ+ youth suicide do not exist. Furthermore, much of the LGBTQ+ youth suicide prevention research we have is focussed on biomedical clinical treatment using feasibility or acceptability pilot RCTs of CBT, and school-based public health suicide prevention. We discuss these both further in the next two sections.

Clinical and Mental Health Services

Given the prevalence of suicidal thoughts and attempts among LGBTQ+ youths, surprisingly few clinical treatment intervention models have been developed and tested for this population (Russon et al., 2022). In a review of the LGBTQI suicide treatment literature, Russon et al. (2022) identify several promising CBT approaches, often web-based, that have been developed and tested. There is a paucity of suicide-specific treatment model interventions, with those found using mainly CBT for depression and other outcomes related to suicidality (Lucassen et al., 2022; McDermott et al., 2021; Russon et al., 2022). Russon et al (2022) conclude that treatment research addressing suicide among LGBTQ+ youth remains in its infancy. The few existing pilot studies have sample sizes too small to demonstrate efficacy and this remains a barrier to developing more robust experimental tests of these interventions.

In addition to the evidence gap on the efficacy of LGBTQ+ suicide prevention, evidence suggests that there can be a stigma to using mental health services and this is particularly prevalent amongst young people and within LGBTQ+ communities. Research demonstrates that LGBTQ+ youth that struggle with suicidal distress and self-harm under-utilize mental health services, do not access them until crisis point and often find them unhelpful due to dismissive attitudes motivated by normative ideas about sexual orientation, gender identity, and emotional maturation (McDermott, 2015; McDermott et al., 2018). This hesitancy to access mental health services can be due to queerphobia, difficulties disclosing sexual and gender identity, or because of fears of being misunderstood or judged; with one UK study finding that only one fifth of participants had sought help from mainstream mental health services for their suicidal distress (McDermott et al., 2018a).

There is also evidence that LGBTQ+ young people have poor overall experiences of mental health services (McDermott et al., 2016; Williams & Chapman, 2011, 2015). Importantly, studies show that LGBTQ+ youth will seek mental health help online and from peers (McDermott, 2015) and would like their health practitioners to have an awareness of LGBTQ+ issues, with a preference for accessing LGBTQ+ specialist mental health support (Johnson et al., 2007; Marzetti, McDaid et al., 2022a). In an integrative review of emergency care for LGBTQ+ youth and suicidal distress, the authors found that youth seeking mental health crisis services chose services over others because the service was LGBTQ+ affirming, the support service was felt to be safe by LGBTQ+ youth, and provided in a timely way (Schultz et al., 2022). These features of LGBTQ+ youth appropriate mental health services have been shown in other research (albeit) early intervention support and not crisis care (McDermott et al., 2021).

School

School is a key focus of suicide prevention, as a site of risk and prevention. In a UK study, the experience of queerphobic abuse doubled the odds of planning or attempting suicide for participants and this abuse occurred most often in the school environment (McDermott et al., 2018). UNESCO's 'Out in the Open' global review reported that a significant proportion of LGBTQ+ young people experience school discrimination and/or violence based on their sexual orientation or gender identity or expression and the harmful impacts to education and mental wellbeing (UNESCO, 2016). UNESCO state that the education sector has a responsibility to provide safe and inclusive learning environments for all young people. However, few countries currently have a comprehensive education sector response in place (UNESCO, 2016).

Systematic reviews clearly indicate that positive school climate can lower the risk of suicide for LGBTQ+ youth (Ancheta et al., 2021; Gorse, 2022; Marraccini et al., 2022). There is now a substantial body of literature that examines factors that promote safe and positive school environments for LGBTQ+ youth (Hackimer & Proctor, 2015; Whitaker et al., 2016). School based LGBTQ+ support groups, such as Gay-Straight Alliances (GSAs), inclusive curricula and comprehensive LGBTQ+ anti-bullying and anti-harassment school policies have all been proposed to improve the academic performance (Kosciw et al., 2013), school safety and the mental health of LGBTQ+ youth through facilitating belonging and connectedness (Heck et al., 2011), reducing homophobia and victimisation (Ioverno et al., 2016; Kosciw et al., 2013) and helping students to identify supportive school staff (GLSEN, 2007; Kosciw et al., 2013).

Marraccini and colleagues (2022) ecological or systems model outlines a strengths-based, culturally responsive framework for approaching school-based suicide prevention among LGBTQ+ youth that includes (a) supporting positive identity development and self-advocacy in LGBTQ+ students, while acknowledging the heterogeneity; (b) fostering healthy and positive relationships and creating safe spaces (e.g., GSA) that celebrate the diversity of LGBTQ+ and ethnic and racial minoritized students within schools; (c) developing school-family and school-community partnerships; (d) building safe communities for schools and students and (e) cultivating social norms of acceptance of LGBTQ+ individuals. They argue that upstream approaches that foster a school climate of understanding, acceptance, and celebration of LGBTQ+ identities could prevent and reduce suicidality. Unfortunately, this is a model that has not been employed in any evaluated intervention.

Similarly, McDermott et al. (forthcoming, forthcoming) argue in their realist synthesis that school-based interventions that directly tackle dominant cisgender and heterosexual norms can improve LGBTQ+ pupils' mental health. The programme theory produced from this review posits three broad multilevel causal pathways in which the interventions might improve mental health: (1) interventions that promoted LGBTQ+ visibility and facilitated the 'usualising' of school belonging, and recognition; (2) interventions for talking and support that developed safety and coping and; (3) interventions that addressed institutional school culture (staff training and inclusion polices) that fostered school belonging, empowerment, recognition and safety. Overall, the evidence suggests that interventions that seek to make the school environment more inclusive for LGBTQ+ young people can improve mental health outcomes by both reducing poor mental health e.g., suicidal feelings, and increasing factors associated with good mental health such as self-esteem and coping.

Frameworks for LGBTQ+ Youth Suicide Prevention

Significantly, the WHO (2021) and UN (2016) recognise that LGBTQ+ youth are vulnerable to suicidal risk in comparison to their peers and advocate that national suicide prevention strategies specifically tackle this inequality. However, to prevent deaths by suicide, the World Health Organization (2021) has suggest a raft of suicide prevention measures that include awareness raising and advocacy around suicide prevention; capacity raising in professionals who work in roles that are likely to come into frequent contact with people in suicidal distress; resourcing for suicide prevention; restriction of access to lethal means; responsible reporting of suicide in the media; fostering socio-emotional life skills amongst children and young people; and enhancing population surveillance to improve the identification of people considered 'at risk' of suicide. These suicide prevention approaches have been criticised for taking a pathologising approach to suicide, individualising risk and viewing suicidal distress as a solely psychological problem, without sufficient consideration of social context. As a result the proposed prevention measures focus on overly narrow methods of 'death prevention' without considering ways to improve the social and material conditions for living (East et al., 2021; Marzetti, Oaten et al., 2022b).

Understanding suicide as a purely pathological problem narrows the potential ways we can intervene to prevent suicide. If we understand the roots of distress as beginning in the foundations of society around the individual and solidifying in the interactions between the individual and their social context, we open up the possibility that suicide prevention practices should not play into pathological ideas about suicidal people's *distorted perceptions* and should instead pay attention to their socio-economic positioning as well as the more individual, psychological contributors (Marzetti et al., 2022a, b). Increasingly, there are now alternatives to individual, pathologizing approaches to LGBTQ+ youth suicide prevention that draw on social and cultural framings of suicide prevention (McDermott et al., 2021): such as public health models, systems-approaches, socio-ecological and human rights framings.

The systems or ecological approach has been developed in a series of systematic reviews (Marraccini et al., 2022; McDermott et al., forthcoming; Poštuvan et al., 2019) of suicide prevention for LGBTQ+ youth suicide, demonstrating that suicidal distress originates in the social environment in which LGBTQ young people live. Poštuvan et al. (2019) in their model of the role of non-acceptance in LGBTIQ youths' development of suicidal behaviour shows how negative social environments (such as a non-inclusive school climate), inadequate support within the closest social network, and an absence of LGBTQ support in communities can contribute to the development of suicidality in young people. The authors of these reviews argue that for suicide prevention efforts to be effective, interventions must address specifically the marginalisation, silence, victimization and misrecognition that LGBTQ+ pupils experience within the dominant cis-heteronormative school, family, peer, digital environments (McDermott et al., forthcoming).

Public health models designed to promote public mental wellbeing and prevent suicide, provide a way of thinking that goes beyond just individual distress. These models, such as the biopsychosocial model and the socio-ecological model highlight the importance of identifying individuals, community and populations with heightened vulnerability to suicidality. Equally critical is the identification of broader socio-cultural environmental or individual protective factors which may reduce a person's vulnerability to suicidal behaviours. Marshall (2016) utilizes the socio-ecological approach to LGBTQ+ youth suicide prevention and argues that it addresses the complex interplay between multiple levels of influence, including individual, relationship, community, and societal factors. Socio-ecological models allows us to understand the range of factors that put individuals at risk of suicide or protect them from experiencing suicidal distress. This approach is often conceived as a 3-tier approach to suicide prevention. The primary level describes interventions targeting universal/general population and aims to modify the social determinants associated with suicidality (e.g. school victimization) including strengthening protective processes (e.g. social connectedness). The secondary level includes interventions which are focusing on particular at-risk populations, in this case LGBTQ+ youth, who may not yet have made a suicide attempt. The tertiary level interventions target specific vulnerable individuals within the population who have made a suicide attempt.

While it is encouraging that there are emerging models of LGBTQ+ suicide prevention that go beyond an individual approach, we remain concerned that worldwide there are very few attempts to prevent suicide in LGBTQ+ young people. We argue that a human-rights approach to LGBTQ+ suicide prevention may be a solution to the inertia currently evident across global suicide prevention policy and practice.

Human-Rights Approach to LGBTQ+ Youth Suicide Prevention

The 2021 WHO 'Helping Adolescents Thrive' document identifies LGBTQ+ young people as vulnerable to poor mental health and advocates a socio-ecological and human rights approach to promoting positive mental health in young people, addressing risk factors at individual, family, community & societal levels to protect and promote young people's mental health. This human-rights approach is echoed by the UN in the UNCRC (2016) implementation of the rights of the child during adolescence. LGBTQ+ and ethnic minority/indigenous young people are identified as those who commonly face difficulties because their age and identities can expose them to discrimination, social exclusion, marginalization, bullying, social injustice and non-inclusion in public spaces. This increases their vulnerability to poverty, mental health issues, including disproportionately high suicide rates, homelessness, poor educational outcomes and high levels of detention within the criminal justice system. They advocate emphasis of ensuring non-discrimination (article 2) and the necessity of an 'intersectional' (UNCRC, 2016, p. 7) approach to improve these injustices and mental health. WHO concur:

> Children and adolescents with mental disorders should be provided with early intervention through evidence-based psychosocial and other non-pharmacological interventions based in the community, avoiding institutionalization and medicalization. Furthermore, interventions should respect the rights of children in line with the United Nations Convention on the Rights of the Child and other international and regional human rights instruments. (Comprehensive Mental Health Action Plan 2013–2030, p. 11) (WHO, 2021)

An example of this 'upstream' approach is in Australia where a systems approach to suicide prevention has been implemented. This strategy utilised a suite of interventions aimed at different elements of the system to reduce suicidality in Aboriginal and Torres Strait Islander people and LGBTQ+ people (WHO, 2021). This included prevention efforts such as cultural-strengthening activities, mental health-awareness, school-based programmes, aftercare support after suicide/attempt. Another example, also in Australia, is a LGBTQI specific programme to promote creating inclusive and safe training workshops for LGBTIQ communities, by LGBTIQ communities; and strengthening the capacity of LGBTIQ organizations to become suicide-safer communities (WHO, 2021, p. 92). This directly addresses concerns regarding a LGBTQ+ youth 'suicide consensus' (Bryan and Mayock, 2017). Unfortunately, these are rare examples of suicide prevention efforts to reduce suicidality in LGBTQ+ young people.

What Is Hindering Policy and Practice Attempts to Reduce LGBTQ+ Youth Suicide?

The absence of international or national suicide prevention strategies for LGBTQ+ young people (or any LGBTQ+ age group) can be explained, in our view, in a number of ways. The exclusion of sexual orientation and gender identity from explanatory models of health inequality, such as the WHO 'equity framework for the Social Determinants of Health' contributes to as Fish and colleagues state: (Fish et al., 2021) 'the subordinate status of SOGI in international policy-making, practice developments and the funding of research to inform evidence-based decision-making' (p. 1). In addition, we would argue that LGBTQ+ mental health inequality is depoliticised by existing public health explanatory theories, models and frameworks that exclude sexual orientation and gender diversity as dimensions of power that interlock with those of socio-economic, race and ethnicity. Furthermore, the framing of national policy discussions of LGBTQ+ youth suicidality within a depoliticised 'it's getting better' narrative, and an unwillingness to adequately acknowledge the unjust social and economic relations that produce LGBTQ+ mental health inequalities side-steps the development of policy, programmes and interventions that can successfully prevent LGBTQ+ youth suicidality.

Perhaps most concerning is the continuation of discriminatory pathologizing histories and legacies that present challenges to LGBTQ+ equality and human rights legislation especially in terms of gender recognition. There is an absence of attention to the social circumstances in which young people are unable to express freely their identity without discrimination, feel safe in education, and develop without fear, which are all contraventions of the UN Convention on the Rights of the Child. The neoliberal state reluctance to address multiple social and economic issues such as isolation due to cis-heteronormativity that exclude and push diverse LGBTQ+ people to the margins act, as Marzetti, Oaten et al. (2022b, p. 11) argue, to manoeuvre suicide 'outside of the public and political sphere and into the private realm of individual pathology' and thus avoids framing LGBTQ+ youth suicidality as a human rights issue.

The UN and the WHO identify the fundamental relationship between human rights and mental health. Both argue that the most effective way to improve young people's mental health should be based on a human rights approach (UNCRC, 2016, p. 16). UNICEF (UK) argue that 'it is key that local government, services and professionals frame good mental health as a basic human right, one all children and young people are entitled to' (UNICEF, 2021). The UN Convention on the Rights of the Child states that young people have a right to good mental health and mental health services (Article 24), alongside rights to non-discrimination (Article 2), and identity (Article 8), and the right to education (Article 28). However, the integration of human rights commitments for children and young people into law, policy and practice worldwide has been slow and inconsistent (Lundy et al., 2012). Globally, the absence of policy attention to the discriminatory experiences of LGBTQ+ pupils in schools and wider life and the consequences to their mental health is a human rights concern.

Conclusion

The 2016 UN Convention on the Rights of Child Committee General Comment no.20 (UNCRC, 2016) on the implementation of child rights during adolescence specifically emphasize that nation states should take effective action to protect lesbian, gay, bisexual, transgender and intersex adolescents from all forms of violence, discrimination or bullying and to improve mental health. We argue from a queer critical suicidology perspective that LGBTQ+ young people's suicide prevention must be approached from a human rights perspective. Current approaches that individualize, pathologise and depoliticize LGBTQ+ youth suicide, avoid acknowledging that LGBTQ+ youth suicide is a human rights issue. This means nation states do not recognise that young people with diverse genders and sexualities may be subject to daily contraventions of their rights at school, home, online and from those around them.

LGBTQ+ young people worldwide continue to confront active legislative and policy attacks on their human rights. For example, the UK, despite protective legislation, was identified alongside Hungary and Poland in a 2021 Council of Europe report condemning attacks on LGBTQ+ human rights, particularly for trans people (Ben Chikha, 2021). The ongoing attacks on LGBTQ+ young people's rights, and the uncertainty surrounding global LGBTQ+ rights suggest more than ever that LGBTQ+ youth suicide should be viewed as a human rights issue.

While national governments and the academy are willing to superficially acknowledge suicide as a biopsychosocial issue, the emphasis is still about preventing the 'moment of death' rather than a focus on the rights of LGBTQ+ young people to live in an environment in which they can thrive (Russon et al., 2022). In our view LGBTQ+ suicide prevention needs a human rights approach to address the multiple marginalisation, isolation, and stigmatisation that LGBTQ+ young people may experience. A human-rights approach to suicide prevention means ensuring the right to freedom of safe self-expression to be upheld and enabling LGBTQ+ young people to envision a more optimistic future and one worth living.

References

Almeida, J., Johnson, R. M., Corliss, H. L., Molnar, B. E., & Azrael, D. (2009). Emotional distress among LGBT youth: The influence of perceived discrimination based on sexual orientation. *Journal of Youth & Adolescence, 38*, 1001–1014. https://doi.org/10.1007/s10964-009-9397-9

Ancheta, A. J., Bruzzese, J. M., & Hughes, T. L. (2021). The impact of positive school climate on suicidality and mental health among LGBTQ adolescents: A systematic review. *Journal of School Nursing, 37*(2), 75–86. https://doi.org/10.1177/1059840520970847

Bailey, E., Alvarez-Jimenez, M., Robinson, J., D'alfonso, S., Nedeljkovic, M., Davey, C. G., Bendall, S., Gilbertson, T., Phillips, J., Bloom, L., Nicholls, L., Garland, N., Cagliarini, D., Phelan, M., McKechnie, B., Mitchell, J., Cooke, M., & Rice, S. M. (2020). An enhanced social networking intervention for young people with active suicidal ideation: Safety, feasibility and acceptability outcomes. *International Journal of Environmental Research and Public Health, 17*. https://doi.org/10.3390/ijerph17072435

Bailey, E., Rice, S., Robinson, J., Nedeljkovic, M., & Alvarez-Jimenez, M. (2018). Theoretical and empirical foundations of a novel online social networking intervention for youth suicide prevention: A conceptual review. *Journal of Affective Disorders, 238*, 499–505. https://doi.org/10.1016/j.jad.2018.06.028

Ben Chikha, F. (2021). *Combating rising hate against LGBTI people in Europe.* Retrieved from Strasbourg: https://assembly.coe.int/LifeRay/EGA/Pdf/Tex tesProvisoires/2021/20210921-RisingHateLGBTI-EN.pdf

Bryan, A., & Mayock, P. (2017). Supporting LGBT lives? Complicating the suicide consensus in LGBT mental health research. *Sexualities, 20,* 65–85. https://doi.org/10.1177/1363460716648099

Button, M. E. (2016). Suicide and social justice: Toward a political approach to suicide. *Political Research Quarterly, 69,* 270–280. https://doi.org/10.1177/1065912916636689

Calear, A. L., Christensen, H., Freeman, A., Fenton, K., Busby Grant, J., van Spijker, B., & Donker, T. (2016). A systematic review of psychosocial suicide prevention interventions for youth. *European Child and Adolescent Psychiatry, 25,* 467–482. https://doi.org/10.1007/s00787-015-0783-4

Canetto, S. S., Antonelli, P., Ciccotti, A., Dettore, D., & Lamis, D. A. (2021). Suicidal as normal—A lesbian, gay, and bisexual youth script? *Crisis, 42,* 292–300. https://doi.org/10.1027/0227-5910/a000730

Cash, S. J., & Bridge, J. A. (2009). Epidemiology of youth suicide and suicidal behavior. *Current Opinion Pediatrics, 21,* 613–619. https://doi.org/10.1097/MOP.0b013e32833063e1

Chandler, A., & Simopoulou, Z. (2020). Self-harm as an attempt at self-care. *European Journal for Qualitative Research in Psychotherapy, 10,* 110–120.

Clements-Nolle, K., Lensch, T., Baxa, A., Gay, C., Larson, S., & Yang, W. (2018). Sexual identity, adverse childhood experiences, and suicidal behaviors. *Journal of Adolescent Health, 62,* 198–204. https://doi.org/10.1016/j.jadohealth.2017.09.022

Cover, R. (2012). *Queer youth suicide, culture and identity: Unliveable lives?* Ashgate Publishing.

Crenshaw, K. (1989). Demarginalizing the intersection of race and sex: A black feminist critique of antidiscrimination doctrine, feminist theory and antiracist policies. In *The University of Chicago Legal Forum* (pp. 139–167). https://doi.org/10.1525/sp.2007.54.1.23.

Davy, Z. (2015). The DSM-5 and the politics of diagnosing transpeople. *Archives of Sexual Behavior, 44,* 1165–1176. https://doi.org/10.1007/s10508-015-0573-6

Davy, Z., & Toze, M. (2018). What is gender dysphoria? A critical systematic narrative review. *Transgender Health, 3,* 159–169. https://doi.org/10.1089/trgh.2018.0014

de Lange, J., Baams, L., van Bergen, D. D., Bos, H. M., & Bosker, R. J. (2022). Minority stress and suicidal ideation and suicide attempts among

LGBT adolescents and young adults: A meta-analysis. *LGBT Health, 9*(4), 222–237. https://doi.org/10.1089/lgbt.2021.0106

di Giacomo, E., Krausz, M., Colmegna, F., Aspesi, F., & Clerici, M. (2018). Estimating the risk of attempted suicide among sexual minority youths. *JAMA Pediatrics*, 1–8. https://doi.org/10.1001/jamapediatrics.2018.2731.

Dube, S. R., Anda, R. F., Felitti, V. J., Chapman, D. P., Williamson, D. F., & Giles, W. H. (2001). Childhood abuse, household dysfunction, and the risk of attempted suicide throughout the life span: Findings from the adverse childhood experiences study. *Journal of the American Medical Association, 286*, 3089–3096. https://doi.org/10.1001/jama.286.24.3089

East, L., Dorozenko, K. P., & Martin, R. (2021). The construction of people in suicide prevention documents. *Death Studies, 45*, 182–190. https://doi.org/10.1080/07481187.2019.1626938

Eliason, M. (2010). Introduction to special issue on suicide, mental health, and youth development. *Journal of Homosexuality, 58*, 4–9. https://doi.org/10.1080/00918369.2011.533622

Evans, E., Hawton, K., & Rodham, K. (2004). Factors associated with suicidal phenomena in adolescents: A systematic review of population-based studies. *Clinical Psychology Review, 24*, 957–979. https://doi.org/10.1016/j.cpr.2004.04.005

Fish, J., Almack, K., Hafford-Letchfield, T., & Toze, M. (2021). What are LGBT+ inequalities in health and social support—Why should we tackle them? *International Journal of Environmental Research and Public Health, 18*(7), 3612. https://doi.org/10.3390/ijerph18073612

Formby, E. (2017). *Exploring LGBT spaces and communities. Contrasting identities, belongings and wellbeing*. Routledge.

Formby, E. (2015). Limitations of focussing on homophobic, biphobic and transphobic 'bullying' to understand and address LGBT young people's experiences within and beyond school. *Sex Education, 15*, 626–640. https://doi.org/10.1080/14681811.2015.1054024

GLSEN. (2007). *Gay-straight alliances: Creating safer schools for LGBT students and their allies*. https://www.glsen.org/sites/default/files/2020-04/Gay-Str aight%20Alliances.pdf.

Gorse, M. (2022). Risk and protective factors to LGBTQ plus youth suicide: A review of the literature. *Child and Adolescent Social Work Journal, 39*(1), 17–28. https://doi.org/10.1007/s10560-020-00710-3

Gould, M. S., & Kramer, R. A. (2001). Youth suicide prevention. *Children, Violence and Bullying: International Perspectives, 31*, 271–281. https://doi.org/10.1521/suli.31.1.5.6.24219

Hacking, I. (2006). Making up people. *London Review of Books, 28.*

Hackimer, L., & Proctor, S. L. (2015). Considering the community influence for lesbian, gay, bisexual, and transgender youth. *Journal of Youth Studies, 18*(3), 277–290. https://doi.org/10.1080/13676261.2014.944114

Hatchel, T., Polanin, J. R., & Espelage, D. L. (2021). Suicidal thoughts and behaviors among LGBTQ youth: Meta-analyses and a systematic review. *Archives of Suicide Research, 25*(1), 1–37. https://doi.org/10.1080/13811118.2019.1663329

Hatzenbuehler, M. L. (2009). How does sexual minority stigma "get under the skin"? A psychological mediation framework. *Psychological Bulletin, 135,* 707–730. https://doi.org/10.1037/a0016441

Hawton, K., Saunders, K. E. A., O'Connor, R. C. (2012). Suicide 1 self-harm and suicide in adolescents. *The Lancet, 379,* 2373–2382. https://doi.org/10.1016/S0140-6736(12)60322-5.

Heck, N. C., Flentje, A., & Cochran, B. N. (2011). Offsetting risks: High school gay-straight alliances and lesbian, gay, bisexual, and transgender (LGBT) youth. *School Psychology Quarterly, 26*(2), 161–174. https://doi.org/10.1037/a0023226

Hubbard, K. A., & Griffiths, D. A. (2019). Sexual offence, diagnosis, and activism: A British history of LGBTIQ psychology. *American Psychologist, 74,* 940–953. https://doi.org/10.1037/amp0000544

Ioverno, S., Belser, A. B., Baiocco, R., Grossman, A. H., & Russell, S. T. (2016). The protective role of gay–straight alliances for lesbian, gay, bisexual, and questioning students: A prospective analysis. *Psychology of Sexual Orientation and Gender Diversity, 3*(4), 397. https://doi.org/10.1037/sgd0000193

Johnson, K., Faulkner, P., Jones, H., & Welsh, E. (2007). *Understanding suicidal distress and promoting survival in lesbian, gay, bisexual and transgender (LGBT) communities.* University of Brighton.

Joiner, T. E. (2007). *Why people die by suicide.* Harvard University Press.

Jowett, A. (2017). Representing the history of LGBT rights: Political rhetoric surrounding the 50th anniversary of the Sexual Offences Act 1967. *Psychology and Sexuality, 8,* 306–317. https://doi.org/10.1080/19419899.2017.1383303

King, C. A., Arango, A., & Ewell Foster, C. (2018). Emerging trends in adolescent suicide prevention research. *Current Opinion in Psychology, 22,* 89–94. https://doi.org/10.1016/j.copsyc.2017.08.037

Kosciw, J. G., Palmer, N. A., Kull, R. M., & Greytak, E. A. (2013). The effect of negative school climate on academic outcomes for LGBT youth and the role of in-school supports. *Journal of School Violence, 12*(1), 45–63. https:// doi.org/10.1080/15388220.2012.732546

LeCloux, M., Maramaldi, P., Thomas, K., & Wharff, E. (2017). Health care resources and mental health service use among suicidal adolescents. *Journal of Behavioral Health Services and Research, 44*, 195–212. https://doi.org/10. 1007/s11414-016-9509-8

Lucassen, M. F. G., Nunez-Garcia, A., Rimes, K. A., Wallace, L. M., Brown, K. E., & Samra, R. (2022). Coping strategies to enhance the mental well-being of sexual and gender minority youths: A scoping review. *International Journal of Environmental Research and Public Health, 19*(14). https://doi.org/ 10.3390/ijerph19148738.

Lundy, L., Kilkelly, U., Byrne, B., & Kang, J. (2012). *The UN Convention on the Rights of the Child: A study of legal implementation in 12 countries.* Retrieved from Belfast: https://www.unicef.org.uk/wp-content/uploads/ 2012/11/UNICEFUK_2012CRCimplementationreport-FINAL-PDF-ver sion.pdf

Marchi, M., Arcolin, E., Fiore, G., Travascio, A., Uberti, D., Amaddeo, F., Converti, M., Fiorillo, A., Mirandola, M., Pinna, F., Ventriglio, A., & Italian Working Group on LGBTIQ Mental Health. (2022). Self-harm and suicidality among LGBTIQ people: a systematic review and meta-analysis. *International Review of Psychiatry, 34*(3-4), 240-256. doi:https:// doi.org/10.1080/09540261.2022.2053070.

Marraccini, M. E., Ingram, K. M., Naser, S. C., Grapin, S. L., Toole, E. N., O'Neill, J. C., Chin, A. J., Martinez, R. R., & Griffin, D. (2022). The roles of school in supporting LGBTQ plus youth: A systematic review and ecological framework for understanding risk for suicide-related thoughts and behaviors. *Journal of School Psychology, 91*, 27–49. https://doi.org/10.1016/ j.jsp.2021.11.006.

Marshal, M. P., Dietz, L. J., Friedman, M. S., Stall, R., Smith, H. A., McGinley, J., Thoma, B. C., Murray, P. J., D'Augelli, A. R., & Brent, D. A. (2011). Suicidality and depression disparities between sexual minority and heterosexual youth: A meta-analytic review. *Journal of Adolescent Health, 49*, 115–123. https://doi.org/10.1016/j.jadohealth.2011.02.005

Marshall, A. (2016). Suicide prevention interventions for sexual & gender minority youth: An unmet need. *Yale Journal of Biology and Medicine, 89*, 205–213.

Marzetti, H. (2018). Proudly proactive: Celebrating and supporting LGBT+ students in Scotland. *Teaching in Higher Education, 23*, 701–717. https:// doi.org/10.1080/13562517.2017.1414788

Marzetti, H., Chandler, A., Jordan, A., & Oaten, A. (in press). The politics of LGBT+ suicide and suicide prevention in the UK: Risk, responsibility and rhetoric. *Culture, Health & Sexuality*.

Marzetti, H., McDaid, L., & O'Connor, R. (2022a). "Am I really alive?": Understanding the role of homophobia, biphobia and transphobia in young LGBT+ people's suicidal distress. *Social Science and Medicine, 298*, 114860. https://doi.org/10.1016/j.socscimed.2022.114860.

Marzetti, H., Oaten, A., Chandler, A., & Jordan, A. (2022b). Self-inflicted. Deliberate. Death-intentioned. A critical policy analysis of UK suicide prevention policies 2009–2019. *Journal of Public Mental Health, 21*, 4–14. https://doi.org/10.1108/JPMH-09-2021-0113

Marzetti, H., Chandler, A., Jordan, A., & Oaten, A. (2023). The politics of LGBT+ suicide and suicide prevention in the UK: Risk, responsibility and rhetoric. *Culture, Health & Sexuality*, 1–18. https://doi.org/10.1080/13691058.2023.2172614

Marzetti, H., McDaid, L., & O'Connor, R. (2023). A qualitative study of young people's lived experiences of suicide and self-harm: Intentionality, rationality and authenticity. *Child and Adolescent Mental Health*. https://doi.org/10.1111/camh.12641

Marzetti, H. L. (2020). *Exploring and understanding young LGBT+ people's suicidal thoughts and attempts in Scotland*.

McDermott, E. (2015). Asking for help online: Lesbian, gay, bisexual and trans youth, self-harm and articulating the "failed" self. *Health, 19*, 561–577. https://doi.org/10.1177/1363459314557967

McDermott, E., Hughes, E., & Rawlings, V. (2016). *Queer futures. Understanding lesbian, gay, bisexual and trans (LGBT) adolescents' suicide, self-harm and help-seeking behaviour* (Final Report).

McDermott, E., Hughes, E., & Rawlings, V. (2018a). Norms and normalisation: Understanding lesbian, gay, bisexual, transgender and queer youth, suicidality and help-seeking. *Culture, Health and Sexuality, 20*, 156–172. https://doi.org/10.1080/13691058.2017.1335435

McDermott, E., Hughes, E., & Rawlings, V. (2018b). The social determinants of lesbian, gay, bisexual and transgender youth suicidality in England: A mixed methods study. *Journal of Public Health, 40*(3), E244–E251. https://doi.org/10.1093/pubmed/fdx135

McDermott, E., Eastham, R., Hughes, E., Pattinson, E., Johnson, K., Davis, S., Pryjmachuk, S., Mateus, C., & Jenzen, O. (2021). Explaining effective mental health support for LGBTQ+ youth: A meta-narrative review. *SSM-Mental Health, 1*, 100004. https://doi.org/10.1016/j.ssmmh.2021.100004.

McDermott, E., Kaley, A., Kaner, E., Limmer, M., McGovern, R., McNulty, F., Nelson, R., Geijer-Simpson, E., & Spencer, L. (2022a). Reducing LGBTQ+ adolescent mental health inequalities: A realist review of school-based interventions. *BMC Public Health* (forthcoming).

McDermott, E., Kaley, A., Kaner, E., Limmer, M., McGovern, R., McNulty, F., Nelson, R., Geijer-Simpson, E., & Spencer, L. (2022b). Understanding how school-based interventions can tackle LGBTQ+ youth mental health inequality: A realist approach. *International Journal of Public Health Environment Research* (forthcoming)

McDermott, E., & Roen, K. (2016). *Queer youth, suicide and self-harm troubled subjects, troubling norms*. Palgrave Macmillan.

McDermott, E., Roen, K., & Scourfield, J. (2008). Avoiding shame: Young LGBT people, homophobia and self-destructive behaviours. *Culture, Health & Sexuality, 10*, 815–829. https://doi.org/10.1080/136910508023 80974

Meyer, I. (2003). Prejudice, social stress, and mental health in lesbian, gay, and bisexual populations: Conceptual issues and research evidence. *Psychological Bulletin, 129*, 674–697. https://doi.org/10.1037/0033-2909.129.5.674.

Meyer, I. H. (1995). Minority stress and mental health in gay men. *Journal of Health and Social Behavior, 36*, 38–56. https://doi.org/10.2307/2137286

Miller, D. N., & Eckert, T. L. (2009). Youth suicidal behavior: An introduction and overview. *School Psychology Review, 38*, 153–167.

Miranda-Mendizábal, A., Castellví, P., Parés-Badell, O., Almenara, J., Alonso, I., Blasco, M. J., Cebrià, A., Gabilondo, A., Gili, M., Lagares, C., Piqueras, J. A., Roca, M., Rodríguez-Marín, J., Rodríguez-Jiménez, T., Soto-Sanz, V., Vilagut, G., & Alonso, J. (2017). Sexual orientation and suicidal behaviour in adolescents and young adults: Systematic review and meta-analysis. *British Journal of Psychiatry, 211*, 77–87. https://doi.org/10.1192/bjp.bp.116.196345

O'Connor, R. C. (2023). *When it is darkest*. Vermillion.

O'Connor, R. C., & Kirtley, O. J. (2018). The integrated motivational–volitional model of suicidal behaviour. *Philosophical Transactions of the Royal Society B: Biological Sciences, 373*(1754), 20170268. https://doi.org/10.1098/rstb.2017.0268

Owens, D., Horrocks, J., & House, A. (2002). Fatal and non-fatal repetition of self-harm: Systematic review. *British Journal of Psychiatry, 181*, 193–199. https://doi.org/10.1192/bjp.181.3.193

Platt, S. (2016). Inequalities and suicial behavior. In R. C. O'Connor, & J. Pirkis (Eds.), *The international handbook of suicide prevention* (pp. 258–283). Wiley Blackwell.

Poštuvan, V., Podlogar, T., Zadravec Šedivy, N., & De Leo, D. (2019). Review suicidal behaviour among sexual-minority youth: A review of the role of acceptance and support. *The Lancet Child and Adolescent Health*, 1–9. https://doi.org/10.1016/S2352-4642(18)30400-0

Puckett, J. A., Horne, S. G., Surace, F., Carter, A., Noffsinger-Frazier, N., Shulman, J., Detrie, P., Ervin, A., & Mosher, C. (2017). Predictors of sexual minority youth's reported suicide attempts and mental health. *Journal of Homosexuality, 64*, 697–715. https://doi.org/10.1080/00918369.2016.119 6999

Riggs, D. W., Pearce, R., Pfeffer, C. A., Hines, S., White, F., & Ruspini, E. (2019). Transnormativity in the psy disciplines: Constructing pathology in the diagnostic and statistical manual of mental disorders and standards of care. *American Psychologist, 74*, 912–924. https://doi.org/10.1037/amp000 0545

Robinson, J., Cox, G., Malone, A., Williamson, M., Baldwin, G., Fletcher, K., & O'Brien, M. (2013). A systematic review of school-based interventions aimed at preventing, treating, and responding to suicide-related behavior in young people. *Crisis, 34*, 164–182. https://doi.org/10.1027/0227-5910/a000168

Robinson, J., Hetrick, S. E., & Martin, C. (2011). Preventing suicide in young people: Systematic review. *Australian & New Zealand Journal of Psychiatry, 45*(1), 3–26.

Russon, J., Washington, R., Machado, A., Smithee, L., & Dellinger, J. (2022). Suicide among LGBTQIA plus youth: A review of the treatment literature. *Aggression and Violent Behavior, 64*. https://doi.org/10.1016/j.avb.2021.101578.

Savin-Williams, R. C. (2001). A critique of research on sexual-minority youths. *Journal of Adolescence, 24*, 5–13. https://doi.org/10.1006/jado.2000.0369

Schnarrs, P. W., Stone, A. L., Salcido, R., Baldwin, A., & Nemeroff, C. B. (2019). Differences in adverse childhood experiences (ACEs) and quality of physical and mental health between transgender and cisgender sexual minorities. *Journal of Psychiatric Research, 119*, 1–6. https://doi.org/10.1016/j.jpsychires.2019.09.001

Schultz, T. R., Zoucha, R., & Sekula, L. K. (2022). The intersection between youth who identify as LGBTQ plus and emergency care for suicidality: An integrative review. *Journal of Pediatric Nursing-Nursing Care of Children & Families, 63,* E82–E94. https://doi.org/10.1016/j.pedn.2021.10.008

Scourfield, J., Roen, K., & McDermott, L. (2008). Lesbian, gay, bisexual and transgender young people's experiences of distress: Resilience, ambivalence and self-destructive behaviour. *Health and Social Care in the Community, 16,* 329–336. https://doi.org/10.1111/j.1365-2524.2008.00769.x

Surace, T., Fusar-Poli, L., Vozza, L., Cavone, V., Arcidiacono, C., Mammano, R., Basile, L., Rodolico, A., Bisicchia, P., Caponnetto, P., & Signorelli, M. S. (2021). Lifetime prevalence of suicidal ideation and suicidal behaviors in gender non-conforming youths: A meta-analysis. *European Child & Adolescent Psychiatry, 30,* 1147–1161. https://doi.org/10.1007/s00787-020-01508-5.

UNCRC. (2016). *General comment No. 20 (2016) on the implementation of the rights of the child during adolescence.*

UNESCO. (2016). *Out in the open: Education sector responses to violence based on sexual orientation and gender identity/expression.* UNESCO.

UNICEF. (2021). *Children's rights in the new normal: Mental health.* Retrieved from London: https://www.unicef.org.uk/child-friendly-cities/wp-content/uploads/sites/3/2021/10/Mental-health_UNICEF-UK-New-Normal-series.pdf

Waidzunas, T. (2012). Young, gay, and suicidal: Dynamic nominalism and the process of defining a social problem with statistics. *Science Technology and Human Values, 37,* 199–225. https://doi.org/10.1177/0162243911402363

Whitaker, K., Shapiro, V. B., & Shields, J. P. (2016). School-based protective factors related to suicide for lesbian, gay, and bisexual adolescents. *Journal of Adolescent Health, 58*(1), 63–68. https://doi.org/10.1016/j.jadohealth.2015.09.008

Williams, A. J., Jones, C., Arcelus, J., Townsend, E., Lazaridou, A., & Michail, M. (2021). A systematic review and meta-analysis of victimisation and mental health prevalence among LGBTQ+ young people with experiences of self-harm and suicide. *PLoS One, 16*(1), e0245268. https://doi.org/10.1371/journal.pone.0245268.

Williams, K. A., & Chapman, M. V. (2011). Comparing health and mental health needs, service use, and barriers to services among sexual minority youths and their peers. *Health & Social Work, 36*(3), 197–206. https://doi.org/10.1093/hsw/36.3.197

Williams, K. A., & Chapman, M. V. (2015). Mental health service use among youth with mental health need: Do school-based services make a difference for sexual minority youth? *School Mental Health, 7*(2), 120–131. https://doi.org/10.1007/s12310-014-9132-x

WHO. (2021). Live life: An implemetation guide for suicide prevention in countries. WHO. https://www.who.int/publications/i/item/WHO-MSD-UCN-MHE-22.02

World Health Organisation (WHO). (2021a). *Comprehensive Mental Health Action Plan 2013–2030*. Retrieved from Genever: https://www.who.int/publications/i/item/9789240031029

World Health Organisation (WHO). (2021b). *Helping adolescents thrive toolkit: Strategies to promote and protect adolescent mental health and reduce self-harm and other risk behaviours*. WHO Geneva

Wozolek, B., Wootton, L., & Demlow, A. (2017). The school-to-coffin pipeline: Queer youth, suicide, and living the in-between. *Cultural Studies—Critical Methodologies, 17*, 392–398. https://doi.org/10.1177/1532708616673659

Ybarra, M. L., Mitchell, K. J., Kosciw, J. G., & Korchmaros, J. D. (2015). Understanding linkages between bullying and suicidal ideation in a national sample of LGB and heterosexual youth in the United States. *Prevention Science, 16*, 451–462. https://doi.org/10.1007/s11121-014-0510-2

17

Sexual Minority Mental Health: A Public Health Perspective

Joanna Semlyen and Jim McManus

In this conversation (audio recorded and transcribed), Jim McManus and Joanna Semlyen talk about trauma, love, and public health in sexual minority mental health.

Joanna: Sexual minority mental health is an enduring and compelling public health issue. About this, we both agree, and strongly agree at that. I would like to explore this with you, for the reader. Thus, can we talk about your perspective about mental health in this population from your position as someone who is both a psychologist, and a public health director?

Jim: I think the benefit of taking a public health approach to the mental health of sexual minorities is that you can focus on both the

J. Semlyen (✉)
Norwich Medical School, University of East Anglia, Norwich, UK
e-mail: j.semlyen@uea.ac.uk

J. McManus
Association of Directors of Public Health, London, UK
e-mail: Jim.McManus@hertfordshire.gov.uk

© The Author(s), under exclusive license to Springer Nature Switzerland AG 2023
J. Semlyen and P. Rohleder (eds.), *Sexual Minorities and Mental Health*,
https://doi.org/10.1007/978-3-031-37438-8_17

421

antecedents and the determinants of poor mental health and of good mental health. So, it forces you to look above an individual lens to the lens of looking at population exposure. Now when you combine that socio-epidemiological perspective with the benefits of being also a chartered psychologist, you can start to take what I think some people who in the 1990s were trying to call a 'public health psychology approach' or a 'public mental health approach'. So, you can begin to look at the fact that the mental health of LGB people is not something which is either purely biological or purely psychological, or purely about them as individuals. There are social causes, there are institutional causes, and there are structural causes. And that gives you a scientific perspective on actions to change it. So, for example, if you are being homophobically bullied at work, as I think most of us have had experience in our lives (I certainly have), giving you a bit of counselling is a 'Band-Aid' when what needs to change is the organization's culture, policies and behaviour.

Joanna: In an ideal world, we would intervene at the structural level, wouldn't we? Do you think that there is a chance that we can make inroads into our current, still homophobic society and effect the changes we need to?

Jim: Yes. So, I'm a great fan of the old 1990 edition of the *Oxford Textbook of Public Health*, the great big, thick thing that does great services as a doorstop but is a wonderful resource. Detels and colleagues, talked about levels of public health: that most public health interventions are not at the biological level, but they also require the psychological level, the social level of interaction between groups, the organizational level and the structural or environmental or political level (Holland et al., 1997). And if you look at something like public mental health, actually, working at a biological level or a psychological level to strengthen the individual is all very well, but you need to also work up to the institutional level. School anti bullying policies are a good example. Changing organizational cultures are a good example. Training sexual minority leaders not to be the heroes who go in and become sacrificial and harm themselves, but to become cool producers of a culture which is supportive of sexual minorities in leadership, is another way, because you are engaging at an organizational level to change culture or policy. And from a public health perspective, I would say you will not get good mental health for lesbian, gay and bisexual people until you do it at a cultural level and an organizational level. The individual level only is essential to support those individuals, but if you don't do the cultural stuff, you really are not going to change society.

Joanna: You've been in public health for 30 years. Would you say that society has become more welcoming and less homophobic in that time?

Jim: I think some bits have. I think some bits have got worse. Similarly with some faith groups, there is still huge prejudice. I've worked with people recently who have a problem with me as a gay man and I've been attacked for it. So, I think it is it is very mixed, and the progress is fragile because it only takes one person to hate, or try to undermine you, to move progress back. That is why the structural level is as important as the individual attitudinal level and strengthening people.

Joanna: That example of a single incident setting you back is a really powerful narrative, and it strikes me that we know from lots of research that sexual minorities are either avoiding altogether or delaying in presenting with mental health conditions to health services. Do you feel that there are things to learn from broader public health under-standings of minority groups that are not yet being adopted that perhaps should be adopted by mainstream mental health services, so that they're more inclusive for sexual minorities?

Jim: Oh yes, and I think there's huge riches and there's a book in there by itself. To start with, the kind of methodological issue, we often talk about interdisciplinary work, which is great but often what happens is you take a discipline, you sit it next to another discipline and you go "OK, that's interesting". And what I'm really interested in, and I think this has come about from engineering science, is what we might call *transdisciplinary* work, which is, you dialogue critically different sets of knowledge to the point where you actually produce some new synthe-sized knowledge out of it. So, if we were going for this idea of "what can public health psychology say about access to health services for lesbian, gay, bisexual people?", for a starter there's the level of welcoming that you give people. I know people think the pride (rainbow) badge was a nice gesture for the NHS, but actually it does make a difference for some LGB people. But if you then get discrimination, that can actually become counterproductive. I think there are lessons from trauma, because if you have been beaten up for being gay or lesbian or bisexual in your past, or you've had a really bad employment experience, or a really judgemental health service experience, it is very easy, I think, to have that trauma reopened, if it happens again. So, there are lessons there from trauma psychology, for example, about re-traumatizing people, particularly with hate crime.

So I think there are huge lessons. Even if it's just co-producing with people who use services for trauma; there are multiple lessons that we can learn from a public health perspective of: "look at this population, this population has already been traumatized, they are more open to being harmed further. What makes them vulnerable to that? What can we structurally do about that? What mechanisms can we put in place and how do we protect them from being further harmed?"

So, the public health lens is a very powerful one and something I often see about public health is, it's a bit like the scavenger of the science world. We actually nick lots of stuff from other peoples' sciences. Epidemiology was a social science in Germany in the 1700s. You could also say that statistics and data is a biomedical science that public health nicked. Planning policy, well, public health got involved in that too. I'd love more psychologists and more policy people to take that public health lens and make it their own in their own work.

Joanna: I wonder if you had a view on the lived experience of sexual minorities… and, when you're talking about trauma, and perhaps this idea of re-traumatization in this population, whether you feel that that might be one of the reasons (because we don't fully know the reasons), why people consider mainstream mental health services as something that they are not that confident about or feel that safe with?

Jim: I remember in 2002 doing some work with Ian Rivers for the Home Office on a toolkit on addressing homophobic violence and we created a set of standards and tips then for the Home Office and the police to use. And one of the sections of that document, if I remember rightly, because it was 20 years ago, was 'things that the police service needs to do not to make it worse'. I think we phrased it like that because actually, if you walk into a police station and you feel dismissed or judged or unwelcome because of the banter that's around (and that's a loaded word), that can retraumatize you and make it worse. So, if you take that lens and apply it to mental health services, undoubtedly, the top line for me about trauma is most people grow beyond it and get beyond it, but some people don't. And it doesn't mean, even if your trauma is resolved, that it goes away and will never come back again. So, if you go to a mental health service where you've been judged before, you can feel judged again. If you go to a mental health service and your partner is unwelcome, you can be judged again.

There are different layers. We had an experience in our Hospice of a woman whose wife died in our Hospice, who came to our Hospice because she had been treated very homophobically in an NHS hospital and you don't need that at end of life care. You don't need that in mental health care. Why would you go to services that don't want to welcome you? So that's one layer. I think the next layer is whether the service actually understands you. The power of kinship; and the meaning of 'family' for sexual minorities, in terms of friends, not biological family, is something I think a lot of services still struggle with. And you'd have thought, during the years of AIDS, you know, so many of us who were family to people who we lost. Uh, not biological family, but every bit as important, and sometimes more important than biological family, would mean the health service had learned that.

And when you look at the mental health impact of Monkey Pox, the stigma of the lesions, the stigma of having to self-isolate, the stigma of people finding out about your sexuality, the stigma of being talked about... I think we failed an awful lot of people as a system because we didn't take seriously the mental health issue. We treated it as yet another Health Protection issue. The beauty of sexual health services is they love people. I think if public health is anything, it is an exercise in love at a population level. Sandro Galea, the American epidemiologist, talks about public health being an exercise in love (Galea, 2020). Avedis Donabedian, the founder of healthcare quality science also talked about good quality healthcare being an exercise in love (Best & Neuhauser, 2004). So, we have to apply that quality, and that love, to sexual minorities because actually they pay their taxes. They have a right and expectation to it. And the public health lens would say *because* they are more likely to be victimized and harmed, we should go out of our way to make sure that they find those services accessible and loving. That's a principle of equity I think that public health has at its heart, even if it doesn't always live it. I have to get the love word in; there's no point doing the job otherwise.

Joanna: We know individual level services are not meeting the needs of the LGB community's own mental health needs, and that change at the structural level is so important. Can we talk about that a little further, perhaps breaking it down into examples that help structural interventions make sense to our readers?

Jim: I would say probably there's two things there, keeping the structural public health lens in mind, the world of education and the world of work. In the world of education, we spend an awful lot of our youth at school and in childhood, and I'm often staggered by the lack of policy application to make sure LGB children are not disadvantaged by hostile and homophobic educational environments because it ruins their attainment. So, if the best things you can do for a child from a public health perspective are to get them vaccinated, get their eyesight and hearing tested, and get their developmental milestones checked so that they can do maximum educational attainment. That means if the child is going to be lesbian, gay or bisexual, or even just questioning or unsure about who they are, you need to actually create an environment as such that they flourish in school. So that they have the maximum potential in life. That's a public health task and it's a structural task that requires school policies.

You translate that to work. Derek Mowbray would say, the primary task of an employer is actually to build a positive psychosocial environment in the workplace for your employees (Mowbray, 2014), and in English employment law there is a something which is called a fundamental covenant of trust and confidence between employer and employee. If you don't have that, your employment contract is broken, either by you or your employer. So being comfortable and included as a sexual minority in that employment environment is really crucial. That's why the world of work has to be accepting and enabling and inclusive, because you get more productivity. So consequently, that needs to follow through in how you recruit, how you manage LGB staff, but also how you build leaders and managers.

If you are building diverse leaders, we need to be careful—thing is, we expect them to be heroes and go out there and be campaigners, and that requires people to be very kenotic—to be self-emptying—and, if they're self-emptying, what's going to fill them up? And why should they have to self-empty when nobody else has to? That's structurally unfair. So, we're building into workplace diversity champions, a program that actually can harm people. So I think we need much more of a public health mindset applied to the world of work and the world of education, and therefore to health services. I would say a taking a public health approach to inclusion and not an individualized approach is key.

Joanna: We are talking about people avoiding mainstream services, and why they may not be meeting needs, by taking a heteronormative, individualised approach. Community-led organizations are providing an excellent alternative to mainstream mental health services for LGB people, such as MindOUT, London Friend, LGBT Foundation. Why do you think they are so successful for LGB populations?

Jim: There are multiple reasons why community-led organizations are so successful. And there are a few of them that strike me immediately. The first is they're ours. They understand us, they understand me. There are people like me running them and working in them who've had my challenges in ways that all those mainstream staff/services might not understand. And however empathetic a straight person in the mental health services might be, sometimes you just need to talk to somebody who actually instinctively knows what you've been through.

And you know, we knew that through HIV. We knew that through Monkey Pox. It wasn't what the statutory sector did, however much we may want to claim that. So that's the first thing; it's identity, it's family, it's something tribal and it's about safety.

I think the second thing is there's all sorts of cultural norms and ways of understanding and working and language that our community organizations understand that the big mainstream organizations may not understand. And that can be healing and welcoming in and of itself. If you need someone to reach you where you're hurting and feel safe, it can feel safer.

I think the third thing is I would often see many of the people in LGB organizations are themselves wounded healers, and there is something in the evidence that's very powerful about people who've been where you are, showing you that it is a possible to find healing. I would say I think that lesbian, gay, bisexual organisations often underestimate the value that they do. Mainstream organisations do their jobs very well, but the foundational layer, that mainstream organizations will never, ever, ever replicate, is the sheer love that comes from them for our own tribe, our own 'family', if you like. And I'm not sorry to put it that way because we shouldn't apologise; an LGB person can understand my grief and my issues better than many heterosexuals, however empathetic, and that's just the way it is. We need to see that as an as an inescapable value, so these community agencies don't become second best. And we know you have to provide mainstream services, but these community organizations are valued in and of themselves because they do something different and something above what the mainstream organizations do, and that's a foundation that, however intangible, it's a bit like providing a safe space that no other organization can. Now we need to try to capture that and operationalise that and the benefit from it. But it's blindingly obvious that it's there to anybody who's experienced it.

Joanna: Public health is often described as being science and art. What are the lessons for LGB communities?

Jim: Public health is one of those things where it is flavour of the month. So, we got public health approaches to everything. The government's claiming to take a public health approach to a number of things right now, and it isn't really. A public health approach is not 'let's do prevention'. A public health approach is actually 'let's understand the population'. Understand the exposures and harms that the population experiences, and understand both the determinants of that and the antecedents. I think that's the first bit that a public health approach; does is it really seeks to understand the population? And I don't think you can do that without the population and their expertise.

I think the second pillar of a public health approach is really understanding the layers as we've talked about elsewhere in this, from the biological layers, of exposure to harm and response to harm, right up to the kind of social, structural, political and environment ones. So, if you took smoking cessation as an example, you can't have a public health approach if you're only doing one thing, which is publishing a leaflet which we all know doesn't work. There's a range of things from, you know, offering access to services, access to nicotine replacement therapy and other good quality services, services that people want to use, right up to things like smoking bans in public places, which arguably have had far more impact on the prevalence of smoking than anything else. So, if you're going to have a public health approach and you haven't got either that understanding of the population or the understanding of risk, harms, determinants, or the levels from the individual to the social, then it's not a public health approach and it's not taking either public health or that population seriously.

One of the problems I have with an awful lot of approaches to LGB populations are those that have claimed to take a public health approach, but actually haven't been. Those that claim to take those populations seriously haven't been actually taking the exposure seriously. It's often focused on the individual stuff. Including employers and hate crime, and as we know, what we need to do is not just work on individual level because you then put the problem back on the community that's experiencing the problem. Now if we continue in this vein, there's a very good definition of public health as the art and science of the organized efforts of society to promote and protect the health of the population. I think this has significance for any work on LGB population health because actually you need to do both the science and the art. And by the art I mean in politics, influencing advocacy, organizational change, because if you just do the science alone, it would just kind of sit there. It might not get used. It might actually be dangerous if you just do the advocacy without the science. How do you know that what you're advocating for is any good?

Joanna: In public health, the Joint Strategic Needs Assessment is so important for funding and resources. Do you have any reflections on that in relation to LGB mental health?

Jim: I will give you an example. In the 1990s, an awful lot of us were running around doing gay and bisexual men, and men who have sex with men (MSM) needs assessments and they were absolutely the right thing to do at the time, because you demonstrated to Commissioners that the population had particular needs that were not being met. And now, needs assessments in England are a statutory requirement. The Joint

Strategic Needs Assessment is a requirement to assess the needs of the population, and a number of areas have produced LGB needs assessments or various other things. Sometimes those needs assessments have been purely driven by the data that the services have, and we all know how variable services are at collecting data, and LGB populations have been traditionally invisible in many public services. So, the current level of measurement doesn't mean that we've got an accurate picture because a lot of people won't declare for all sorts of reasons, even if the question's being asked (see more on measurement in Chapter 2).

I think the other thing is that if you purely go from the evidence that you have. There is now a massive amount of evidence on LGB health, thanks to pioneers, but it's still a relatively under researched and under evidenced topic. And a lot of research is still based on convenience sample surveys, whereas you know, people like you Joanna, have been actually doing work based on national data and national services, which is what we need. We should be benchmarking with others. So even in that bit of the science, there are significant challenges that mean that your product will be at risk.

There's another problem in that if you go and produce a whole load of quantitative data but don't overlay it with the experience of communities, it's neither use nor ornament sometimes, and so the quality of the science has methodological challenges. Ethnicity data recording for most NHS services is very, very poor still, despite 40 years of trying to do it and that actually we need to take into account when we are looking at measuring LGB populations. So, you have to go that extra mile to get the science right.

So, I think that the science and art of public health is something LGB communities could really grab for ourselves and advocate on. But there are several problems. One is, as I've alluded to elsewhere, when we train LGB populations in leadership we often use, I think, a model of turning people into heroes that actually expects them to be very kenotic and self-giving and self-sacrificial in their leadership, which can actually predispose some people to harm, and means that the individual has to do all the running and there is no risk for the organization. I think we have to ditch that.

I think the second thing is building a critical mass. Individual heroes are all very well, but what you need to do is build a critical mass through networks if you're going to influence systems. So, the hero model of leadership I think is out-dated because it can be harmful, but it's also outdated because it doesn't work for the modern systems.

The final thing I would say is that system leaders are very good at stonewalling people who want to come for funding by saying "you haven't got enough data, you haven't got enough evidence". And what I have seen consistently, particularly when it comes to NHS commissioning, is that third sector agencies and LGB agencies will be held to a higher standard of evidence for money from the NHS than internal NHS cases.

Joanna: That is so disappointing but not that surprising to be honest.

Jim: Sometimes the NHS doesn't want to spend the money on the voluntary sector and as we know, the NHS is not as good as local government spending the money. But also, sometimes because they don't particularly want to because it's too much effort to readjust and it's a good way of saving money. Some Commissioners, when they don't want to spend money, will take people through governance and evidence games rather than actually make the decision to spend money. And it's not just LGB populations I've seen this happen to. Head injury charities and hospices are put through the "give us the evidence, give us the evidence, give us the evidence". And I guess the upshot of that is if you are really going to develop the next era of LGB equality and equity, we need to really develop that kind of public health approach and that brings me to one final point. There is a very nerdy tool in public health which I love, which is about using data to create equity analyses of, you know, "actually 8% of the people with a particular type of mental health may be from the LGB population but only 1% of them are getting into services. Why is that?" And then you can begin to systematically analyse the tools and the barriers and the obstacles. Is it about information? Is it about acceptability? Is it about attitude? Is it about the services being seen to be irrelevant? And that can then introduce a whole load of stuff that I think we really need to work on in LGB health, which is health care quality improvement science. Now, I would say that, wouldn't I, as somebody who has been trained in it, but actually this is, I think is the time when we are building an evidence base on LGB health. We really, I think, have lots of tools from public health that we could appropriate and, in many cases, have. And we also, I think, need to appropriate things like leadership science and health care quality improvement science for the next generation of work to be done. How you do that with communities is a whole separate set of challenges. And I think there's a whole lot of work to be done there, but I think one of the pillars of really improving population health for LGB populations, is public health and quality improvement sciences.

Joanna: Music to my ears, Jim. Of course, we need the data to create these steps. So, there was a recent development of a monitoring standard for sexual minorities in order to allow us to capture ongoing data across all health outcomes as part of standard daily practice in healthcare (NHS England, 2017). It appears that this has been very poorly implemented and I wonder if you had any thoughts on how can we encourage our NHS colleagues across primary care, secondary care and tertiary care to adopt this monitoring standard as part of their daily practice?

Jim: I think it is important to monitor for several reasons. The first is if you don't get monitored, you're invisible in services and you can't do the research on differential access, differential equity, differential exposure and differential outcomes. So, for example, how do you know that LGB people are coming out of drug and alcohol services worse or better than heterosexual people or faring the same, if you don't monitor?

So, I think it is worth persevering with from the fundamental principle of equity of access and equity of outcome. Also, if you don't measure it, you're invisible in the commissioning system so you don't get money and you don't get flows, and if you don't measure it how can the NHS meet its health inequalities obligation and local authorities meet their health improvement obligations. I'm taking an English context here, but for every nation of the United Kingdom there is a statutory duty to reduce health inequalities incumbent upon the public sector. And how do you do that if you don't monitor it?

I think what causes us to be disheartened is here we are in 2023, and we have had to set up a race and health observatory because our public system isn't collecting enough data about race and health outcomes. And yet we've been trying to monitor ethnicity, supposedly, for 40 years. And there's a whole literature around why things don't get done in health and care services, but we are not anywhere near as good as we ought to be, even though there have been improvements in monitoring race and ethnicity. So, it doesn't surprise me that that sexual orientation has got some considerable way to go outside things like sexual health services, who typically lead the field. But even they would say they could improve, and everybody could improve, but once you get that good level of detail, it enables you to ask more questions.

Then, if I might take the example of suicide audits. Suicide audits are no longer statutory in England. A suicide audit was when the director of Public Health or somebody on their behalf, went into the coroner's office and various other places and physically audited every suicide file and every potential suicide file. And it's a harrowing thing to do. I've done it myself. But you get data from that that you don't get from other things. And I have moved to do much more work to kind of look to see if there's any evidence of sexual orientation in suicide. Why is that important? It's important because it will give you a bit more information about suicide in the LGB populations. That's part of a jigsaw of building up a picture of a LGB populations more at risk of suicide and more likely to end their life by suicide because they feel that there is no alternative.

Joanna: This is of course in the wider context, that as part of the systematic review I did with Michael King, that no data on completed suicides and LGB identity was included in the analysis as only three papers even existed (King et al., 2008). It is worth noting here, for the purposes of wider context, that the national suicide strategy was changed to include sexual orientation identity as a specific risk factor because of that review. Although little has changed...

Jim: And if you look at the national review of suicide plans for England, working on the mental health of sexual minorities to reduce and prevent suicide is really crucial. You can't do that effectively without data and thus knowing what the challenge is.

This is a marathon of marathons, not a sprint, sadly, but the work that has been done has made us better able to serve LGB people than we were ten years ago. It is, I think, saddening that we are taking so long to progress. But I think we have to keep at it. Otherwise, I think we betray our professionalism as psychologists and, personally speaking, as a public health professional, and we betray our populations and their best interests if we don't. And I have often felt like we should just give up on the monitoring cause, it's never got anywhere, and I think that's a council of despair. There are things you can do without monitoring, but there are things that you *cannot* do without monitoring, and you know, we have to do better at that.

Joanna: So, yes, how do we get our colleagues to ask the bloody question about sexual orientation! We know anyway in society people have a fear of causing offence, so they don't ask the question, which is why they didn't include it in the 2011 Census, which was such a wasted opportunity. But we now know from the census that as many as 93% of the population were happy to answer the voluntary question about sexual orientation identity. Do you think this evidence might work in encouraging our colleagues in the health service to start to ask this question of their patients, to allow us to be able to monitor sexual minority health?

Jim: I think what you find is that there are a number of aspects to getting people to feel comfortable to asking questions that they may feel are intrusive. The first is getting the questions right. And the second is the way you collect it. You know many places do it by giving people a tablet with questions on it and the monitoring forms and say 'please do it'. The third is the confidence in the staff and the training in this staff to ask the question sensitively and appropriately. Our sexual health services have been doing that for years, but actually a number of services are very good at asking sensitive questions. And I think the fourth thing is the environment. So are there strong cues when you come into the environment, you know, do you make it routine and dull, boring, unexceptional and fairly standard in a way? I mean, do you make it so boring that nobody even remarks about it, is one thing that some people do with diversity monitoring, and no, we still make it special. We still make it, like, you know, almost as if it's a 'Les Dawson' question of you. We need to, you know, make it so dull and boring that that nobody cares, and this I think is one of the lessons about monitoring diversity data while at the same time creating an atmosphere of respect.

Joanna: Yes. The Census 2021 made the sexual orientation question voluntary.

Jim: And here the questions are in the census and actually the vast majority of people couldn't care less. You know there's some of us really happy they're being asked. There's some people, a very small number really, upset they're being asked, and the vast majority of the public couldn't care. That's a good sign. And if you get to that point, you've won.

Joanna: I think that's right. I think it's where the word 'usualises' comes in. We just need to 'usualise' it. But I do think the person asking the question is the gate keeper and we still need to reach our colleagues and say nobody really minds about this. And if you make it as ordinary and dull and as uninteresting as you as described, then I think all of a sudden it just becomes run-of-the-mill.

Jim: Yeah, and absolutely. And you know, and if you can get nurses during Monkey Pox vaccinations to ask, you know, "are you having, you know, quite a lot of multiple partner anonymous sex", for example, or other things in sexual health, if you can ask that in a way that's anonymous and respectful, you can ask a question about whether one might be gay.

Joanna: I think our sexual health colleagues are absolute trailblazers in this work of getting our other health service colleagues to reduce their own level of embarrassment or, as I say, gatekeeping behaviour, because to me, they have become the one safe space for LGB people to go to. And I suspect you may have similar knowledge about this. But I have a sense that anecdotally anyway, we know that very often the one place that LGB people feel safe to go to is the sexual health clinic and not necessarily for sexual health reasons, but that they find the staff to be non-judgmental, very often LGB themselves, and a very comfortable environment for perhaps addressing issues that don't belong in sexual health, and this is something I'm very, very interested in. And I wondered if you had knowledge yourself from your position in wider public health that this (use of sexual health clinics for non STI input) is actually happening across the country?

Jim: Yes, I would say that's absolutely true. I mean, I think there are some sexual services where people have felt they haven't been welcomed, but that's by far the minority and very small. So, we're not perfect, but by and large, I think you're absolutely right, because you look at sexual health services and it's very often it's often easy for us to take for granted what they do. They work in a very kind of intimate place where people can feel stigma and shame and pain, and they reach in, and they try to bring healing into that environment. I often talk about what sexual health services do is being a bit of an ordinary miracle of healing people. When they're hurting in all sorts of different ways. And it might be psychological as well as physical and emotional and what we saw, particularly during Monkey Pox is things like, they were referring people on for cost of living advice for help with financial support for the emotional support of the trauma of having Monkey Pox and the disfigurement, and just listening to people. I've never seen a sexual health service that hasn't had some element of just kind of empathy and support around it for the person and that's really special for opening up. So, I think there's lots of evidence about what you're saying and lots of evidence about how they support people and that means I think there's a great deal that we could take out of their book and mainstream.

I remember a colleague who's just turned 20 and he said "well, you know, I, I've just had an experience in a sexual health clinic" and I'm thinking, "oh Lord, here we go. What? What, what's coming now?" I'm hoping this won't be bad. And he said "well I went in because I picked up an STI and I was really upset and worried by it and they were wonderful. You know, really, they were really supportive. They were really supportive around the fact this is the first time I've had a... I was quite shocked and upset. It also, I mean, I actually said well, you know I wasn't that comfortable being gay and still had problems with my family". And he said they were really supportive, and they listened and that the health advisor made him a cup of tea and came back and sat and talked and gave him details on other support groups. So, it was a kind of an all-round intervention. I could tell you other stories of where people have gone to sexual health clinics mentioned they were being bullied in the workplace and ended up being advised to contact the Union and passported into the Union and all sorts of added value. So absolutely.

Joanna: So, there's something there about thinking outside the box. Looking at our colleagues and drawing in best practice from wherever we can to try and improve mainstream services for our sexual minority service users.

So, Jim, my final question is, we've talked a lot about population level provision, mainstream services. We've also touched on community-led services, and we have evidence of differential outcomes in mainstream mental health services, for example, the work around CBT provision, which is covered in Chapter 11. Do you have a view on whether we should direct our energies into improving the LGB accessibility of our mainstream services or whether we should instead be developing tailored, bespoke LGB specific services?

Jim: This is the thing we've all been wrestling with for about 30 years, haven't we? I think the best approach is a mixed economy. And there are three reasons to that. One is innovation. The second is population distribution, and access. And the third is there being no wrong door.

If you look at population innovations, e.g. if you look at chemsex services as one example of innovation to deal with non-sexual health issues that were impacting on sexual health from alcohol and drugs, in a particular set of populations, the innovation there came from sexual health clinicians plus mental health clinicians plus community organizations, and working together. That kind of innovation came from a place where a number of people from different types of services came together. So, I think in the interest of innovation, the more you have a mixed economy of services doing stuff, the more you can take strength from everybody.

I think the second reason I gave was about population access and distribution. I think there are some places where you could easily produce parallel services, if you had the money, or dedicated services. I think for some populations you need dedicated services because either their needs are so specific, or they have been so traumatized by mainstream services or you got such a dense concentration of population with a particular issue—chemsex in bits of London for example and other cities—that it makes perfect sense to have those specialist services. But in rural areas like Cumbria, the Highlands of Scotland; if you purely go down the specialist service model, does somebody have to travel from north of Inverness to Aberdeen to access the nearest service for them? That in itself will put a massive disincentive on them accessing services and may worsen their health. So, 'there should be no wrong door' would be the answer. So, it's kind of a both. And I go back to the D word which is the 'discernment' word. What you need is a group of people to sit down; the commissioners, the director of public health, the local community, the services and discern what model works best for the population and what model works best for which issue that people are coming up with.

So, providing a generic mental health counselling service for people who've experienced really bad homophobia in the workplace. Umm, probably not a great idea. You might want the specialist ones, but actually making people have to travel 60 miles to a specialist sexual health service to talk about their alcohol and sex use or whatever, is also not a good idea. So, I think it has to be that kind of mixed economy of 'horses for courses' if you genuinely want equity. I used to believe the answer to everything was mainstreaming. Umm, but I don't think that's right, and I don't think similarly the answer to everything is specialized services.

Joanna: I completely agree. I think it's a mixture and I think both things have to happen in parallel, because it's a complex picture and not everybody wants the same thing or can deliver the same thing.

Jim: Yeah, absolutely. And if you have a government that is making policy choices that are about funding mainstream and everything else, no amount of evidence will persuade a government which is decided its policy choice is to give people what they think they're going to give people, you know. I mean the current government has cut public health, bangs on regularly, issues lots of rhetoric about value in public health and yet has taken a billion pounds out of the public health grant over five years. So, you know, that's a policy choice. That's a deliberate policy choice, not to prioritize prevention by successive governments.

Joanna: That seems very worrying when so much around mental health is around prevention work and it's such a short-sighted approach, Jim. I'm going to stop on us holding government to account on this.

References

Best, M., & Neuhauser, D. (2004). Avedis Donabedian: Father of quality assurance and poet. *BMJ Quality & Safety, 13*(6), 472–473.
Galea, S. (2020). *How health is threatened by hate* [video]. TEDMED Talks.

Holland, W. W., Detels, R., & Knox, E. G. (1997). *Oxford textbook of public health*. Oxford University Press.

King, M., Semlyen, J., Tai, S. S., Killaspy H., & Nazareth, I. (2008). A systematic review of mental disorder, suicide, and deliberate self harm in lesbian, gay and bisexual people. *BMC Psychiatry* 8.

Mowbray, D. (2014). Psychological responsibility. *Clinical Psychology Forum*.

NHS England. (2017). *DCB2094: Sexual orientation monitoring standard*. NHS England.

Index

© The Editor(s) (if applicable) and The Author(s), under exclusive
license to Springer Nature Switzerland AG 2023
J. Semlyen and P. Rohleder (eds.), *Sexual Minorities and Mental Health*,
https://doi.org/10.1007/978-3-031-37438-8

Milton Keynes UK
Ingram Content Group UK Ltd.
UKHW020646211123
432967UK00004B/120